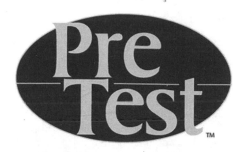

Biochemistry and Genetics

PreTest™ Self-Assessment and Review

Notice

Medicine is an ever-changing science. As new research and clinical experience broaden our knowledge, changes in treatment and drug therapy are required. The authors and the publisher of this work have checked with sources believed to be reliable in their efforts to provide information that is complete and generally in accord with the standards accepted at the time of publication. However, in view of the possibility of human error or changes in medical sciences, neither the authors nor the publisher nor any other party who has been involved in the preparation or publication of this work warrants that the information contained herein is in every respect accurate or complete, and they disclaim all responsibility for any errors or omissions or for the results obtained from use of the information contained in this work. Readers are encouraged to confirm the information contained herein with other sources. For example and in particular, readers are advised to check the product information sheet included in the package of each drug they plan to administer to be certain that the information contained in this work is accurate and that changes have not been made in the recommended dose or in the contraindications for administration. This recommendation is of particular importance in connection with new or infrequently used drugs.

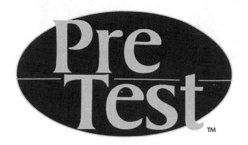

Biochemistry and Genetics

PreTest™ Self-Assessment and Review

Fourth Edition

Golder N. Wilson MD, PhD
Clinical Professor of Pediatrics, Obstetrics & Gynecology
Texas Tech University
KinderGenome Pediatric Genetics
Dallas, Texas

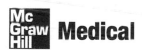 **Medical**

New York   Chicago   San Francisco   Lisbon   London   Madrid   Mexico City   Milan
New Delhi   San Juan   Seoul   Singapore   Sydney   Toronto

The McGraw·Hill *Companies*

Biochemistry and Genetics: PreTest™ Self-Assessment and Review, Fourth Edition

Copyright © 2010 by The McGraw-Hill Companies, Inc. All rights reserved. Printed in the United States of America. Except as permitted under the United States Copyright Act of 1976, no part of this publication may be reproduced or distributed in any form or by any means, or stored in a database or retrieval system, without the prior written permission of the publisher.

Previous editions copyright © 2007, 2005, and 2002 by The McGraw-Hill Companies, Inc.

PreTest™ is a trademark of The McGraw-Hill Companies, Inc.

1 2 3 4 5 6 7 8 9 0   DOC/DOC   14 13 12 11 10

ISBN 978-0-07-162348-3
MHID 0-07-162348-5

This book was set in Berkeley by Glyph International.
The editors were Kirsten Funk and Cindy Yoo.
The production supervisor was Sherri Souffrance.
Project management was provided by Somya Rustagi, Glyph International.
The cover designer was Maria Scharf.
RR Donnelley was printer and binder.

This book is printed on acid-free paper.

Library of Congress Cataloging-in-Publication Data

Wilson, Golder.
  Biochemistry and genetics : PreTest self-assessment and review / Golder N. Wilson.—4th ed.
    p. ; cm.
  Includes bibliographical references and index.
  ISBN-13: 978-0-07-162348-3 (pbk. : alk. paper)
  ISBN-10: 0-07-162348-5 (pbk. : alk. paper)
  1. Biochemistry—Examinations, questions, etc.   2. Genetics—Examinations, questions, etc.   I. Title.
  [DNLM: 1. Biochemistry—Examination Questions.   2. Genetics, Medical—Examination Questions.   QU 18.2 W748b   2010]
  QP518.5.P74   2010
  612'.015076—dc22

2009047849

McGraw-Hill books are available at special quantity discounts to use as premiums and sales promotions, or for use in corporate training programs. To contact a representative please e-mail us at bulksales@mcgraw-hill.com.

Student Reviewers

Daniel Eskenazi
University of Washington School of Medicine
Medical Scientist Training Program
Entering Class of 2005

TeSha English
SUNY Upstate Medical University
Class of 2010

David Scoville
University of Kansas School of Medicine
MD/PhD candidate
Class of 2011

Andrew Degnan
George Washington University School of Medicine
Class of 2011

Contents

Bioenergetics and Energy Metabolism

Lipid, Amino Acid, and Nucleotide Metabolism

Vitamins and Minerals

Hormones and Integrated Metabolism

Inheritance Mechanisms/Risk Calculations

Genetic and Biochemical Diagnosis

Preface

The new edition of *Biochemistry and Genetics: PreTest™ Self-Assessment and Review* is based in part on earlier editions prepared by Golder N. Wilson, MD, PhD, Department of Pediatrics, Texas Tech University Health Sciences Center; Cheryl Ingram-Smith, PhD; Kerry S. Smith, PhD, Department of Genetics, Biochemistry, and Life Science Studies Clemson University Clemson, South Carolina; and by Francis J. Chlapowski, PhD, Department of Biochemistry and Molecular Biology, University of Massachusetts Medical School. All questions are in single-best-answer format and a large number are analogous to those of the United States Medical Licensing Examination (USMLE), Step 1. Questions are updated to the most current editions of leading textbooks in medical biochemistry and medical genetics.

Introduction

Biochemistry and Genetics: PreTest™ Self-Assessment and Review, Fourth Edition, allows medical students to comprehensively and conveniently assess and review their knowledge of microbiology and immunology. The 500 questions provided here have been written with the goal to parallel the topics, format and degree of difficulty of the questions found in the United States Medical Licensing Examination (USMLE) Step 1.

The High-Yield Facts in the beginning of the book are provided to facilitate a rapid review of biochemistry. It is anticipated that the reader will use these High-Yield Facts as a "memory jog" before proceeding through the questions.

Each question in the book is followed by four or more answer options to choose from. In each case, select the one best response to the question. Each answer is accompanied by a specific page reference to a text that provides background to the answer, and a short discussion of issues raised by the question and answer. A bibliography listing all the sources can be found following the last chapter. Over 100 clinical disorders or processes are discussed and related to biochemical and/or genetic mechanisms (see the Appendix for a list of disease examples). For genetic disorders, a McKusick number is included (eg, MIM*154700 for Marfan syndrome) that allows the reader to immediately access information about the disorder using the Online Mendelian Inheritance in Man Internet site *(http://www.ncbi.nlm.nih.gov/omim/)*.

To simulate the time constraints imposed by the licensing exam, an effective way to use this book is to allow yourself 1 minute to answer each question in a given chapter. After you finish going through the questions in the section, spend as much time as you need verifying your answers and carefully reading the explanations provided. Special attention should be given to the explanations for the questions you answered incorrectly; however, you should read every explanation even if you've answered correctly. The explanations are designed to reinforce and supplement the information tested by the questions. For those seeking further information about the material covered, consult the references listed in the bibliography or other standard medical texts.

Note Concerning Disease Examples

This book provides over 100 disease examples (see Appendix) to illustrate the broad application of biochemistry and genetics to medicine. These include more common chromosomal or multifactorial disorders (Down syndrome, cleft palate, diabetes mellitus) that have incidences ranging from 1 in 200 to 1 in 3000 to less common single gene disorders (cystic fibrosis, glycogen storage diseases) with incidences of 1 in 1600 to 1 per million individuals. Students can ignore clinical information about these rare diseases since such knowledge is not tested in first/second-year biochemistry/genetic courses or USMLE I examinations. The examples are provided to place basic science knowledge in clinical context and to demonstrate the broad range of organ systems and medical specialties that are impacted by genetic/biochemical disease. More relevant to examination are much-used disease prototypes like diabetes, cleft palate, Down/Turner syndromes, sickle cell anemia, phenylketonuria (PKU): students may need to match them with underlying biochemical/genetic mechanisms.

Abbreviations

ACAT	acyl-CoA—cholesterol acyl transferase
ACTH	adrenocorticotropic hormone
ADP	adenosine diphosphate
AMP	adenosine monophosphate
ATP	adenosine triphosphate
ATPase	adenosine triphosphatase
CDP	cytidine diphosphate
CMP	cytidine monophosphate (cytidylic acid)
CoA	coenzyme A
cyclic AMP	adenosine 3′,5′-cyclic monophosphate (3′,5′-cyclic adenylic acid)
DHAP	dihydroxyacetone phosphate
DNA	deoxyribonucleic acid
DNP	2,4-dinitrophenol
DPG	diphosphoglycerate
dTMP	deoxythymidine monophosphate
dUMP	deoxyuridine monophosphate
EF	elongation factor
EGF	epidermal growth factor
EGFR	epidermal growth factor receptor
FAD (FADH)	flavin adenine dinucleotide (reduced form)
FMN	flavin mononucleotide
FSH	follicle-stimulating hormone
GDP	guanosine diphosphate
GMP	guanosine 5′-monophosphate (guanylic acid)
GTP	guanosine triphosphate
hCG	human chorionic gonadotropin
HDL	high-density lipoprotein
HGPRT	hypoxanthine-guanine phosphoribosyl-transferase
HMGCoA	3-hydroxy-3-methylglutaryl-Coenzyme A
hnRNA	heterogeneous RNA of the nucleus
IDL	intermediate density lipoprotein
IMP	inosine 5′-monophosphate (inosinic acid)
IP_3	inositol 1,4,5-triphosphate
LDH	lactate dehydrogenase

LDL	low density lipoprotein
LH	luteinizing hormone
mRNA	messenger RNA
MSH	melanocyte-stimulating hormone
NAD (NADH)	nicotinamide adenine dinucleotide (reduced form)
NADP (NADPH)	nicotinamide adenine dinucleotide phosphate (reduced form)
PGH	pituitary growth hormone
P_i	inorganic orthophosphate
PP_i	inorganic pyrophosphate
PRPP	5-phosphoribosylpyrophosphate
RNA	ribonucleic acid
RQ	respiratory quotient
rRNA	ribosomal RNA
TMP	thymidine monophosphate
TPP	thymidine pyrophosphate
tRNA	transfer RNA
TSH	thyroid-stimulating hormone
TTP	thymidine triphosphate
UDP	uridine diphosphate
UMP	uridine monophosphate
UTP	uridine triphosphate
VLDL	very low density lipoprotein

High-Yield Facts in Biochemistry and Genetics

DNA STRUCTURE, REPLICATION, AND REPAIR

Key concepts: DNA structure (Murray, pp 302-311. Scriver, pp 3-45. Lewis, pp 168-181.)

- Deoxyribonucleic acid (DNA) is the chemical basis of genes and chromosomes, its structure providing information for cell division, embryogenesis, and heredity. Changes in DNA structure cause human variation and genetic disease, providing the basis for DNA diagnosis.
- Each DNA strand is a sequence of the GATC deoxyribonucleotide units shown in Fig. 1A; the DNA strands are directional and are diagrammed with the free triphosphate of the 5'-sugar-carbon (5'-end) at the left and the 3'-end to the right (Fig. 1B). The 2-deoxyribose in DNA contrasts with the 2' and 3' hydroxyls of ribose in ribonucleic acid (RNA) that are susceptible to base hydrolysis.
- DNA in eukaryotic cells is a double helix with the strands oriented in opposite directions (antiparallel—Fig. 2A), with sugar-phosphate links on the outside and complementary base pairing on the inside (Fig. 2B). DNA duplex that is not compacted by histone/RNA binding has a length of 3.4 nm per 10 base pairs (bp).
- DNA duplexes can be denatured or "melted" into component single strands at a temperature (T_m) that is proportionate to the fidelity of A-T or G-C base pairing and the percentage of G-C pairs that confer higher melting temperatures due to their three hydrogen bonds (Fig. 2B). The reverse process of renaturation underlies DNA replication, transcription, or repair in that one DNA strand serves as guide or template for its complementary strand.
- The human haploid genome contains 3×10^9 bp of which 70% is unique or low-copy DNA that forms *euchromatin*— less compacted chromatin that is hypersensitive to deoxyribonuclease digestion. Euchromatin contains the estimated 25,000 transcribed genes and stains lightly with standard chromosome banding techniques. The remaining 30% of human

Base Formula	Base X = H	Nucleoside X = ribose or deoxyribose	Nucleotide, where X = ribose phosphate
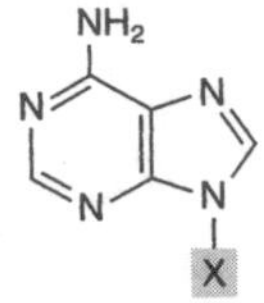 *(adenine structure, NH$_2$, X)*	Adenine A	Adenosine A	Adenosine monophosphate AMP
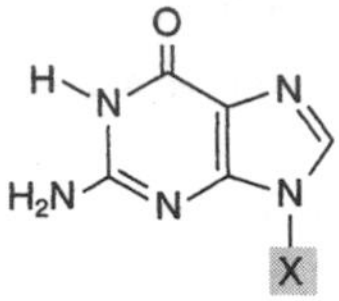 *(guanine structure, O, H-N, H$_2$N, X)*	Guanine G	Guanosine G	Guanosine monophosphate GMP
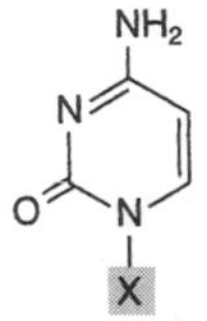 *(cytosine structure, NH$_2$, O, X)*	Cytosine C	Cytidine C	Cytidine monophosphate CMP
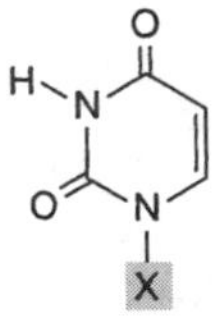 *(uracil structure, O, H-N, O, X)*	Uracil U	Uridine U	Uridine monophosphate UMP
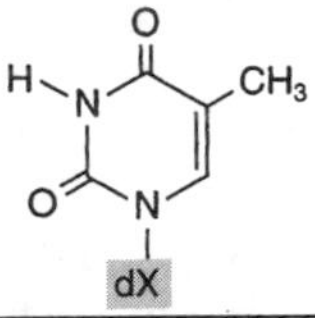 *(thymine structure, O, H-N, CH$_3$, O, dX)*	Thymine T	Thymidine T	Thymidine monophosphate TMP

Figure I (A)

Bases, nucleotides, and nucleosides. *(Reproduced, with permission, from Murray RK, Bender DA, Botham KM, et al. Harper's Illustrated Biochemistry. 28th ed. New York, NY: McGraw-Hill; 2009:287.)*

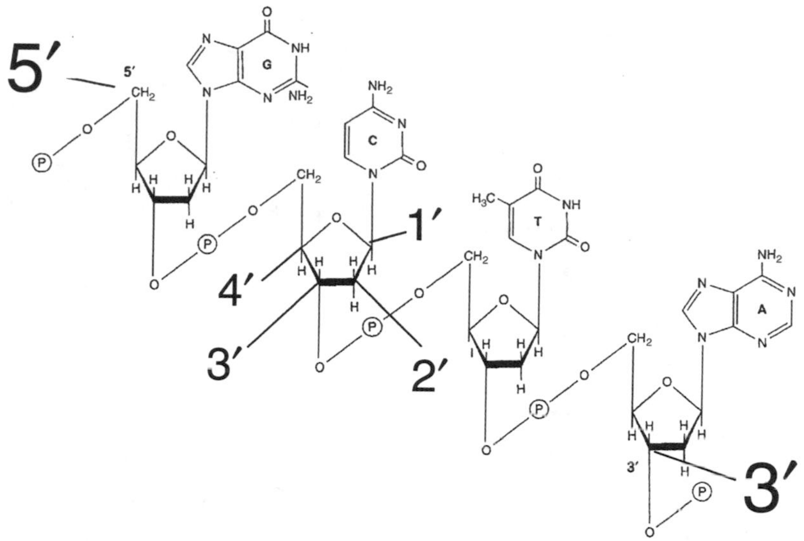

Figure 1 (B)
DNA strand showing 5' to 3' direction of phosphodiester linkages. The pictured strand could also be diagramed as pGpCpTpA. (Adapted, with permission, from Murray RK, Bender DA, Botham KM, et al. Harper's Illustrated Biochemistry. 28th ed. New York, NY: McGraw-Hill, 2009·306.)

genomic DNA contains repetitive DNA sequences that compose *heterochromatin*. Heterochromatin is more compacted chromatin that is less transcribed but important for the structure of chromosome centromeres, telomeres, and satellites.

- Heterochromatin structures evident in the standard Giemsa (G)-banded, metaphase karyotype include densely stained centromeres that anchor chromosomes to the meiotic/mitotic spindle and separate short (p) from long (q) arms. Satellites are regions of heterochromatin that may extend like snail eyes from the p arms of certain chromosomes, their stalks containing ribosomal RNA genes preferentially stained with silver (nucleolar organizer regions or NOR). Telomeres form the ends of chromosomes and have special replication properties. Telomere lengths shorten with age and expand in some neoplastic cells.

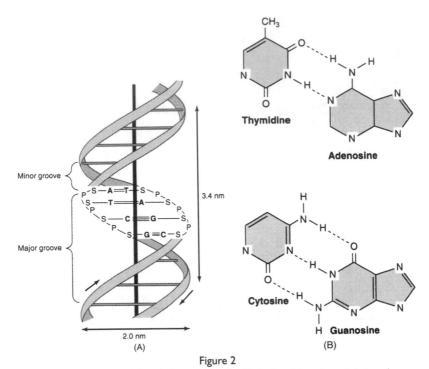

Figure 2

(A) Structure of DNA (B form) showing the double helix with antiparallel strands (arrows). One complete turn (3.4 nm) includes 10 base pairs (bp) A, adenine; C, cytidine; G, guanine; T, thymine; P, phosphate; S, deoxyribose sugar; (B) Base pairing showing two hydrogen bonds (broken lines) between A and T and three bonds between C and G. *(Reproduced, with permission, from Murray RK, Bender DA, Botham KM, et al. Harper's Illustrated Biochemistry. 28th ed. New York, NY: McGraw-Hill; 2009:304.)*

- DNA is compacted some 8000-fold in eukaryotic cells, associating with histone octamers (two H2A-H2B dimers plus two H3/H4 dimers) and histone H1 to form nucleosomes (10 nm), chromatin fibrils (30 nm), chromosome loops (300 nm), and chromosomes; the average human chromosome (haploid number 23) contains a DNA duplex of 1.3×10^8 bp (4 cm compacted to 1.4 mm) and about 1000 genes.
- DNA can be modified by several chemical reactions including methylation at CpG dinucleotides during genomic imprinting and some types of oncogenesis. The associated histones can also be modified by acetylation,

phosphorylation, methylation, etc, often at basic amino acids like lysine and arginine where cationic ammonium side chains form ionic bonds with DNA phosphate groups. Such modifications together with binding of small RNAs constitute a "second code" of genetic regulation that is known as epigenesis.

Key concepts: DNA replication and repair (Murray, pp 334-347. Scriver, pp 3-45. Lewis, pp 171-184.)

- Copying of DNA is synchronous during cell division (DNA replication) and continuous when needed to replace altered bases or broken strands (DNA repair).
- DNA replication is effected by DNA polymerase I, a complex of helicases and topoisomerases for duplex DNA unwinding, primase for initiating DNA copying with RNA primer, DNA single-strand binding proteins (SSBs) for maintenance or proofreading, and ligase for sealing nicks between nascent strands and Okazaki fragments (Fig. 3).
- DNA synthesis occurs during the synthetic or S phase of the cell cycle, after the growth or gap 1 (G1) phase and before the gap 2 (G2) and mitosis (M) phases. The cycle is coordinated by a protein cascade of cyclin-dependent protein kinases (CDKs), cyclins (cyclin D1 is a product of the *bcl* or B-cell lymphoma oncogene), and transcription factors including E2F and Rb (retinoblastoma protein).
- Maintenance of the primary DNA code responsible for accurate protein synthesis and function requires proofreading at the time of DNA replication and DNA repair. Since there are 10^{16} cell divisions per lifetime with 6×10^9 bp replicated for each cell division, more than 6×10^{25} bp of DNA must be replicated during each human lifetime. Extremely low DNA error or damage rates must be enforced because even one error per 10^{20} bp replicated would yield almost a million mutations per individual lifetime.
- Specific DNA repair processes (Table 1) exist for each of the four types of DNA damage: (1) depurination or other modification of DNA bases (radiation, chemical agents), (2) two-base alterations (thymine-thymine dimers with ultraviolet light), (3) strand breaks (radiation, free radicals), and (4) cross-linkage of DNA with its associated proteins (chemical agents)
- Four checkpoint controls monitor DNA and chromosome integrity during the cell cycle—checks for damaged DNA at G1 and G2, incomplete replication in S, and improper spindle alignment at M. Irreparable damage halts cell cycle progression and initiates cell death (apoptosis). The tumor suppressor gene p53, mutated in Li-Fraumeni tumor syndrome and several human cancers, has a key role in G1/G2 checkpoint controls.

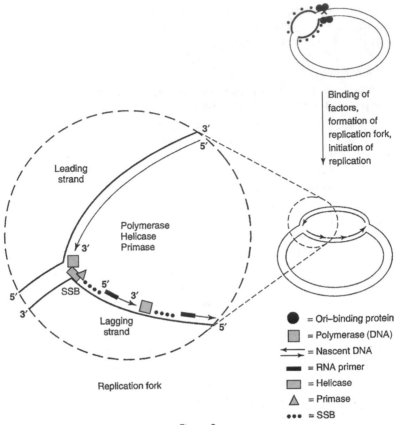

Figure 3

DNA replication fork demonstrating asymmetry with continuous DNA polymerization (long arrow) on the leading strand and discontinuous DNA polymerization/ligation of Okazaki fragments on the lagging strand (short arrows). The asymmetry is necessary for unidirectional replication along antiparallel DNA strands because nature provides only 5′ to 3′ DNA polymerases. Specific binding of the ori-binding protein begins unwinding of the DNA helix, maintained in single-stranded conformation by single-strand-binding proteins (SSBs). The diagram shows circular bacterial or mitochondrial DNA, but can be extrapolated to linear chromosomes by imagining the same steps of origin recognition, denaturation of AT-rich regions, and asymmetric DNA synthesis at multiple chromosomal origins. *(Modified, with permission, from Murray RK, Bender DA, Botham KM, et al. Harper's Illustrated Biochemistry. 28th ed. New York, NY: McGraw-Hill; 2009:323.)*

TABLE I. TYPES OF DNA REPAIR		
Types of Repair	Types of DNA Damage	Mechanism (*Associated Processes*)
Mismatch repair	Copying errors—single base or 2- to 5-base unpaired loops*	Exonuclease digestion of damaged strand relative to methylated A within GATC site; strand replaced by DNA polymerase and ligase (*defective in heredi tary nonpolyposis colon cancer-HNPCC*)
Base excision repair	Chemical or radiation change/removal of a base as in depurination or cytosine to uracil*	N-Glycosidases remove abnormal bases, apurinic or apyrimidinic endonuclease recognizes damaged sites and removes the sugar, and a new nucleotide is inserted using DNA polymerase and ligase.
Nucleotide excision repair	Chemical or radiation damage to DNA segment*	A special exonuclease excises 27-29 nucleotides from the damaged strand followed by special DNA polymerases and ligase (*damage by UV light, cigarette smoking; defective in xeroderma pigmentosum*)
Double-strand break repair	Ionizing radiation, chemotherapy, oxidative free radicals	Proteins bind to and unwind the duplex DNA ends. These are joined by uneven base pairing, trimmed by exonuclease, and sealed by ligase (*part of the physiologic process of immunoglobidin gene rearrangement*)

*These processes can occur spontaneously or in response to agents, exposures, and specific genetic conditions. (*Modified, with permission, from Murray RK, Bender DA, Botham KM, et al. Harper's Biochemistry. 28th ed. New York: McGraw-Hill; 2009:331.*)

• Enzymes for DNA synthesis and repair are used in vitro for DNA engineering, using restriction enzymes to create DNA segments with "sticky ends," ligase enzymes to link DNA segments from different sources, and DNA/RNA polymerase or reverse transcriptase enzymes to synthesis labeled DNA/RNA "probes" that detect specific gene segments. DNA engineering allows isolation or "cloning" of DNA segments from complex genomes (humans, mammals, fruit flies) by placing them in simpler, rapidly replicating bacterial or viral genomes.

GENE EXPRESSION AND REGULATION

Key concepts: Gene expression (Murray, pp 369-387. Scriver, pp 3-45. Lewis, pp 182-201.)

• RNA is polymerized (transcribed) using one strand of DNA as template, RNA polymerase enzyme, DNA sequence signals (promoters, enhancers), and DNA-binding or polymerase-associated proteins (transcription factors). Alterations in DNA sequence or its expression produce genetic disease.
• Three major RNA polymerases in eukaryotic cells transcribe product RNAs as summarized in Table 2. Primary transcription of heterogenous

TABLE 2. EUKARYOTIC RNAs AND RNA POLYMERASES

RNAs (Stability)	Types and Abundance (% Total)	RNA Polymerase (α-Amanitin Sensitivity)
Ribosomal (rRNA) (very stable)	28S, 18S, 5.8S, 5S (80%)	I (insensitive)
Messenger (mRNA) (unstable to very stable)	>100,000 species (2%-5%)	II (very sensitive)
Transfer (tRNA) (very stable)	~60 species (~15%)	III (slightly sensitive)
Small nuclear (snRNA) (very stable)	~30 species (<1%)	III (slightly sensitive)
Micro (miRNA) (stable)	100-1000 species (<1%)	II (very sensitive)

(Modified, with permission, from Murray RK, Bender DA, Botham KM, et al. Harper's Illustrated Biochemistry. 28th ed. New York, NY: McGraw-Hill; 2009:336.)

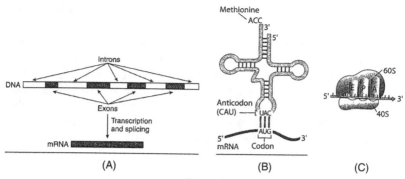

Figure 4
(A) RNA splicing removes introns from the HnRNA primary transcript to produce mRNA for export to the cytoplasm; (B) Specific tRNAs are "charged" with their specific amino acid using aminoacyl-tRNA synthetase and ATP, mediating code-specific insertion of amino acids through binding of their specific anticodon to mRNA codons on the ribosome; (C) Ribosomes composed of 60/40s ribosomal RNAs and multiple proteins provide exit (E), peptidyl (P) and aminoacyl (A) sites that accomplish protein synthesis using energy from GTP hydrolysis. *(Reproduced, with permission, from Le T, Bhushan V, Rao D. First Aid for the USMLE Step 1. New York, NY: McGraw-Hill; 2008:85-86.)*

(Hn) RNA is followed by RNA processing, involving RNA splicing to remove introns, 7-methyl-guanine capping on the 5′-end, polyadenylation to add approximately 200 adenosines at the 3′-end, and transport to the cytoplasm, yielding a contiguous mRNA template for protein translation (Fig. 4A).

• Small nuclear RNAs (SnRNAs) are often processed from double-stranded or hairpin (stem-loop) structures. Certain U SnRNAs plus more than 60 proteins from a small ribonucleoprotein complex (snurp) that binds to the primary transcript to form a spliceosome. Splicing begins with a cut after the 3′G of the upstream exon (GU splice donor site) and proceeds with lariat formation of the intronic RNA, cleavage of the 3′A of the intron (AG splice acceptor site), and joining of the 3′G from the upstream exon with the 5′G from the downstream exon (see Figs. 4A and 5).

- RNA polymerase II transcription involves a ribonucleoprotein complex and includes (1) transcription factors and (2) activators/coactivators that chemically modify the polymerase (phosphorylation or dephosphorylation is common). Transcription elements and factors control RNA polymerase binding (Table 3), while small molecules may change RNA polymerase specificity through transcription factor activation/deactivation (signal transduction).

- Transfer RNAs are 75 to 90 nucleotide single strands with clover-leaf shapes that include specific 3-bp anticodon sites and 3'-CCA ends that are charged with specific amino acids using aminoacyl-tRNA synthetase and ATP (Fig. 4B).

- Translation involves conversion of processed mRNA into protein using transfer RNA intermediaries (Fig. 4A and B), catalytic sites on ribosomes (Fig. 4C), and the genetic code (Table 4).

- The genetic code (Table 4) is unambiguous, degenerate (more than one codon per amino acid), nonoverlapping (sequential codon reading),

TABLE 3. EXAMPLES OF TRANSCRIPTION CONTROL ELEMENTS AND ASSOCIATED TRANSCRIPTION FACTORS

Element	Consensus Sequence	Factors
TATA box	TATAAA	TBP/TFII
CAAT box	CCAATC	C/EBP, NF-Y
GC box	GGGCGG	Sp1
	CAACTGAC	MyoD
	T/CGGA/CN5GCCAA	NF1
AP1	TGAG/CTC/AA	Jun, Fos, ATF

C/EBP-CCAAT Enhancer-binding protein, active in adipose and myeloid tissues, mutated in some leukemias; NF-Y, nuclear factor binding protein binds CCAAT in the Y box of major histocompatibility complex (MHC) genes; Sp1, specificity protein 1 that acts as a transcription factor in the fruit fly and in human brain where it inhibits cell death mediated by huntingtin protein in Huntington disease (MIM*143100); MyoD, myogenic factor that stimulates transcription and differentiation in myocytes; NF1, tumor suppressor gene that is ablated in neurofibromatosis-1 (MIM*162200) and negatively regulates the p21-ras member of rat sarcoma/human bladder cancer gene family; Jun (from Japanese ju-nana for 17—the transforming factor from avian sarcoma virus 17) and Fos (transcription factor from murine osteosarcoma virus) are part of the AP-1 (activator protein-1) transcription factor complex that regulates gene expression in brain and other tissues; ATF (also known as CRE-cAMP response element-binding protein), a family of transcription factors mediating cellular responses to cyclic AMP. (*Adapted, with permission, from Murray RK, Bender DA, Botham KM, et al. Harper's Illustrated Biochemistry. 28th ed., New York, NY: McGraw-Hill; 2009:344.*)

and universal (with exceptions of mitochondria, mycoplasma, and archaeobacteria that have unusual tRNAs).

- Initiation of protein synthesis involves binding of ribosomes, mRNA, and over 10 initiation factors such as eIF-1, eIF-2, eIF-3. The factor eIF-2 is a control point for protein synthesis initiation and is phosphorylated on its α-subunit by several protein kinases activated when the cell is under stress; factor eIF-2 is inhibited by diphtheria toxin.

- Initiation involves successive steps including (1) binding of GTP to eIF-2 and one of the tRNAs for methionine, (2) binding of this complex and

TABLE 4. THE GENETIC CODE (CODON ASSIGNMENTS IN MESSENGER RNA)

First Nucleotide	Second Nucleotide				Third Nucleotide
	U	C	A	G	
	Phe(F)	Ser(S)	Tyr(Y)	Cys(C)	U
	Phe	Ser	Tyr	Cys	C
U	Leu(L)	Ser	Stop	Stop	A
	Leu	Ser	Stop	Trp(W)	G
	Leu	Pro(P)	His(H)	Arg(R)	U
	Leu	Pro	His	Arg	C
C	Leu	Pro	Gln(Q)	Arg	A
	Leu	Pro	Gln	Arg	G
	Ileu(I)	Thr(T)	Asn(N)	Ser	U
	Ileu	Thr	Asn	Ser	C
A	Ileu	Thr	Lys(K)	Arg	A
	Met(M)	Thr	Lys	Arg	G
	Val(V)	Ala(A)	Asp(D)	Gly(G)	U
	Val	Ala	Asp	Gly	C
G	Val	Ala	Glu	Gly	A
	Val	Ala	Glu	Gly	G

Three-letter amino acid codes are shown with single-letter codes in parentheses.
(Reproduced, with permission, from Murray RK, Bender DA, Botham KM, et al. Harper's Illustrated Biochemistry. 28th ed. New York, NY: McGraw-Hill; 2009:354.)

the 40S ribosomal subunit to form a 43S preinitiation complex, (3) binding to the capped 5'-terminus of mRNA to form a 48S preinitiation complex (after the cap mRNA region has been unwound by eIF-4 factors and ATP-dependent helicase), and (5) scanning for the initiator codon AUG that specifies methionine (usually the first AUG but determined by Kozak consensus sequences). The poly (A) tail of the mRNA is important for protein synthesis initiation.

- Elongation of protein (peptide bond) synthesis involves successive binding and shifting of aminoacyl-tRNAs from A (aminoacyl), to P (peptidyl) to E (exit) sites on the ribosome; these translocation steps are powered by GTP hydrolysis (Fig. 4C).

Key concepts: Gene regulation (Murray, pp 369-387. Scriver, pp 3-45. Lewis, pp 202-213.)

- DNA sequence elements that regulate transcription efficiency include promoters (eg, the TATA box), enhancers, repressors or silencers, and RNA termination signals (eg, the AAUAAA DNA sequence).

- Most mammalian genes have a TATAAA (TATA box) promoter located 25 to 30 bp upstream from the transcription start site that directs RNA polymerase II to the proper location; TATA binding protein (TBP) and its associated factors (TAFs) comprise transcription factor TFIID that is instrumental in forming the transcription initiation complex (see Table 3).

- Genes without a TATA box have other promoter elements up- or downstream of the initiator site. Many have elements 50 to 70 bp upstream such as the CCAAT box that influence the frequency of transcription initiation (see Table 4).

- Alternative processing can produce different mRNAs and different proteins by using different combinations of splice donor, splice acceptor, and polyadenylation sites (see Fig. 5).

- Changes in the primary genetic code (mutations) can occur as single bp substitutions (silent, missense, nonsense mutations) or as 1 to 3 bp insertions/deletions that can change the frame of codon reading (frameshift mutations—see Fig. 6). Mutations that change the reading frame of the primary genetic code can produce nonsense codons that terminate translation and result in truncated proteins.

- Single bp substitutions at the third position of codons may cause silent mutations with no amino acid change due to tRNA "wobble," while

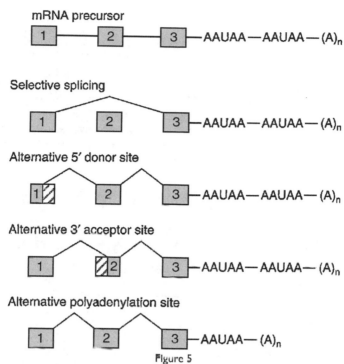

Figure 5

Alternative processing of messenger RNA precursors through use of selective 5'-donor, 3'-acceptor, or polyadenylation sites. *(Reproduced, with permission, from Murray RK, Granner DK, Rodwell VW. Harper's Illustrated Biochemistry. 27th ed. New York, NY: McGraw-Hill; 2006:362.)*

those at first or second codon positions may change the coded amino acid (missense mutations—see Fig. 6).

- Human disease can result from (1) mutations that alter the primary genetic code with resulting changes in gene and protein sequence or (2) mutations that alter the complex "second code"—epigenetic changes in chromatin (DNA/histone) structure/conformation, small RNAs, or the numerous protein factors that regulate RNA transcription, RNA processing, and protein synthesis.

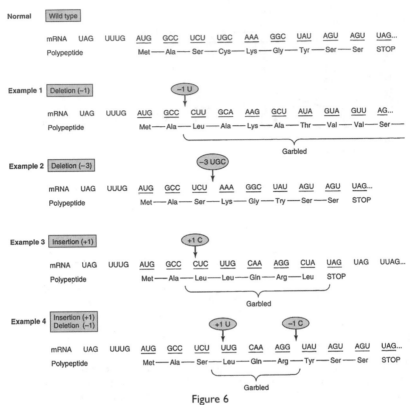

Figure 6

Effects of gene mutation on mRNA and protein products. *(Reproduced, with permission, from Murray RK, Bender DA, Botham KM, et al.* Harper's Illustrated Biochemistry. *28th ed. New York, NY: McGraw-Hill; 2009.)*

ACID-BASE EQUILIBRIA, AMINO ACIDS, AND PROTEIN STRUCTURE/FUNCTION

Key concepts: Acid-base equilibria and protein structure (Murray, pp 6-13. Scriver, pp 3-45. Lewis, pp 194-199.)

- Water has a dipolar structure that solvate organic molecules through formation of hydrogen bonds.
- The polar environment of aqueous solutions stabilizes organic molecules by hydrogen bonding (eg, CHO–H–OH), electrostatic interaction (eg,

R–NH3$^+$—$^-$OOC–CHR), hydrophobic interactions (eg, bases inside DNA helix), and van der Waal forces (transient dipolarity over short atomic distances).

- Solvated organic molecules (eg, amino acids of proteins, nucleotide bases of DNA, RNA; lipids and complex carbohydrates) interact with water as acids (proton or H$^+$ donors) or bases (proton acceptors like hydroxyl ion OH$^-$).

- The tendency of acids to dissociate into anion (A$^-$) and proton (H$^+$) is measured by the dissociation constant (K_a); this equilibrium can be arranged as the Henderson-Hasselbach equation (brackets [ ] indicate concentrations):

$$HA \leftrightharpoons H^+ + A^- \quad \text{and} \quad K_a = \frac{[H^+][A^-]}{[HA]}$$

$$\text{Rearranging: } [H^+] = \frac{K_a[HA]}{[A^-]}$$

Taking the –log of both sides of the equation yields:

$$-\log[H^+] = -\log K_a - \frac{\log[HA]}{[A^-]}$$

Using the symbol pN for –log$_{10}$ [N]:

$$pH = pK_a + \log \frac{[A^-]}{HA}$$

(Note that the unprotonated form is up.)

- Weak acids with low dissociation constants (eg, $H_2CO_3 \rightarrow HCO_3^-$) with pK of 6.4 act to buffer changes in pH in biological fluids like that outside of cells (pH range 7.35-7.45).

- Amino acids are Zwitterions with dual charges from carboxyl (COO$^-$) and amino (NH$_3^+$) groups that react to form peptide bonds (RCO–NHR); peptides (short amino acid chains) and longer polypeptide proteins are also important buffers through their amino acid side groups (Table 5).

- Interaction of side groups and other factors convert linear amino acid sequences (primary structures) into α-helical or β-sheet segments (secondary structures) to three-dimensional conformations (tertiary structures) with functional regions (domains—see Fig. 7).

TABLE 5. L-α-AMINO ACIDS PRESENT IN HUMAN PROTEINS

Name	Symbol	Structural formula	Name	Symbol	Structural formula
With apliphatic side chains			**With side chains containing basic groups**		
Glycine	Gly [G]	$H-CH-COO^-$ $\mid$ NH_3^+	Arginine	Arg [R]	$H-N-CH_2-CH_2-CH_2-CH-COO^-$ $\mid$ $\qquad\qquad\qquad\quad\mid$ $C=NH_2^+ \qquad\quad NH_3^+$ $\mid$ NH_2
Alanine	Ala [A]	$CH_3-CH-COO^-$ $\mid$ NH_3^+			
Valine	Val [V]	H_3C $\quad\diagdown$ $\qquad CH-CH-COO^-$ $\quad\diagup \qquad\quad\mid$ $H_3C \qquad\qquad NH_3^+$	Lysine	Lys [K]	$CH_2-CH_2-CH_2-CH_2-CH-COO^-$ $\mid \qquad\qquad\qquad\qquad\mid$ $NH_3^+ \qquad\qquad\qquad\quad NH_3^+$
Leucine	Leu [L]	H_3C $\quad\diagdown$ $\qquad CH-CH_2-CH-COO^-$ $\quad\diagup \qquad\qquad\mid$ $H_3C \qquad\qquad\quad NH_3^+$	Histidine	His [H]	$\qquad\qquad\qquad CH_2-CH-COO^-$ $HN\diagup\diagdown N \qquad\qquad\mid$ $\qquad\qquad\qquad\qquad NH_3^+$
			Containing aromatic rings		
			Histidine	His [H]	See above.
Isoleucine	Ile [I]	$\qquad CH_3$ $\qquad\mid$ $\qquad CH_2$ $\qquad\mid$ $\quad CH-CH-COO^-$ $\quad\mid \qquad\mid$ $\quad CH_3 \quad NH_3^+$	Phenylalanine	Phe [F]	$\langle\bigcirc\rangle-CH_2-CH-COO^-$ $\qquad\qquad\qquad\mid$ $\qquad\qquad\qquad NH_3^+$
With side chains containing hydroxylic (OH) groups					
Serine	Ser [S]	$CH_2-CH-COO^-$ $\mid \qquad\mid$ $OH \quad NH_3^+$	Tyrosine	Tyr [Y]	$HO-\langle\bigcirc\rangle-CH_2-CH-COO^-$ $\qquad\qquad\qquad\qquad\mid$ $\qquad\qquad\qquad\qquad NH_3^+$
Threonine	Thr [T]	$CH_3-CH-CH-COO^-$ $\qquad\mid \qquad\mid$ $\qquad OH \quad NH_3^+$	Tryptophan	Trp [W]	$\qquad\qquad\qquad\quad CH_2-CH-COO^-$ $\qquad\qquad\qquad\qquad\qquad\mid$ $\qquad\qquad\qquad\qquad\qquad NH_3^+$
Tyrosine	Tyr [Y]	See below.			
With side chains containing sulfur atoms			**Imino acid**		
Cysteine	Cys [C]	$CH_2-CH-COO^-$ $\mid \qquad\mid$ $SH \quad NH_3^+$	Proline	Pro [P]	
Methionine	Met [M]	$CH_2-CH_2-CH-COO^-$ $\mid \qquad\qquad\mid$ $S-CH_3 \quad NH_3^+$			
With side chains containing Acidic groups or their amides					
Aspartic acid	Asp [D]	$^-OOC-CH_2-CH-COO^-$ $\qquad\qquad\qquad\mid$ $\qquad\qquad\qquad NH_3^+$			
Asparagine	Asn [N]	$H_2N-C-CH_2-CH-COO^-$ $\quad\;\;\mid\mid \qquad\qquad\mid$ $\quad\;\; O \qquad\qquad NH_3^+$			
Glutamic acid	Glu [E]	$^-OOC-CH_2-CH_2-CH-COO^-$ $\qquad\qquad\qquad\qquad\mid$ $\qquad\qquad\qquad\qquad NH_3^+$			
Glutamine	Gln [Q]	$H_2N-C-CH_2-CH_2-CH-COO^-$ $\quad\;\;\mid\mid \qquad\qquad\qquad\mid$ $\quad\;\; O \qquad\qquad\qquad NH_3^+$			

(Modified, with permission, from Murray RK, Bender DA, Botham KM, et al. Harper's Illustrated Biochemistry. 28th ed. New York, NY: McGraw-Hill; 2009:15-16.)

16

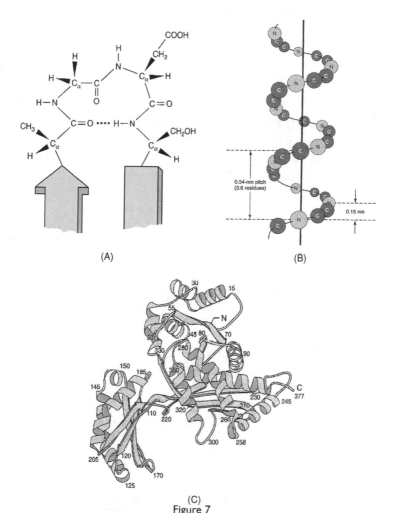

(A)

(B)

(C)
Figure 7

Levels of protein structure: (A) Primary structure of O=C-NHC peptide bond (top center) shown as a turn within a secondary structure of antiparallel β sheets. The four residue segment Ala-Gly-Asp-Ser is stabilized by a hydrogen bond (dotted line—center); (B) Orientation of the core C and N atoms within a peptide segment with α-helical secondary structure; (C) Tertiary structure of a bacterial enzyme illustrating the folding of sequential amino acid molecules (numbers) to form a three-dimensional protein scaffold with helical and β-sheet domains. (Reproduced, with permission, from Murray RK, Bender DA, Botham KM, et al. Harper's Illustrated Biochemistry. 28th ed. New York, NY: McGraw-Hill; 2009:32-35.)

- Tertiary protein structures comprising one peptide chain can associate with other peptide chains (subunits) to form quaternary structures.
- Tertiary and quaternary structures are stabilized by hydrogen bonds (discussed earlier) and by covalent links like disulfide (-S-S-) bonds.

PROTEIN STRUCTURE/FUNCTION

Key concepts: Protein structure/function (Murray, pp 31-42. Scriver, pp 3-45. Lewis, pp 194-199.)

- The folding of proteins into tertiary and quaternary structures is stepwise, thermodynamically favored, and assisted by auxiliary proteins like chaperones, disulfidases, and proline *cis-trans* isomerases.
- Protein conformation provides a diversity of protein function illustrated by the fibrils of collagen or fibrillin, ligand binding like heme/bisphosphoglycerate with hemoglobin, and assembly of catalytic sites for enzymes.
- Influence of small molecules on protein conformation/function is exemplified by the Bohr effect on the hemoglobin saturation curve (Fig. 8) or initiation of signal transduction cascades by molecules like cyclic adenosine monophosphate (cAMP).
- Amounts of proteins may be measured by reaction with specific antibodies (eg, Western blotting or enzyme-linked immunosorbent assays [ELISA]) or, for enzyme proteins, by their rates of conversion of substrates to products (enzyme catalysis).
- Enzymes lower the activation energy for reactions of substrates (precursors) to products; the amino acid side groups within enzyme catalytic sites lower energy by forming substrate-enzyme intermediates (transition states).
- Enzyme assays use initial rate conditions with excess substrate such that the initial velocity (V_i) of substrate reaction is proportionate to enzyme concentration.
- For a given amount of enzyme, the relation between reaction velocity V and substrate concentration S is given by the Michaelis-Menton equation and its reciprocal (plotted in Fig. 9):

$$V_i = \frac{V_{max}[S]}{K_m + [S]} \text{ and } \frac{1}{V_i} = \frac{K_m + [S]}{V_{max}[S]} \text{ or } \frac{1}{V_i} = \frac{K_m}{V_{max}} \times \frac{1}{[S]} + \frac{1}{V_{max}}$$

- The Michaelis constant K_m is defined as the substrate concentration giving one-half the maximal reaction velocity, and can be viewed as a binding constant—substrates with high affinity for the enzyme catalytic site have low K_m values and vice versa.

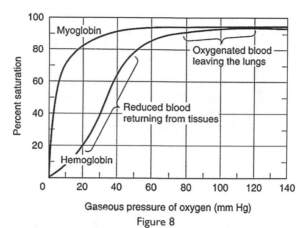

Figure 8

Oxygen binding curves of both hemoglobin and myoglobin. The arterial oxygen tension of blood leaving the lungs is about 100 mm Hg compared to 40 mm for veins returning blood from tissues or 20 mm within capillary beds of actively metabolizing tissues like muscle. The contrast in percent oxygen saturation between hemoglobin (~30%) and myoglobin (~90%) in the 20 to 40 mm Hg oxygen tension region of the curve (the oxygen tension of peripheral tissues) illustrates that greater release of oxygen at low tensions made possible by the subunit structure of hemoglobin via cooperativity. *(Reproduced, with permission, from Murray RK, Bender DA, Botham KM, et al. Harper's Illustrated Biochemistry. 28th ed. New York, NY: McGraw-Hill; 2009:45.)*

As S increases and becomes much greater than the K_m, V approaches its maximal velocity V_{max}:

$$V = \frac{V_{max}[S]}{[S]} = V_{max}$$

Substrates with higher affinity (lower K_m) will thus saturate enzyme catalytic sites and achieve V_{max} at lower concentrations.

- Because the Michaelis-Menton equation shows that attainment of V_{max} is a hyperbolic curve (Fig. 9A), use of the reciprocal Lineweaver-Burk equation shown above provides an easy graphical determination of V_{max} and K_m as shown in Fig. 9B. The reciprocal of velocity $1/V$ is plotted on the y axis against the reciprocal of substrate concentration $1/S$ on the x axis. Direct graphic determination of V_{max} is made by measuring the y intercept (= $1/V_{max}$ when $1/S = 0$). Direct graphic measurement of the K_m is made by measuring the x intercept (= $\sim 1/K_m$ when $1/V = 0$). The slope is K_m/V_{max}.

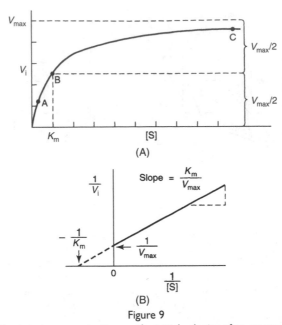

Figure 9
(A) Effect of substrate concentration on the initial velocity of an enzyme-catalyzed reaction. (B) Double reciprocal or Lineweaver-Burk plot of $1/V_i$ versus $1/[S]$ that can be used to evaluate K_m and V_{max}. *(Reproduced, with permission, from Murray RK, Bender DA, Botham KM, et al. Harper's Illustrated Biochemistry. 28th ed. New York, NY: McGraw-Hill; 2009:67-68.)*

- The reciprocal Lineweaver-Burk plot constructed by measuring enzyme velocities with and without inhibitor distinguishes competitive inhibition from noncompetitive inhibition (Fig. 10). A competitive inhibitor will have similar structure to the substrate and compete for enzyme catalytic sites, changing the effective K_m but not the V_{max} (Fig. 10A). A simple noncompetitive inhibitor does not resemble substrate in structure and will not compete for its binding at the enzyme catalytic site, binding instead to an allosteric site. Noncompetitive inhibitors thus change V_{max} but not K_m (Fig. 10B).

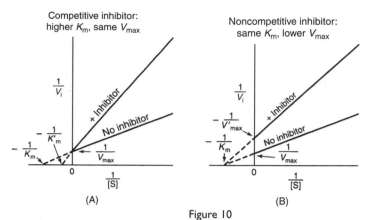

Figure 10

(A) Lineweaver-Burk plot of competitive inhibition. Note the complete relief of inhibition at high [S] (ie, low 1/[S] concentrations); (B) Lineweaver-Burk plot for simple noncompetitive inhibition. Note the change in V_{max} with identical K_m. *(Reproduced, with permission, from Murray RK, Bender DA, Botham KM, et al. Harper's Illustrated Biochemistry. 28th ed. New York, NY: McGraw-Hill; 2009:71.)*

- Categories of enzymes include:
  1. Oxidoreductases that add oxygen or remove hydrogens (oxidases, dehydrogenases) or add hydrogens (reductases) to substrates.
  2. Transferases that move chemical groups (glycosyl, methyl, phosphoryl) from one substrate to another.
  3. Hydrolases that cleave substrate bonds using water (adding H or OH to the cleavage products); many subtypes including peptidases, lipases, etc.
  4. Isomerases that rearrange substrate molecules to form a different isomer.
  5. Synthases that join substrates by forming new bonds.
  6. Phosphatases that remove phosphate groups and phosphorylases or kinases that add phosphate groups to substrates.

INTERMEDIARY METABOLISM

Key concepts: Intermediary metabolism (Murray, pp 132-144. Scriver, pp 3-45.)

- Metabolism involves breakdown (catabolism) of dietary carbohydrates, fat, and protein to glucose, fatty acids/glycerol, and amino acids, respectively, providing energy for biosynthesis (anabolism) and organ function.

- Common metabolic diseases involve nutrient, vitamin, or hormone deficiencies that reflect interaction of genes and environment (multifactorial determination), exemplified by marasmus, rickets, or diabetes mellitus.
- Rarer metabolic diseases (inborn errors of metabolism) result from specific enzyme deficiencies and exhibit autosomal or X-linked recessive inheritance; accumulation or deficiency of small molecules often produces acute catastrophic disease (acidosis, seizures, coma) while accumulation of larger molecules often produces chronic disease (storage disease).
- The enzyme and cofactor deficiencies of inborn errors of metabolism can be defined in terms of substrate excess and product deficit, guiding diagnostic tests (blood amino acids, urine organic acids) and therapies (substrate avoidance and product or vitamin supplementation through the diet).
- Metabolic pathways are highly compartmentalized as enzyme complexes (eg, the pyruvate dehydrogenase with >30 peptides) or organelles (eg, citric acid cycle enzymes in the mitochondrial matrix); even the cytoplasm is a liquid crystal of heterogenous enzyme associations rather than a homogenous protein solution.
- The entry and flow (flux) of metabolites in pathways is controlled through compartmentalization, irreversibility of certain enzyme steps, binding of substrates by low K_m, first-step pathway enzymes, and regulatory/rate-limiting enzymes that are activated or inhibited by small molecules (allosteric modifiers) or hormones.

CARBOHYDRATE AND GLYCOGEN METABOLISM

Key concepts: Carbohydrate structures and glycoproteins (Murray, pp 113-120. Scriver, pp 1407-1666.)

- Carbohydrates (sugars), and particularly glucose, are important metabolic fuels for mammals, particularly during fetal development.
- Glucose is the common currency of carbohydrate metabolism, synthesized in plant photosynthesis, ingested and absorbed into animal bloodstreams, and converted from other sugars in the liver (Fig. 11).
- Monosaccharides include 3-carbon trioses (glyceraldehyde), 5-carbon pentoses (ribose, arabinose, xylose), and 6-carbon hexoses (glucose, galactose, mannose); each group has many isomers (same structural formulas but different arrangement of CHO groups).

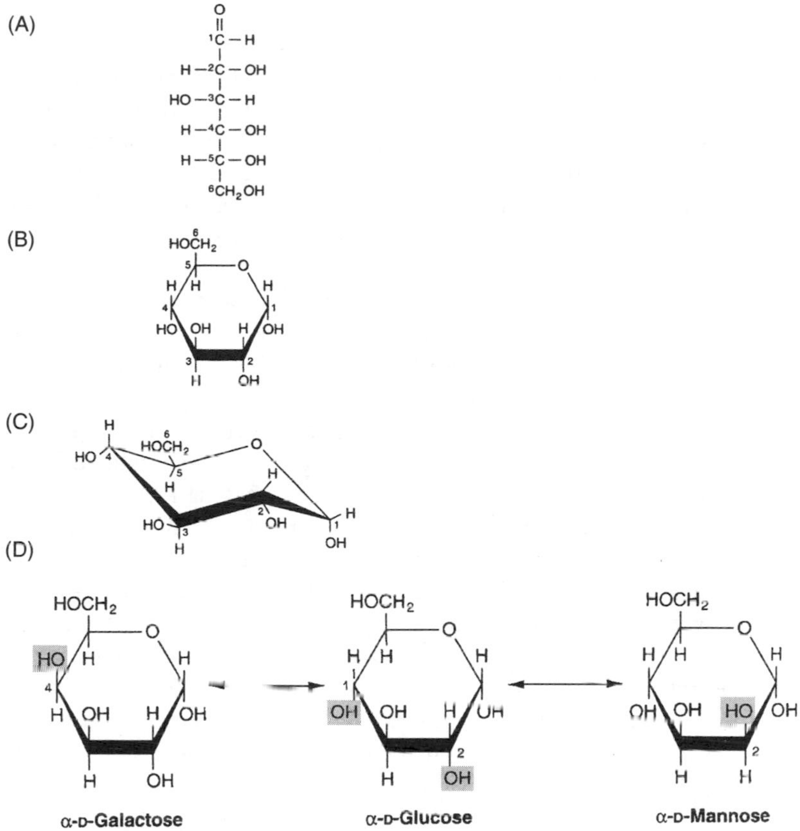

Figure 11

D-Glucose in (A) straight chain form; (B) With C1-O-C5 ring formation to yield C1 hydroxyl orientation (arrow) as α-anomer; (C) Actual structural conformation of α-D-glucose as Haworth projection showing –OH (and –CH₂OH) groups in most stable position (in plane with ring) except for C1 α-hydroxyl (arrow—note that C1 β-hydroxyl would be in plane, accounting for 62% β, 38% α-anomers of D-glucose in water solution); (D) Biologically important epimers of D-glucose shown as α-anomers (galactose and mannose) will include hydroxyls out of ring plane in Haworth projection, accounting for decreased stability and potential energy release when converted to glucose as "ground state" of animal metabolism. *(Reproduced, with permission, from Murray RK, Bender DA, Botham KM, et al. Harper's Illustrated Biochemistry. 28th ed. New York, NY: McGraw-Hill; 2009:114-115.)*

- The four optically active carbons of hexoses with CH = O (aldehyde group) at carbon 1 (C1) produce 16 isomers including glucose; these include dextro (D) or levo (L) conformations at C4 (optical isomers), formation of 4 carbon (furan) or 5 carbon (pyran) rings through C1-O-C4 or C1-O-C5 bonds, and upward (β) or downward (α) conformations of the C1-hydroxyl group after ring formation (anomers).
- Important monosaccharides with a C = O group at C2 (ketoses) include fructose (6 carbons), xylulose or ribulose (5 carbons), and dihydroxyacetone (3 carbons).
- Disaccharides can be formed between various sugar isomers, including lactose (β-D-galactose-C1-O-C4-β-D-glucose = β-D-galactose-[1 → 4]-β-D-glucose), maltose (α-D-glucose-[1 → 4]-α-D-glucose), or sucrose (α-D-glucose-[1 → 2]-β-D-fructose).
- Longer sugar chains (polysaccharides) are composed of single sugars (eg, starch, amylopectin, and glycogen with α-D-glucose 1 → 4 links and 1 → 6 branches) or multiple sugars (eg, mucopolysaccharides or heparin with glucuronic acid, acetylglucosamine, iduronic acid groups, etc).
- Sugars may be added to amino acid side chains on proteins to form glycoproteins, illustrated by influenza virus hemagglutinins, coagulation proteins (like thrombin), surface antigens (like the ABO blood groups), or glycosylated hemoglobin A_{1c} formed during hyperglycemia from uncontrolled diabetes mellitus. The latter modification is extremely important in monitoring diabetic control and outcomes since the 120-day life span of red blood cells and their component hemoglobin reflects average glucose levels over that time period.

Key concepts: Carbohydrate metabolism (Murray, pp 113-120, 131-142. Scriver, pp 1407-1666.)

- Major themes of human carbohydrate metabolism include the distribution of glucose to tissues, metabolism to lactate in anaerobic tissues, metabolism to pyruvate and acetyl coenzyme A (acetyl-CoA) in aerobic tissues, and generation of energy (ATP) through the citric acid cycle and oxidative phosphorylation (ox-phos).
- Glucose, fructose, and galactose are the main carbohydrates absorbed from dietary starch, sucrose, and lactose, respectively; fructose and galactose are converted to glucose in liver (mainly) and deficiencies in their conversion cause essential fructosemia and galactosemia.
- Glycolysis (Fig. 12) is the main path of glucose metabolism (and of dietary fructose or galactose), producing lactate in anaerobic tissues

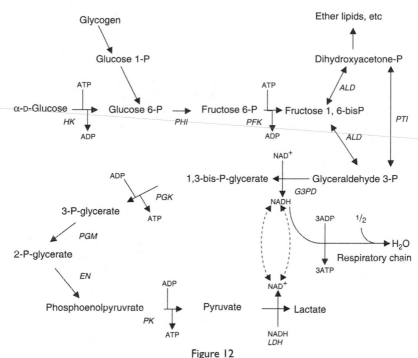

Figure 12

Pathway of glycolysis showing steps yielding ATP (adenosine triphosphate) and NADH (nicotinamide dinucleotide), which is subsequently oxidized in the mitochondrial respiratory chain. P, phosphoro- or phosphate; enzymes in italics: *HK*, hexokinase; *PHI*, phosphohexose isomerase; *PFK*, phosphofructokinase; *ALD*, aldolase; *PTI*, phosphotriose isomerase; *G3PD*, glyceraldehyde-3-phosphate dehydrogenase; *PGK*, phosphoglycerate kinase; *PGM*, phosphoglycerate mutase; *EN*, enolase; *PK*, pyruvate kinase; *LDH*, lactate dehydrogenase. *(Modified, with permission, from Murray RK, Bender DA, Botham KM, et al. Harper's Illustrated Biochemistry. 28th ed. New York, NY: McGraw-Hill; 2009:151.)*

(brain, muscle, gastrointestinal tract, retina, skin, and erythrocytes with no mitochondria).

- Aerobic tissues like heart, liver, or kidney glycolyze glucose to pyruvate, convert pyruvate to acetyl-CoA via pyruvate dehydrogenase (PDH), and effect complete oxidation to carbon dioxide and water using the citric acid cycle (CAC) and ox-phos.

- Aerobic tissues oxidize lactate when oxygen is plentiful and ox-phos is effective, but produce lactic acidosis under circumstances of hypoxia, cardiopulmonary failure, exercise fatigue, or ox-phos interruption (PDH or thiamine cofactor deficiencies), PDH inhibitors (arsenate, mercurate ions), mitochondrial diseases, alcoholism with thiamine deficiency.
- Deficiencies of glycolytic enzymes have predominant effects in anaerobic tissues including hemolytic anemias or myopathies.
- The pentose phosphate pathway is an alternative route for glucose metabolism that generates reducing equivalents of NADPH for steroid/ fatty acid synthesis and ribose for nucleotide formation.
- The citric acid cycle (CAC) is a final common pathway for carbohydrate, lipid, and amino acid metabolism, combining acetyl-CoA with oxaloacetate and cycling through seven intermediates to generate oxaloacetate again (Fig. 13).
- The CAC is channeled within mitochondria, directly generating ATP or substrates such as reduced nicotinamide-NADH or flavin adenine (FADH$_2$) dinucleotides that produce ATP through ox-phos.
- The CAC is amphibolic, involved in catabolism to yield ATP energy and anabolism through gluconeogenesis and fatty acid synthesis.
- The CAC is under respiratory control, being tightly coupled to ox-phos by levels of oxidized cofactors (like NAD$^+$) and by end-product inhibition of PDH (acetyl-CoA, NADH).

Key concepts: Glycogen metabolism and gluconeogenesis (Murray, pp 157-164. Scriver, pp 1521-1552.)

- Glycogen is stored glucose in the form of a branched polysaccharide analogous to starch in plants; it accounts for 6% of liver mass and 1% of muscle mass in fed states.
- Glycogenesis utilizes high energy uridine diphosphate glucose (UDPGlc) formed from glucose 1-phosphate and UTP, forming 1 → 4 links with a synthase and 1 → 6 links with branching enzymes.
- Glycogen synthase adds glucose units to preexisting glucose chains on the primer protein glycogenin; the primer glucose chain is attached to the hydroxyl of a tyrosine residue.
- Glycogenolysis is very different from glycogen synthesis, requiring multiple enzymes such as glycogen phosphorylase that employs phosphate to hydrolyze 1 → 4 links and debranching enzymes that hydrolyze 1 → 6 links. Liberated glucose 1-phosphate is converted to glucose 6-phosphate

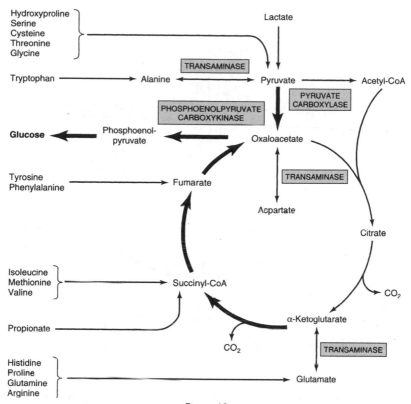

Figure 13

Involvement of the citric acid cycle in transamination and gluconeogenesis. Bold arrows indicate the main pathway of gluconeogenesis. *(Reproduced, with permission, from Murray RK, Bender DA, Botham KM, et al. Harper's Illustrated Biochemistry. 28th ed. New York, NY: McGraw-Hill; 2009:146.)*

and (in liver) to glucose by glucose-6-phosphatase (thus increasing blood glucose—Fig. 14).

- Phosphorylases differ between liver and muscle, activated by phosphorylation of their serine hydroxyl groups (via phosphorylase kinase and protein phosphatase) and by allosteric interactions with cyclic AMP or AMP.
- Cyclic AMP is formed from ATP by adenyl cyclase in response to hormones such as epinephrine, norepinephrine, and glucagon; it is hydrolyzed

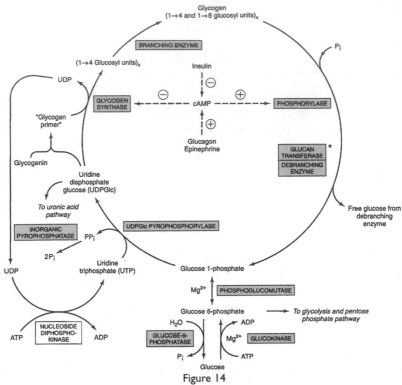

Figure 14

Pathway of glycogenesis and glycogenolysis in the liver. Two mol of high energy phosphates are used in the incorporation of 1 mol of glucose into glycogen. + refers to simulation, − to inhibition. Insulin decreases the level of cAMP only after it has been raised by glucagons or epinephrine—that is, it antagonizes their action. Glucagon is active in heart muscle but not in skeletal muscle. At asterisk; Glucan transferase and debranching enzyme appear to be two separate activities of the same enzyme. *(Reproduced, with permission, from Murray RK, Bender DA, Botham KM, et al. Harper's Illustrated Biochemistry. 28th ed. New York, NY: McGraw-Hill; 2009:158.)*

by phosphodiesterase to produce 5′ AMP, an activator of muscle phosphorylase during fatigue (Fig. 14).

- Insulin slows glycogenolysis by direct stimulation of liver phosphodiesterase (to decrease cAMP) and inhibition of liver glycogen phosphorylase through glucose uptake, increased formation of glucose 6-phosphate, and reduced activity of phosphorylase kinase.

• Inherited enzyme deficiencies produce glycogen storage in liver or muscle according to enzyme location (Table 6); failure of liver glycogenolysis and blood glucose supply cause recurrent hypoglycemia, lactic acidemia, and shift to fatty acid metabolism with hypercholesterolemia and hyperuricemia.

BIOENERGETICS, ENERGY METABOLISM, AND BIOLOGICAL OXIDATION

Key concepts: Bioenergetics and energy metabolism (Murray, pp 92-102. Scriver, pp 2261-2296.)

• Bioenergetics is the study of energy changes that accompany metabolism; biological systems use chemical energy, taking fuel from food.

• Food and micronutrient (vitamins, minerals) availability determine the rate of energy release, modulated by thyroid hormones.

• States of energy depletion (starvation, marasmus) or excess (obesity) are powerful influences in medicine and disease.

• Biochemical reactions are of two types—exergonic (catabolic) that yield energy (eg, conversion of phosphoenolpyruvate to pyruvate) and endergonic (anabolic) that consume energy (eg, conversion of glucose to glucose 6-phosphate and synthesis of biopolymers). Exergonic reaction products (eg, NADH, ATP) are often coupled to endergonic (synthetic) reactions (eg, production of ATP, GTP during fat or glucose oxidation, and GTP hydrolysis during aminoacyl translocation of protein synthesis).

• High energy phosphates are the currency of cellular energy exchange, including ATP and GTP; glycolytic compounds 1,3-bisphosphoglycerate and phosphoenolpyruvate; and creatine phosphate in muscle.

• Other high energy compounds include coenzyme A derivatives, S-adenosylmethionine, and UDP-glucose.

• The ratio of ATP to ADP reflects cellular energy potential and coordinates various processes like oxidative-phosphorylation, glycolysis, and the citric acid cycle.

• Enzymes such as myokinase or adenyl kinase catalyze ATP-ADP-AMP interconversions in response to cellular energy supplies.

Key concepts: Biological oxidation (Murray, pp 98-112. Scriver, pp 2261-2296.)

• Chemical oxidation of a substrate involves removal of electrons while chemical reduction involves a gain in electrons.

TABLE 6. GLYCOGEN STORAGE DISEASES

Glycogenosis (% patients)	Type-Name	Cause of Disorder	Characteristics
Type I (a-c) (25%)	L-von Gierke disease (MIM*232200)	Deficiency of glucose-6-phosphatase catalytic subunit (a), microsomal glucose-6 phosphatase (b), or phosphate transport (c).	Liver cells and renal tubule cells loaded with glycogen. Hypoglycemia, lacticacidemia, ketosis, hyperlipemia.
Type II (15%)	M-Pompe disease (MIM*232300)	Deficiency of lysosomal glucosidase (acid maltase)	Fatal, accumulation of glycogen in lysosomes, heart failure.
Type III (24%)	L-Forbes or Cori disease (MIM* 232400) (limit dextrinosis)	Absence of debranching enzyme	Accumulation of branched polysaccharide in liver with hepatomegaly; hypoglycemia, and growth failure.
Type IV (3.3%)	L-Andersen disease (amylopectinosis— MIM*232500)	Absence of branching enzyme	Accumulation of unbranched polysaccharide. Death due to cardiac or liver failure in first year of life.
Type V (2%)	M-McArdle syndrome (myophosphorylase deficiency— MIM*232300)	Absence of muscle phosphorylase (myophosphorylase)	Diminished exercise tolerance; increased muscle glycogen, decreased lactate after exercise, potential myoglobinuria, and renal failure.
Type VI (30% with IX)	L-Hers disease (MIM*232700)	Deficiency of liver phosphorylase	High glycogen content in liver, tendency toward hypoglycemia.
Type VII (0.2%)	M-Tarui disease (MIM*232800)	Phosphofructokinase deficiency in muscle and erythrocytes	As for type V but also possibility of hemolytic anemia.
Type IX (a-f) (30% with VI)	L-Phosphorylase kinase deficiencies (MIM*306000)	Phosphorylase kinase deficiencies in liver, skeletal, and/or heart muscle; various subunit deficiencies account for subtypes (a-f)	Similar to type VI. Type IXa was formerly called type VIII and is the only X-linked recessive disorder.

• Oxygen provided by animal respiration provides direct oxidation (addition of oxygen to substrates by oxidases, cytochromes P450, etc) or indirect oxidation (removal of hydrogens from substrates to form water by dehydrogenases, etc).
• The generation of energy by oxidation-reduction reactions is proportionate to their redox potential (analogous to battery voltage); the conversion of oxygen to water (last step of the respiratory chain) has the greatest (most positive) redox potential.
• The high redox potential of oxygen to water conversion drives the intermediate reactions of food oxidation/metabolism, generating reducing equivalents that are converted to fuel (ATP, high energy phosphates) by ox-phos.
• Several classes of enzymes catalyze oxidative reactions, using the redox potential to generate high energy compounds or to detoxify drugs or environmental agents (see Table 7).

LIPID, AMINO ACID, AND NUCLEOTIDE METABOLISM

Key concepts: Significant lipids and lipid synthesis (lipogenesis— Murray, pp 121-130, 193-204. Scriver, pp 2705-2716.)

• Lipids, including fats, oils, steroids, and waxes, are related by their insolubility in water and function in energy storage, membrane barriers, and neutral insulation.
• Simple lipids are fatty acids linked with alcohols to form esters, including fats (solid glycerol esters), oils (liquid glycerol esters), and waxes (fatty acids linked to long chain alcohols).
• Complex lipids include links to phosphoric acid (phospholipids), the 18-carbon amino alcohol sphingosine (sphingophospholipids), carbohydrate (glycosphingolipids), and proteins (including lipoproteins).
• Derived lipids include saturated (no double bonds) or polyunsaturated fatty acids (multiple double bonds), polyunsaturated fatty acids with rings (eicosanoids including prostaglandins and leukotrienes, vitamins including E and K), steroids derived from cholesterol including hormones (aldosterone, estrogen, testosterone) or vitamins (vitamin D), and polymers containing ceramide (a sphingosine derivative), carbohydrates (generating cerebrosides), or carbohydrates with sialic acid (gangliosides).
• Amphipathic lipids (eg, glycerophospholipids) contain hydrophobic (water-repelling) and hydrophilic (water-soluble) regions; they form water-lipid interfaces such as bilayer membranes or multilamellar sheaths, micelles (droplets with oil inside), and liposomes (water inside).

TABLE 7. CLASSES OF ENZYMES USED IN OXIDATION REACTIONS

Enzyme Class	Example	Function	Cofactors/Inhibitors
Copper oxidases	Cytochrome oxidase	Last step of mitochondrial respiratory chain	Heme iron, copper/CO, CN
Flavoprotein oxidases	L-Amino acid oxidase	Oxidizes amino acids	FMN, FAD (riboflavin)
NAD^+ dehydrogenases	Respiratory chain carriers	Oxidation of substrates to water	NAD^+, $NADP^+$ (niacin)
FMN, FAD dehydrogenases	Succinate dehydrogenase	Transfer reducing equivalents from CAC to respiratory chain	FMN, FAD (riboflavin)
	Dihydrolipoyl dehydrogenase	Reduces lipoic acid during oxidative decarboxylation of pyruvate, α-ketoglutarate	
	Electron transfer flavoprotein	Acyl-CoA intermediates and respiratory chain	
Hydroperoxidases	Glutathione peroxidase	Protects against peroxides	Reduced glutathione, selenium
	Catalase	Protects by removal of hydrogen peroxide	Heme iron
Oxygenases	Cytochromes P450 (>100 enzymes)	Direct incorporation of oxygen into substrates; detoxification	
Free radical oxidation	Superoxide dismutase	Protects by removal of superoxide radical	Works in concert with antioxidants like vitamin E

(Data from Murray RK, Bender DA, Botham KM, et al. Harper's Illustrated Biochemistry. 28th ed. New York, NY: McGraw-Hill; 9:98-102.)

- Fatty acid synthesis begins in the cytoplasm with biotin-mediated carboxylation of acetyl-CoA to form malonyl-CoA by acetyl-CoA carboxylase (Fig. 15). Initial fatty acyl synthesis is sequestered within a dimeric, 14-enzyme fatty acid synthase complex that transfers the CoA molecules onto pantothenic acid sulfhydryl groups before condensing them to form enzyme-bound acetoacetyl groups.

- A microsomal fatty acid elongase extends C10 and longer fatty acids through direct condensation of fatty acyl- and acetyl-CoA. Fatty acids are thus made using acetyl-CoA building blocks, with similar steps of 2-carbon addition for the synthase or elongation pathways (Fig. 15).

- Linoleic (C18 with two double bonds), α-linolenic (C18 with three double bonds), and arachidonic acids (C20 with four double bonds and precursor to prostaglandins) cannot be synthesized in humans and must be supplied in the diet (essential fatty acids); essential fatty acid deficiencies can occur with intestinal malabsorption (cystic fibrosis, Crohn disease) or liver disease (cirrhosis, alcoholism, immature neonatal liver) while excess trans-unsaturated fatty acids are associated with atherosclerosis.

- Glycerophospholipids (ie, lung surfactant, cholines, inositol second messengers) are synthesized from acyl-CoAs (activated by acyl-CoA synthetase) and glycerol-3-phosphate, while glycerol-ether lipids (platelet activating factor) are analogously synthesized from dihydroxyacetone phosphates.

- Fatty acid synthesis (lipogenesis) is promoted in fed states through supplies of NADPH from the pentose phosphate pathway, allosteric activation of acetyl-CoA carboxylase by citrate (high concentrations when acetyl-CoA is abundant), and inhibition of acetyl-CoA carboxylase and pyruvate dehydrogenase by the products of lipogenesis, long-chain fatty acyl-CoAs.

- Insulin increases lipogenesis by inhibiting phosphorylation and inactivation of acetyl-CoA carboxylase, while epinephrine and glucagon inhibit lipogenesis and promote lipolysis; insulin also decreases cellular cAMP, reducing lipolysis in adipose tissue and decreasing plasma concentrations of free fatty acids.

Key concepts: Lipid catabolism (lipolysis) and transport (Murray, pp 184-204. Scriver, pp 2705-2716.)

- Glycosphingolipid polymers such as ceramides or gangliosides are degraded by lysosomal enzymes that, when deficient, cause lipid storage

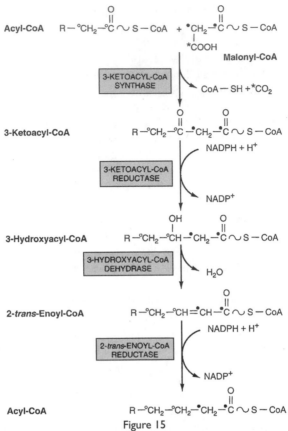

Figure 15

Synthesis and elongation of fatty acids. Initial synthesis of a fatty acid occurs within a fatty acid synthase complex composed of two symmetrical dimmers, each with seven enzymes plus pantothenic acid. Acetyl-CoA is carboxylated using biotin to yield malonyl-CoA, and each molecule is transferred to apposing pantothenic acid sulfhydryl groups within the synthase followed by condensation to make acetoacetyl-CoA (R = H in diagram). Elongation of fatty acids above 10 carbons is performed by a microsomal fatty acid elongase that condenses malonyl and acetyl-CoA directly, followed by similar steps of reduction to hydroxyacyl-CoA, enoyl-CoA, and acyl-CoA. Each cycle of this reaction sequence adds two carbons to the fatty acyl chain, occurring within the synthase complex for C4-C16 and/or within microsomes for C10 and above. *(Reproduced, with permission, from Murray RK, Bender DA, Botham KM, et al. Harper's Illustrated Biochemistry. 28th ed. New York, NY: McGraw-Hill; 2009:197.)*

diseases affecting brain, bones, and the reticuloendothelial system (Tay-Sachs, Gaucher, Niemann-Pick diseases—see table in Appendix for disease descriptions).

- Glycerophospholipids are degraded by phospholipases, some of which occur in snake venom; the combined action of phospholipases with fatty acyl activation and transfer allows remodeling of glycerol lipids through exchange of fatty acid groups.
- Fatty acid oxidation occurs in mitochondria, utilizing NAD^+, FAD, and oxygen to remove 2-carbon blocks and generate ATP (Fig. 16).
- Fatty acid oxidation produces ketone bodies (acetoacetate, 3-hydroxybutyrate, acetone) in the liver through mitochondrial formation of hydroxymethylglutaryl (HMG)-CoA; ketone bodies provide energy for extrahepatic tissues through conversion to acetyl-CoA and accumulate during starvation (ketosis) or insulin deficiency (ketoacidosis in diabetes mellitus).
- "Free" fatty acids are in fact bound to albumin in plasma and binding proteins in the cell, requiring activation to fatty acyl-CoA molecules before oxidation; longer chain fatty acyl CoAs must be converted to acyl-carnitines by carnitine palmitoyltransferase-1 (CPT-1) and transferred into mitochondria for oxidation by carnitine-acylcarnitine translocase.
- CPT-1 activity, the gateway into mitochondria, is an important regulator of fatty acid oxidation that is inhibited by malonyl-CoA; starvation increases levels of free fatty acids and fatty acyl-CoAs that inhibit acetyl-CoA carboxylase and levels of its product, malonyl-CoA.
- Inherited defects of fatty acid oxidation include defects of carnitine transport, CPT deficiencies, and several enzyme deficiencies grouped as long, medium, or short chain disorders with differing symptoms; environmental insults include toxins such as hypoglycin in Jamaican vomiting sickness and nutritional deficiencies of carnitine with prematurity or renal disease.
- Lipid transport involves complexing of amphipathic lipids and proteins to form water-soluble lipoproteins, including chylomicrons (from intestine), very low density lipoprotein (VLDL) from liver, high density lipoproteins (HDLs), and free fatty acid-albumin from adipose tissue (see Table 8).
- Major plasma lipoproteins can be separated by density or lipoprotein electrophoresis, each including specific apolipoproteins as listed in Table 8. Chylomicrons transport fats from the intestine to other tissues and HDL transports cholesterol from the periphery back to the liver.

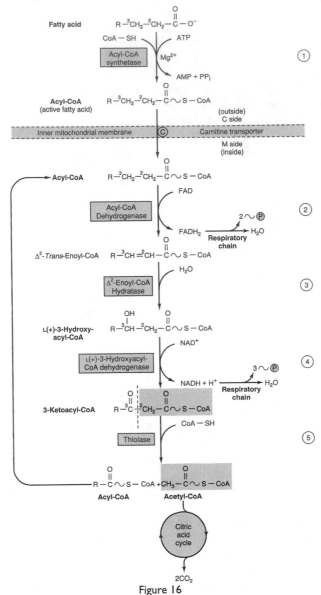

Figure 16

β-oxidation of fatty acids. Long-chain acyl-CoA is cycled through reactions 2 through 5, and one acetyl-CoA moiety is removed with each cycle. *(Reproduced, with permission, from Murray RK, Bender DA, Botham KM, et al. Harper's Illustrated Biochemistry. 28th ed. New York, NY: McGraw-Hill; 2009:186.)*

TABLE 8. HUMAN PLASMA LIPOPROTEINS

Lipoprotein	Source	Density (g/mL)	Main Lipid Components (% as lipid) #	Apolipoproteins
Chylomicrons	Intestine	<0.95	Triacylglycerols (98%-99%)	A-I, A-II, A-IV, B-48, C-I, C-II, C-III, E
Chylomicron remnants	Chylomicrons	<1.006	Triacylglycerols phospholipids cholesterol (92%-94%)	B-48, E
VLDL	Liver (intestine)	0.95-1.006	Triacylglycerol (90%-93%)	B-100, C-I, C-II, C-III
IDL	VLDL	1.006-1.019	Triacylglycerol cholesterol (89%)	B-100, E
LDL	VLDL	1.019-1.063	Cholesterol (79%)	B-100
HDLs*	Liver, intestine, VLDL Chylomicrons	1.063->1.210*	Phospholipids cholesterol (43%-68%)	A-I, A-II, A-IV, C-I, C-II, C-III, D, E
Albumin-FFA	Adipose tissue	>1.281	FFA (1%)	

VL, very low; H, high; I, intermediae; DL, density lipoprotein; FFA, free fatty acids; # the remainder is protein; *several HDL classes including HDL, of density similar to LDL and pre β-HDL with very high density >1.21 (sometimes called VHDL). (Modified, with permission, from Murray RK, Bender DA, Botham KM, et al. Harper's Biochemistry 28th ed. New York, NY: McGraw-Hill; 2009:213).

- Plasma free fatty acids are released from adipose tissue during starvation, stored as triacylglycerol (particularly in heart and muscle), or rapidly metabolized; fatty acid oxidation provides 25% to 50% of energy requirements during fasting.
- Absorbed triacylglycerols are transported as chylomicrons in intestinal lymph and cleaved by lipoprotein lipase within capillary linings to form chylomicron remnants; the liberated fatty acids are absorbed by heart and muscle, while liver receptors (apo E and LDL) absorb remnant lipoproteins.
- Liver has key roles in lipid transport/metabolism including bile synthesis to promote digestion/absorption, oxidation/synthesis of fatty acids and glycerophospholipids, secretion of VLDL for use by other tissues, conversion of fatty acids to ketone bodies (ketogenesis), and the uptake/metabolism of lipoproteins.
- Free or esterified cholesterol is present in most tissues, derived in about equal parts from diet or biosynthesis; all cholesterol carbons are derived from acetyl-CoA, first as the 5-carbon mevalonic acid (by hydroxymethylglutaryl-CoA reductase that is inhibited by statins—Fig. 17), then as successive joining of 5-carbon isoprene units to generate geranyl phosphate (10 carbons), farnesyl phosphate (15 carbons), and squalene (30 carbons) that is oxidized and cyclized to form the four rings of cholesterol.
- The isoprenoid signal transducer dolichol and the respiratory constituent ubiquinone are derived from farnesyl diphosphate, while cholesterol is modified to form steroid hormones or vitamins and excreted as bile acids (cholic acid) and bilirubin.
- Diseases of lipoprotein metabolism include fatty liver due to triacylglycerol accumulation (alcoholism, toxins, diabetes), abetalipoproteinemia (apo B deficiency), atherosclerosis (hypercholesterolemia due to LDL receptor deficiency, high HDL, lipoprotein lipase deficiency), and apo A (HDL) deficiency (Tangier disease).

Key concepts: Amino acid metabolism (Murray, pp 234-270. Scriver, pp 1667-2108.)

- Of 20 amino acids in proteins, humans can synthesize 12 including 3 (cysteine, tyrosine, hydroxylysine) from the eight nutritionally essential amino acids—remembered as the acronym PVT TIM HALL using the single-letter amino acid code (Table 4).
- Nonessential amino acids include glutamate/glutamine from α-ketoglutarate, alanine from pyruvate, aspartate/asparagines from oxaloacetate,

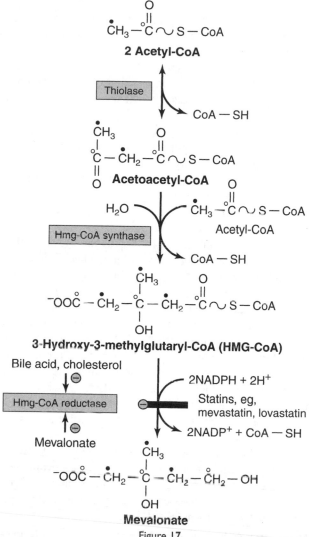

Figure 17

Biosynthesis of mevalonate, showing the critical step of HMG-CoA reductase that is inhibited by statins. The open and solid circles indicate the fates of carbons in acetyl-CoA. *(Reproduced, with permission, from Murray RK, Bender DA, Botham KM, et al. Harper's Illustrated Biochemistry. 28th ed. New York, NY: McGraw-Hill; 2009:225.)*

serine from 3-phosphoglycerate, glycine from glyoxylate/serine/choline, proline from glutamate, cysteine from methionine, and tyrosine from phenylalanine.

- Hydroxylysine and hydroxyproline are hydroxylated after incorporation into protein (mostly collagens); vitamin C and iron-requiring oxygenases add the hydroxyl groups, and ascorbate deficiency causes bone and gum disease (scurvy).

- Normal but aged proteins are cleaved internally by proteases (including lysosomal cathepsins) and the peptides cleaved to amino acids by peptidases; abnormal proteins are targeted by ubiquitin (binding its carboxyl group to amino side groups using ATP) and degraded by a protease complex known as the proteasome.

- Amino acid nitrogen is catabolized to ammonia, which is neurotoxic, and to urea, which is excreted by the kidney.

- Ammonia is converted to glutamine (from glutamate), alanine (from pyruvate), and glutamate (from α-ketoglutarate) in the liver; cirrhosis produces collateral circulation with bypass of portal blood, causing hyperammonemia and neurologic symptoms including cognitive dysfunction, slurred speech, blurred vision, rapid breathing, coma, and death.

- Urea is the major end product of nitrogen metabolism in humans and is synthesized through the urea cycle (Fig. 18); carbamoyl synthetase is rate limiting for urea synthesis and its activity is determined by acetyl-CoA levels through its conversion to N-acetylglutamate cofactor.

- Inherited enzyme deficiencies are associated with each enzyme of the urea cycle, producing severe hyperammonemia, neurotoxicity, and death if the ammonia is not removed by dialysis or salvage agents (eg, glutamate derivatives).

- Catabolism of amino acid carbon chains often yields acetyl-CoA; enzyme deficiencies in the degradation pathways for phenylalanine (phenylketonuria), tyrosine (tyrosinemia, alkaptonuria), branched chain amino acids (maple syrup urine disease), and tryptophan (Hartnup disease) cause specific metabolic diseases.

Key concepts: Porphyrin and nucleotide metabolism (Murray, pp 271-284. Scriver, pp 2961-3104.)

- Porphyrins consist of four pyrrole rings containing a nitrogen and four carbons; porphyrins are synthesized from the condensate of succinyl-CoA and glycine to form aminolevulinic acid, porphobilinogen, protoporphyrin, and (after incorporation of iron) heme.

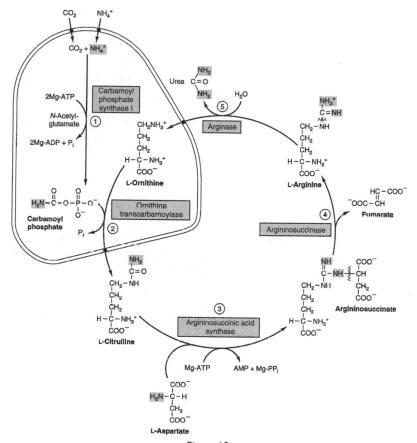

Figure 18

Reactions and intermediates of urea biosynthesis. The nitrogen-containing groups that contribute to the formation of urea are shaded. Reactions 1 and 2 occur in the matrix of liver mitochondria and reactions 3, 4, and 5 in liver cytosol. CO_2 (as bicarbonate), ammonium ion, ornithine, and citrulline enter the mitochondrial matrix via specific carriers (see heavy dots) present in the inner membrane of liver mitochondria. *(Reproduced, with permission, from Murray RK, Bender DA, Botham KM, et al. Harper's Illustrated Biochemistry. 28th ed. New York, NY: McGraw-Hill; 2009:244.)*

- Porphyrias result from deficiencies of the enzymes responsible for porphyrin synthesis; deficiencies of hepatic enzymes (acute intermittent porphyria, porphyria cutanea tarda, variegate porphyria) produce abdominal pain, photosensitivity, and neuropsychiatric symptoms while those of erythrocyte enzymes (X-linked sideroblastic anemia, congenital erythropoietic porphyria, protoporphyria) produce anemia and skin changes with or without photosensitivity.
- Catabolism of heme removes iron and produces bilirubin, which is conjugated with glucuronide in liver, secreted into bile and then the intestine, and converted into urobilinogen by fecal flora; a fraction of urobilinogen is reabsorbed to produce an enterohepatic cycle that can be disrupted by liver disease or immaturity to produce hyperbilirubinemia (jaundice).
- Neonatal jaundice due to liver immaturity produces unconjugated (water insoluble or indirect-reacting) hyperbilirubinemia, while obstruction of the bile duct (gallstones, cancer, biliary atresia) produces conjugated (water soluble or direct-reacting) hyperbilirubinemia; excess unconjugated bilirubin can cross the blood-brain barrier and cause neurotoxicity (kernicterus).
- Enzyme deficiencies can affect liver secretion or conjugation of bilirubin (Crigler-Najjar, Gilbert syndromes with indirect hyperbilirubinemia) or bile excretion (Dubin-Johnson, Rotor syndromes with direct hyperbilirubinemia). Direct (-reacting) bilirubin is conjugated with glucuronide groups, indirect bilirubin is unconjugated as categorized by laboratory methods for bilirubin measurement.
- Purine and pyrimidine nucleotides are not essential nutrients but require considerable energy to synthesize; nucleosides from the diet or cell cycles are often salvaged by conversion to nucleoside phosphates (nucleotides).
- Purine nucleotide synthesis begins with placement of a high energy pyrophosphate at the C1 position of ribose-5-phosphate; phosphoribosylpyrophosphate (PRPP) is the pyrophosphate donor and PRPP synthase catalyzes the rate-limiting initial reaction that is feedback inhibited by the end-products AMP, ADP, GMP, and GTP (Fig. 19). Note that PRPP is required for both purine and pyrimidine synthesis.
- Inosine monophosphate is the product of purine synthesis, converted to adenosine and guanine nucleotides that occur in nucleic acids; the amino acids aspartate, glycine, and glutamate contribute nitrogens to the purine ring, while folate derivatives contribute two carbons.

- Purines are catabolized to uric acid, increased in purine imbalance disorders (eg, mutations increasing PRPP synthase activity), renal disorders (with decreased urate excretion), glycogen storage disorders (that produce increased ribose-5-phosphate), and Lesch-Nyhan syndrome with defects in hypoxanthine-guanine phosphoribosyl transferase (HGPRT—diminishing its role in purine salvage and increasing levels of PRPP); inborn errors or folate antagonists that inhibit purine synthesis impair DNA synthesis and disproportionately impact rapidly dividing cells, illustrated by the immune deficiencies adenosine deaminase or purine nucleoside phosphorylase deficiencies and the use of folate antagonists (eg, methotrexate) in anticancer therapy.

- Pyrimidine synthesis begins with a cytosolic carbamoyl phosphate synthase II that is different from the mitochondrial carbamoyl synthase I of the urea cycle; enzyme complexes (including aspartate transcarbamoylase and orotic acid phosphoribosyl transferase) channel the first steps of pyrimidine synthesis.

- PRPP and folic acid derivatives are also important in pyrimidine synthesis, emphasizing the coordination of purine and pyrimidine synthesis appropriate for their use in nucleic acid; carbamoyl transferase (by UTP) and aspartate transcarbamoylase (by CTP) are inhibited by their product pyrimidines (analogous to purine feedback inhibition shown in Fig. 19).

- Ribonucleoside reductase (using thioredoxin) converts nucleoside diphosphates to deoxyribonucleoside diphosphates and is another step where pyrimidine and purine nucleotide levels are coordinated by cross-inhibition (GDP inhibits reduction of UDP and CDP, dTTP inhibits reduction of UDP but stimulates reduction of GDP, etc); salvage reactions generating nucleotides by phosphoribosylation of nucleosides are also cross-regulated to ensure equal supplies of purine and pyrimidine nucleotides for nucleic acid synthesis.

- Pyrimidine catabolism yields water-soluble products like β-aminoisobutyrate with few consequences for disease (except for a rare anemia due to orotic aciduria); pyrimidine synthetic enzymes do convert analogues like allopurinol (lowers uric acid in treatment of gout) or 5-fluorouracil (anticancer drug) to nucleotides, and thymidylate synthase that converts dUMP to TMP (using methylene tetrahydrofolate) is a prime target for anticancer folate antagonists.

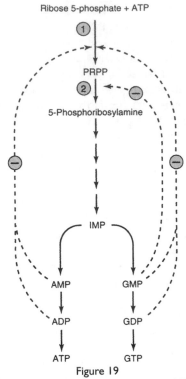

Ribose 5-phosphate + ATP

PRPP

5-Phosphoribosylamine

IMP

AMP   GMP

ADP   GDP

ATP   GTP

Figure 19

Control of the rate of de novo purine nucleotide synthesis. Solid lines represent metabolite flow, and dashed lines show feedback inhibition (0) by end-products of the pathway. Reactions 1 and 2 are catalyzed by PRPP synthase and PPRP glytamylamido-transferase, respectively. (*Reproduced, with permission, from Murray RK, Bender DA, Botham KM, et al.* Harper's Illustrated Biochemistry. *28th ed. New York, NY: McGraw-Hill; 2009:296.*)

NUTRITION

Key concepts: Nutrition (Murray, pp 459-468. Scriver, pp 155-166, 3897-3964.)

- Nutrition (including food availability [diet], ingestion, digestion, and intestinal absorption) provides carbohydrates and lipids as metabolic fuels, proteins for growth and tissue repletion, and the vitamins or minerals that are needed in small amounts for selected metabolic reactions.

- Abnormal diets, with over- or undernutrition, cause or contribute to the majority of human ills; diseases affecting dietary intake (neuromuscular swallowing problems), digestion (deficiency of bile acids in gall bladder disease, intestinal enzymes in cystic fibrosis), or absorption (lactose intolerance, celiac disease, vitamin B_{12} deficiency) are also common.

- Disorders of undernutrition present as "failure to thrive" in infancy and at later stages with feeding or nutritional challenges (puberty, pregnancy, old age).

- Digestion involves enzyme action at various locations in the gastrointestinal tract as illustrated by salivary and pancreatic amylases, lipases, peptidases like pepsin and trypsin (secreted as inactive zymogens), and disaccharidases; the liberated small molecules are absorbed using specific transporters in the intestinal brush border.

- Bile acids are essential for lipid emulsification and absorption, vitamin D for induction of calbindin and calcium absorption, intrinsic factor for vitamin B_{12} absorption, and vitamin C for promoting the limited human iron absorption through binding to mucosal cell ferritin and plasma transferring.

- The basal metabolic rate (BMR) measures body energy requirements at rest, assessed at 12 hours after feeding (morning); charts accounting for weight, age, and gender allow calculation of BMR rather than direct measurement.

- Vigorous activity, hypermetabolic states (AIDS, cancer), and protein catabolism after trauma or inflammatory illnesses can increase the BMR up to eightfold (with skiing, stair climbing, jogging); intake of calories above those needed to maintain the BMR causes the individual to be overweight (BMI >25) or obese (BMI >30) where the BMI (body mass index) is weight in kilograms divided by height in meters squared.

- Poor nutrition can produce specific deficiency diseases (eg, the fragile/misshapen bones of rickets) or more general phenotypes such as marasmus (muscle and tissue wasting, resigned affect), kwashiorkor (reddish hair, swollen liver, subcutaneous swelling = edema), and cachexia (exaggerated symptoms of marasmus with greater protein deficiency) from eating disorders (anorexia nervosa), chronic diseases (AIDS, lupus), or cancers. Kwashiorkor is distinguished from marasmus by its normal caloric intake with deficient protein.

VITAMINS AND MINERALS

Key concepts: Vitamins and minerals (Murray, pp 467-481. Scriver, pp 155-166, 3897-3964.)

- Vitamins and minerals are micronutrients that generally cannot be synthesized by the body; their dietary intake must be between the extremes of low (causing clinical deficiency disease) or high (causing overdose toxicity as with hypervitaminosis A or iron tablet ingestion).
- The lipid-soluble vitamins A, D, E, and K are absorbed with fat, so maintenance of adequate levels requires normal intestinal fat absorption. Disorders causing bile acid/gut enzyme deficiencies (cystic fibrosis) or intestinal transit/brush border dysfunction (inflammatory bowel disease, chronic diarrhea/fatty stools = steatorrhea) can lead to fat-soluble vitamin deficiencies.
- A vitamin is defined as an organic compound needed in small amounts to foster metabolic integrity, usually as a cofactor in enzyme reactions; this definition highlights the illogical use of high-dose vitamin mixtures (megavitamin therapy) for various chronic illnesses (eg, autism, Down syndrome, cancers).
- Vitamin deficiency diseases are listed in Table 9 along with scientific uses of high-dose vitamin therapy (to overcome altered enzyme/cofactor binding in specific genetic disorders or to lower risks for birth defects).
- Essential minerals (Table 10) include those with significant tissue concentrations and dietary requirements (eg, sodium, potassium, calcium chloride) and trace metals required in small amounts that are analogous to vitamins (eg, zinc, iron, copper).

HORMONES AND INTEGRATED METABOLISM

Key concepts: Types of hormones and hormone action (Murray, pp 425-443, 444-458. Scriver, pp 3965-4292.)

- Integrated actions of the endocrine and neural systems produce hormones, acting on distant cells (endocrine), adjacent cells (paracine), or the same cell (autocrine) as agonists (stimulants) or antagonists (inhibitors) of various cell functions.
- The recognition of numerous signaling molecules including growth factors, cytokines, interleukins, etc, places hormone action within the general category of signal transduction. Environmental or internal stimuli are recognized by the organism, releasing signal molecules that trigger adaptive responses. These signal molecules effect sequential changes in

TABLE 9. VITAMIN FUNCTIONS, DEFICIENCY DISEASES, AND HIGH-DOSE THERAPIES

	Vitamin	Functions	Deficiency Disease	High-Dose Therapy
A	Retinols, β-carotene	Retinal pigment, signal transduction, antioxidant	Night blindness, dry eyes (xerophthalmia) with corneal ulcers and blindness, hyperkeratosis (scaly skin)	Contraindicated—causes increased intracranial pressure
D	Calciferol	Calcium absorption/excretion, bone formation	Rickets: poor bone mineralization (osteomalacia) and formation (bowed legs)	Vitamin D-resistant rickets
E	Tocopherols	Antioxidant	Neurologic symptoms (rare); anemia	Common in skin care but not proven effective
K	Phylloquinone	Blood clotting and bone formation; made by intestinal flora	Normal newborns; bleeding and bone changes (stippled epiphyses, short nose)	Routine nursery administration, rare inborn errors
B_1	Thiamin	Coenzyme for pyruvate dehydrogenase (PDH) and other enzymes	Beriberi: burning sensory neuropathy, cardiac failure, edema, Wernicke-Korsakoff dementia in alcoholics	Leigh disease and other mitochondrial disorders with PDH deficiency[*]
B_2	Riboflavin	Coenzyme in redox reactions; precursor to flavoproteins FMN, FAD	Photophobia, stomatitis (irritation at corners of mouth, lips, and tongue), anemia	Mitochondrial enzyme deficiencies having flavin cofactors[*]
B_3	Niacin	Coenzyme in redox reactions as part of NAD(P)/NAD(P)H	Pellagra—photosensitive dermatitis, psychosis	Hartnup disease—defect in neutral amino acid including tryptophan; effective at raising HDL

(*Continued*)

TABLE 9. VITAMIN FUNCTIONS, DEFICIENCY DISEASES, AND HIGH-DOSE THERAPIES (Continued)

	Vitamin	Functions	Deficiency Disease	High-Dose Therapy
B_6	Pyridoxine	Coenzyme for amino acid, glycogen, steroid metabolism	Convulsions; peripheral nerve pain in slow metabolizers with P450 variants and alcoholics	Infantile convulsions of unknown cause; homocystinuria
	Folic acid	Coenzyme for one-carbon transfer as in nucleotide synthesis	Megaloblastic anemia	Megaloblastic anemia; preconceptional therapy to lower risk for neural tube defects
B_{12}	Cobalamin	Coenzyme for one-carbon transfer and in folate metabolism	Pernicious anemia with neuromuscular symptoms	Methylmalonic acidemia, folate metabolism defects
	Pantothenic acid	Part of fatty acyl synthase complex, fatty acid synthesis	Rare, usually with other vitamin deficiencies—irritability, depression, cramps	
H	Biotin	Coenzyme for carboxylation reactions in gluconeogenesis, fatty acid synthesis	Metabolic acidosis, hair loss, skin rashes, failure to thrive	Biotinidase deficiency, propionic acidemia
C	Ascorbic acid	Collagen proline, lysine hydroxylation, antioxidant, enhances iron absorption	Scurvy—poor wound healing, bone tenderness with rib swelling (rachitic rosary), gum disease with tooth loss, hemorrhage with bruising, nosebleeds	Wound healing after surgery; not effective for URI in controlled trials

*Not highly effective; P450, cytochromes P450s responsible for drug detoxification; URI, upper respiratory infections.

TABLE 10. ESSENTIAL MACRO- AND MICROMINERALS

	Mineral	Functions	Deficiency and Toxicity Diseases	Dietary Sources
Essential macrominerals				
Na⁺⁺	Sodium	Main cation of extracellular fluid; water/salt balance; neuromuscular functions	Hypotonic dehydration in children; renal disorders; salt-wasting in chronic illness; *hypertension*	Table salt
K⁺	Potassium	Main cation of intracellular fluid; water/base balance, neuromuscular functions	Muscle weakness, confusion, metabolic alkalosis; *cardiac arrest, intestinal ulcers*	Vegetables, fruits (bananas), nuts
Cl⁻	Chloride	Fluid/electrolyte balance; gastric fluid	Prolonged vomiting (as with pyloric stenosis), causing hypochloremic alkalosis; *hypochloremic alkalosis;*	Table salt
Ca⁺⁺	Calcium	Constituent of bones, teeth; regulates neuromuscular function	Rickets (soft, fragile bones—osteomalacia—and bony deformities) in children; bone pain and osteoporosis in adults; muscle contractions (tetany); *renal disease*	Dairy products, beans, leafy vegetables
P	Phosphorus	Constituent of bones, teeth; high energy intermediates and nucleic acid at cellular level	Rickets in children, osteomalacia in adults; *bone loss by stimulating secondary hyperparathyroidism*	Phosphate food additives

(Continued)

TABLE 10. ESSENTIAL MACRO-AND MICROMINERALS (Continued)

Mineral		Functions	Deficiency and Toxicity Diseases	Dietary Sources
Magnesium	Mg^{++}	Constituent of bones, teeth; enzyme cofactor (kinases, etc)	Muscle contractions; muscle dysfunction with decreased reflexes and respiratory depression	Leafy green vegetables

Selected essential microminerals (silicon, vanadium, nickel, tin, manganese, lithium also thought to be essential)*

Mineral		Functions	Deficiency and Toxicity Diseases	Dietary Sources
Chromium	Cr	Potentiates insulin	Impaired glucose tolerance	Meat, liver, grains, nuts, cheese
Cobalt	Co	Constituent of vitamin B_{12}		
Copper	Cu	Constituent of oxidases, promotes iron absorption	Similar to scurvy; kinky hair and connective tissue defects in Menkes disease; *cerebral and liver toxicity in Wilson disease*	Liver
Iodine	I	Constituent of thyroid hormones	Hypothyroidism, producing low muscle tone, porcine features, and developmental retardation in children (cretinism), enlarged thyroid (goiter), lethargy, myopathy and lower leg swelling (myxedema) in adults; *hyperthyroidism with protruding eyes (exophthalmos), tachycardia, goiter*	Iodized table salt, seafood

Fe	Iron	Constituent of heme cofactor for hemoglobins, cytochromes	Anemia (hypochromic, microcytic) with pallor, fatigue, and heart failure; iron overload (hemosiderosis in cells) with liver and heart failure; those with hereditary hemochromatosis more susceptible	Plants, meat
Se	Selenium	Constituent of glutathione peroxidase	Subtle protein-energy malnutrition; hair loss, dermatitis, irritability	
Zn	Zinc	Cofactor for diverse enzymes, constituent of zinc finger DNA-binding motifs of signal transduction proteins	Acrodermatitis enterohepatica with hair loss, skin rashes, bowel malabsorption; decreased taste and smell acuity; gastrointestinal irritation, vomiting	
F	Fluoride	Can be incorporated into bones and teeth for increased hardness	Dental caries, osteoporosis; dl fluorosis (spotting)	Drinking water where added

*Aluminum, arsenic, antimony, boron, bromine, cadmium, cesium, germanium, lead, mercury, silver, and strontium are known to be toxic in excess.

diverse molecules (transduction of signals) along pathways; small concentration changes in signal molecules are amplified to produce adaptive responses that maintain homeostasis.

- Certain signal molecules, sometimes distinguished as group I hormones, are fat soluble and can cross cell membranes to bind to cytosolic or nuclear receptors. These include steroid hormones (eg, androgens, estrogens, gluco- and mineralocorticoids) as well as retinoic acid and thyroid hormones. Other signal molecules, sometimes distinguished as group II hormones, are water soluble and bind to the external surface of the cell membrane, effecting responses through cytoplasmic "second messengers" (Fig. 20).

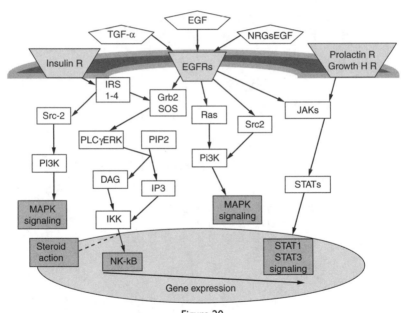

Figure 20

Insulin pathways overlap with EGF/TGF-α pathways that have intrinsic receptor kinases; insulin results in phosphorylation of insulin receptor substrates (IRS 1 to 4) and triggers MAPK anabolic signaling. Growth hormone and prolactin receptors are examples of those without intrinsic kinase activity, activating Janus kinases (JAKs) and STAT (signal transducer and activator of transcription) molecules to alter gene expression.

- The epidermal growth factor (EGF) pathway (Fig. 20) is an example of hormone action/signal transduction. EGF binds to four tyrosine kinase receptors (EGFRs) within the ErbB (erythroblastic leukemia viral oncogene homolog) family. These include EGFR (ErbB1) and Her2/c-neu (ErbB2), the latter an important marker of breast cancer. EGF and other ligands like transforming growth factor-α (TGF-α), or neuroregulins (NRGs) bind to EGFRs, which like the insulin or insulin-like-growth factor receptors, have an intrinsic protein kinase. Binding initiates a kinase cascade with phosphorylation of other signaling proteins like Grb2 (growth factor receptor-bound protein-2), SOS (son of sevenless named from its embryonic role in the fruit fly), phospholipase C (PLCγ), and Ras (an oncogene discovered in rat sarcoma cells). PLCγ cleaves phosphatidylinositol 4.5 bisphosphate (PIP2) to 1,2-diacylglycerol (DAG) and inositol 1,4,5-trisphosphate (IP3), all important second messengers. Kinases like PI3K (phosphatidylinositol 3-kinase) activate anabolic MAPK (mitogen-activated protein kinase) signaling that promotes cell growth and division while IKK (I-kappaB-kinase) facilitates nuclear transfer of NK-kB (nuclear factor-kappaB) transcription factor that promotes growth of inflammatory and immune response cells in the presence of cytokines or infections. Anti-inflammatory glucocorticoids act at several sites including the pathways that transfer NK-kB to the nucleus.
- Second messengers include cAMP (employed by adrenergic catecholamines, ACTH, FSH, glucagon, and TSH), cGMP (employed by atrial natriuretic factor, nitric oxide), calcium and/or phosphatidylinositols (employed by acetylcholine, angiotensin II, oxytocin), and protein kinase/phosphatase cascades (employed by epidermal growth factor, erythropoietin, fibroblast growth factor, growth hormone, insulin). Overlapping actions of the latter category of hormones are illustrated in Fig. 20.
- Chemical types of hormone include cholesterol derivatives (steroid hormones—eg, testosterone, cortisol), tyrosine derivatives (eg, thyroxine, epinephrine), peptides (eg, ACTH), and glycoproteins (eg, TSH, FSH).
- Membrane-soluble signals (including group I hormones) act by diffusing into the cytoplasm or nucleus to form a ligand-receptor complex that interacts with (1) modifying proteins, (2) hormone response elements (HRE) in DNA, and (3) transcription factors to alter cell function.
- Water-soluble signals (including group II hormones) often interact with characteristic 7-membrane-spanning domain receptors and G protein complexes: GTP is exchanged with GDP on the α-subunit, which

activates the effector (adenyl cyclase, potassium/calcium channels, phospholipase, etc). Some receptors have intrinsic kinase domains that are activated by ligand-binding (eg, epidermal growth factor, insulin receptors shown in Fig. 20) while others activate cytosolic kinases to begin the process of signal transduction.

- Signals acting at cell membranes can produce activation-deactivation of over 300 kinases/phosphodiesterases in cascades that use levels of second messengers (cAMP, cGMP, calcium, phosphatidyl inositols) to provide diverse and multifaceted regulatory mechanisms (see Fig. 20).
- The complex pathways illustrated in Fig. 20, considerably simplified for brevity, illustrate three points: (1) hormones, growth factors, and second messengers trigger overlapping pathways that culminate in altered gene expression, (2) many signal transduction intermediates have parallel roles in cancer (Ras, ErbB2-Her2) and embryonic development (SOS, EGFs, TGFs), and (3) defects in primary signal molecules will have multiple secondary effects (eg, the many abnormalities in diabetes mellitus, Cushing disease (cortisol excess), or developmental syndromes. Effective therapies can be envisioned by manipulating stem molecules in these branching pathways (eg, Herceptin antibody against Her2 in breast cancer, Gleevec antibody against the c-bcr/c-abl fusion product in chronic myelogenous leukemia—MIM*189980).

Key concepts: Integrated metabolism (Murray, pp 131-142, 444-458. Scriver, pp 131-142.)

- Many metabolic fuels are interconvertible, with an equilibrium between oxidation/catabolism for energy and reduction/anabolism for synthesis and reserve; an imperative affecting this equilibrium is the need to maintain blood glucose levels to fuel central nervous system and erythrocyte functions.
- Fatty acids and their generated ketones or acetyl-CoA cannot be used for gluconeogenesis (except for odd-carbon chains that generate propionic acid); certain (glucogenic) amino acids can enter the citric acid cycle with net synthesis of oxaloacetate (and thus of glucose through phosphoenolpyruvate phosphokinase, etc) but others (ketogenic amino acids) yield acetyl-CoA.
- The catabolic/anabolic equilibrium is precisely regulated by hormones controlling the level of blood fuels and their delivery to tissues; the primary control hormones of metabolism are insulin and glucagon, with antagonizing effects on blood glucose levels (see Table 11).

TABLE 11. ACTIVITIES OF METABOLIC PATHWAYS IN FED OR FASTED STATES			
	Fed	Fasted	Diabetes
Glycogen synthesis	+	–	–
Glycolysis (liver)	+	–	–
Triacylglyceride synthesis	+	–	–
Fatty acid synthesis	+	–	–
Protein synthesis	+	–	–
Cholesterol synthesis	+	–	–
Glycogenolysis	–	+	+
Gluconeogenesis (liver)	–	+	+
Lipolysis	–	+	+
Fatty acid oxidation	–	+	+
Protein breakdown	–	±	±
Ketogenesis (liver)	–	+	+
Ketone body utilization (non-hepatic tissues)	–	+	+

- After a meal, fuels are abundant with glucose being the principal substrate for oxidation; insulin released from pancreatic β-islet cells allows glucose uptake in muscle and adipose cells (using the GLUT glucose transporter family) and promotes glycogen synthesis in liver and muscle.
- Blood levels of glucose, amino acids, fatty acids, and ketone bodies are maintained by the ratio of insulin/glucagon concentrations; high blood sugars increase this ratio, signaling the fed state and promoting anabolic activities; the ratio decreases as glucagon is secreted from pancreatic α cells in response to falling blood glucose (between meals, during fasting or starvation).
- Glucagon inhibits liver glycogen synthase and activates its glycogen phosphorylase, releasing glucose 6-phosphate that is converted to glucose; falling insulin levels act to preserve blood glucose by diminishing adipose and muscle uptake.
- Glucagon inhibits lipogenesis and stimulates lipase in adipose tissue, causing increased lipid catabolism with increased ketone bodies, free fatty acids, and glycerol; glycerol is an effective substrate for gluconeogenesis in liver.

- Muscle lacks a glucose-6-phosphatase to produce glucose from glycogen catabolism (using glucose-6-phosphate for energy instead); its increased fatty acid oxidation increases acetyl-CoA and citrate levels, inhibits glycolysis (to spare glucose), and yields pyruvate and alanine that travel to liver for gluconeogenesis (the Cori cycle).

- Epinephrine has effects similar to those of glucagon, except that glucagon has a greater effect on the liver, whereas epinephrine has a greater effect on muscle; epinephrine or norepinephrine is released during exercise to promote catabolism of glucose and fat that supports muscular activity.

- Glucagon inhibits lipogenesis in adipose cells. Fat is catabolized during fasting or starvation to supply energy, causing increases in ketone bodies and free fatty acids.

- Uncontrolled diabetes causes blood glucose levels to rise due to lack of or insensitivity to insulin, decreased glucose uptake by adipose/muscle tissue, and increased liver gluconeogenesis from amino acids; increased lipolysis in adipose tissue produces fatty acids for liver ketogenesis (distributing ketone bodies as fuel) with progressive ketosis and acidosis (acetoacetic acid and β-hydroxybutyrate are strong acids).

- The increased osmolarity of hyperglycemic blood plus increased lipids and cholesterol produce chronic vascular and nerve damage in diabetes (leading to hypertension, coronary artery disease, and retinal hemorrhage with blindness); acute hyperosmolarity (exacerbated by polyuria/dehydration) and ketoacidosis can lead to fatal diabetic coma unless insulin is provided.

INHERITANCE MECHANISMS AND BIOCHEMICAL GENETICS

Key concepts: Inheritance mechanisms/Risk calculations (Lewis, pp 69-89. Scriver, pp 3-45.)

- Human gametes have 23 chromosomes (haploid chromosome number n = 23), while most somatic cells have 46 chromosomes (diploid chromosome number 2n = 46).

- Genes occupy sites on chromosomes (loci) and occur in alternative forms (alleles); interaction of these alleles determine inheritance patterns of disease that can be recognized using standard family history (pedigree) symbols (Fig. 21).

Pedigree symbols

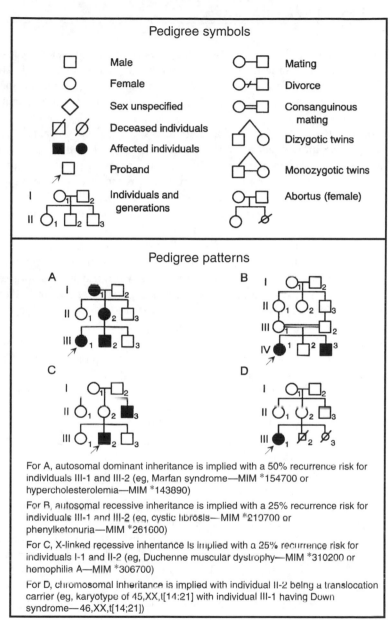

□	Male
○	Female
◇	Sex unspecified
▨ ⦸	Deceased individuals
■ ●	Affected individuals
▱ (proband)	Proband
○—□	Mating
○⁄□	Divorce
○═□	Consanguinous mating
□ ○ (twins)	Dizygotic twins
□ ○ (twins)	Monozygotic twins
○—□	Abortus (female)

Pedigree patterns

For A, autosomal dominant inheritance is implied with a 50% recurrence risk for individuals III-1 and III-2 (eg, Marfan syndrome—MIM *154700 or hypercholesterolemia—MIM *143890)

For B, autosomal recessive inheritance is implied with a 25% recurrence risk for individuals III-1 and III-2 (eg, cystic fibrosis—MIM *219700 or phenylketonuria—MIM *261600)

For C, X-linked recessive inheritance is implied with a 25% recurrence risk for individuals I-1 and II-2 (eg, Duchenne muscular dystrophy—MIM *310200 or hemophilia A—MIM *306700)

For D, chromosomal inheritance is implied with individual II-2 being a translocation carrier (eg, karyotype of 45,XX,t[14:21] with individual III-1 having Down syndrome—46,XX,t[14;21])

Figure 21
Pedigree symbols and pedigree patterns.

- Rarer Mendelian diseases exhibit autosomal dominant, autosomal recessive, or X-linked inheritance, while more common disorders like birth defects (spina bifida), diabetes mellitus, schizophrenia, or hypertension are caused by multiple genes plus environmental factors (multifactorial determination).

- Characteristics of autosomal dominant diseases include a vertical pattern of affected individuals in the pedigree, affliction of both males and females, variable expressivity (variable severity among affected individuals), frequent new mutations, and a 50% recurrence risk for offspring of affected individuals (see pedigree A of Fig. 21). Corollary: Germ-line mosaicism may produce affected siblings with autosomal dominant disease when neither parent is affected.

- Characteristics of autosomal recessive diseases include a horizontal pedigree pattern, affliction of males and females, frequent consanguinity (inbreeding), frequent carriers (heterozygotes without manifestations of disease), and a 25% recurrence risk for carrier parents (see pedigree B of Fig. 21). Corollary: Normal siblings of individuals with autosomal recessive disease have a two-third chance of being carriers.

- Characteristics of X-linked recessive diseases include an oblique pedigree pattern, affliction of males only, frequent female carriers, and a 25% recurrence risk for carrier females (see pedigree C of Fig. 21). Corollary: Haldane law predicts a two-third chance that the mother of an affected male with X-linked recessive disease is a carrier (and a one-third chance the affected male represents a new mutation).

Key concepts: Genetic and biochemical diagnosis (Lewis, pp 379-394. Scriver, pp 3-45. Murray, pp 388-405.)

- Certain ethnic groups have higher frequencies of particular Mendelian disorders illustrated by cystic fibrosis in Caucasians, sickle cell anemia in African Americans, β-thalassemia in Italians and Greeks, α-thalassemia in Asians, and Tay-Sachs disease in Ashkenazi Jews.

- Advanced maternal age is associated with higher risks for chromosomal disorders (eg, Down syndrome or trisomy 13), while advanced paternal age is associated with higher risks for new mutations (eg, those producing achondroplasia or Marfan syndrome).

- The Hardy-Weinberg law predicts allele frequencies in an idealized population according to the formula $p^2 + 2pq + q^2 = 1$. Applied to cystic fibrosis, the law predicts that homozygotes (q^2) have a frequency of 1 in 1600, predicting that carriers ($2pq$) have a frequency of 1 in 20.

- A karyotype is an ordered arrangement of chromosomes that is described by cytogenetic notation. A karyotype can be obtained from dividing cells (blood leukocytes, bone marrow, fibroblasts, amniocytes), but not from frozen or formalin-fixed cells.
- Cytogenetic notation includes the chromosome number (usually 46), description of the sex chromosomes (usually XX or XY), and indication of missing, extra, or rearranged chromosomes. Examples include 47,XY, +21 (male with Down syndrome); 47,XX,13 (female with trisomy +13); 45,X (female with monosomy X or Turner syndrome); 46,XX,del(5p) (female with deletion of the chromosome 5 short arm).
- DNA diagnosis examines specific regions of genes for altered nucleotide sequences or deletions that affect gene expression and function; techniques include Southern blotting, gene amplification with the polymerase chain reaction (PCR), and mutant allele detection by hybridization with allele-specific oligonucleotides (ASOs). Chromosome microdeletions encompass several genes and are detected by fluorescent in situ hybridization (FISH).
- Non-Mendelian inheritance mechanisms include mitochondrial inheritance (exhibiting maternal transmission), expansion of triplet repeats (exhibiting anticipation in pedigrees as in the fragile X syndrome), and genomic imprinting (exhibiting different phenotypes according to maternal or paternal origin of the aberrant genes).
- Prenatal diagnosis can include fetal ultrasound, maternal serum studies, or sampling of cells from the fetoplacental unit by chorionic villus sampling (CVS at 10-12 weeks, amniocentesis at 15-18 weeks, or percutaneous umbilical sampling [PUBS] from 16 weeks to term).

DNA Structure, Replication, and Repair

Questions

I. A 3-year-old boy is evaluated for symptoms of autism including poor eye contact and severe speech delay. Family history indicates that his mother had trouble in school due to "attention deficit," that he has an older brother with mental disability, and that another older brother and older sister are normal. The figure below diagrams the results of genetic analysis of the boy (lane 4), his mother (lane 5), and his siblings (lanes 1-3) for fragile X syndrome (MIM*309550). Which of the following best describes the results of this genetic analysis?

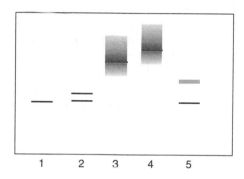

a. Immunoblot analysis reveals the boy is not affected with fragile X syndrome but one brother is.

b. Northern blot analysis reveals the boy is affected with fragile X syndrome and that his mother is a carrier.

c. Southern blot analysis reveals the boy is affected with fragile X syndrome as is one brother.

d. Western blot analysis reveals that the boy and his siblings do not have fragile X syndrome.

e. Reverse transcriptase-PCR amplification reveals no aberrant RNA transcription in this family.

2. A 2-year-old Scottish-American girl presents with deeply pigmented and scarred skin and her growth is delayed. Her dermatologist obtains a skin biopsy, suspecting the xeroderma pigmentosum group of diseases (MIM*278730); these have decreased ability to repair thymine-thymine dimers in DNA that are caused by ultraviolet light (sunlight exposure). Which of the following strategies would best measure unscheduled DNA synthesis (DNA repair) in the patient's skin fibroblasts?

a. Cell synchrony, then incubation with labeled iodine in G phase to complex with newly created hydroxyl groups in deoxyribose residues

b. Incubation with labeled purines to replace newly synthesized bases on the outside of the DNA duplex

c. Cell synchrony, then incubation with labeled deoxyribonucleotides in G phase to measure extension of single DNA strands in the 3′ to 5′ direction

d. Incubation with labeled deoxyribonucleotide triphosphates to measure extension of both strands in the 5′ to 3′ direction

e. Incubation with labeled deoxyribonucleotide triphosphates to measure extension of both strands in the 3′ to 5′ direction

3. The most common mutation causing cystic fibrosis (MIM*219700) in Caucasians is ΔF508, accounting for 70% of mutations—ΔF508 refers to deletion of a phenylalanine residue (F in single-letter amino acid code) at the 508th amino acid of the cystic fibrosis transmembrane regulator (CFTR) protein. Which of the following would best describe DNA diagnosis of cystic fibrosis patients who are homozygous for the ΔF508 mutation?

a. Polymerase chain reaction using primers surrounding nucleotide #1522 of the normal cystic fibrosis DNA coding sequence; positive hybridization only with an oligonucleotide specific for the ΔF508 allele.

b. Northern blotting of sputum RNA samples developed with CFTR gene probes, yielding two abnormally sized RNA transcripts.

c. Southern blotting using restriction endonucleases that yield 100 bp fragments containing nucleotide #508 of the normal cystic fibrosis DNA coding sequence; hybridization with a DNA probe for this region, yielding two CFTR gene fragment sizes.

d. Western blotting of sputum proteins developed with antibody to CFTR protein, yielding two abnormally sized bands.

e. Polymerase chain reaction using primers that amplify a 100 bp fragment surrounding nucleotide #508 of the normal cystic fibrosis DNA coding sequence, agarose gel electrophoresis demonstrates a single, abnormal fragment size using ultraviolet light.

4. A research project examines multiple chromosome regions in Italian families selected because several individuals are affected with insulin-dependent diabetes mellitus (IDDM, MIM*222100). The results reveal a single nucleotide change from A to G in a noncoding region of chromosome 10 that is present in 9 of 10 diabetics and only 6 of 30 nondiabetics. The conclusion is best described by which of the following statements?

a. Mutations in a gene on chromosome 10 cause diabetes in Italians, allowing DNA diagnosis by Southern blot with a 90% sensitivity.

b. Mutations in a gene on chromosome 10 cause diabetes in Italians, allowing DNA diagnosis by PCR amplification and DNA sequencing with a 60% positive predictive value.

c. A single nucleotide polymorphism on chromosome 10, detected by PCR amplification and DNA sequencing, is associated with IDDM in Italian families (sensitivity is 90%).

d. A single nucleotide polymorphism on chromosome 10, detected by PCR amplification and DNA sequencing, is now available for worldwide screening of diabetes susceptibility.

e. Association of a chromosome 10 gene mutation with IDDM in Italian families suggests that HLA loci may exist outside of chromosome 6.

5. A 55-year-old Caucasian male becomes exhausted after jogging 2 miles despite a prior schedule of jogging 30 miles per week. Evaluation discloses severe anemia with elevated white blood cell count, and bone marrow examination suggests a diagnosis of chronic myeloid leukemia (MIM*608232). Which of the following results would be most diagnostic of chromosome 22 deletion that can be seen in this leukemia?

a. Increased incorporation of labeled acetate into histones of chromatin regions on chromosome 22

b. Altered DNA restriction patterns of chromosome 22 regions with methylation-sensitive endonucleases

c. Altered pattern of small RNAs along leukemic chromatin

d. Altered DNA sequence for at least one chromosome 22 locus

e. Decreased transcription from loci on chromosome 22

6. A newborn Caucasian girl exhibits extreme hypotonia (low muscle tone) after an unremarkable pregnancy and delivery. The hypotonia is so severe that tube feeding is required, and the physician notes facial changes (almond-shaped eyes, down-turned corners of the mouth) and underdevelopment of the labia that suggest a diagnosis of Prader-Willi syndrome (MIM*176270). It can involve changes in gene structure or modification. The physician orders chromosome testing to look for the characteristic chromosome 15 deletion in Prader-Willi syndrome and DNA testing to evaluate an alteration of genomic imprinting. Which of the following processes occurs at the fifth position of cytidine and often correlates with gene inactivation?

a. Gene conversion
b. Sister chromatid exchange
c. Pseudogene
d. Gene rearrangement
e. DNA methylation

7. A 25-year-old Caucasian female is evaluated because her father, paternal grandfather, and uncle developed colon cancer before age 40. Examination has revealed an unusually dark complexion similar to that of her father and supernumerary (extra) teeth with multiple caries. Her past medical history indicates she had bony cysts noted on her tibia after x-rays for a fracture, and her physician suspects a diagnosis of autosomal dominant Gardner syndrome (MIM*175100) that has dark complexion, tooth changes, bony tumors (osteomas), and multiple colonic polyps with high rates of colon cancer. DNA testing for the causative adenomatous polyposis coli (APC) gene revealed a nucleotide substitution that changed the DNA sequence from CAGAGGT to CAGGGGT. This mutation ablated the splice junction at the border of exon 7 and its adjacent intron. A partial sequencing result is shown in the figure below, and supports which of the following conclusions about the female's APC genotype and expression?

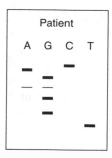

a. Homozygous for the normal Gardner allele, some smaller mRNA molecules
b. Heterozygous for normal and mutant Gardner allele, some larger mRNA molecules
c. Heterozygous for normal and mutant Gardner allele, some smaller mRNA molecules
d. Homozygous for mutant Gardner allele, no change in mRNA molecules
e. Homozygous for mutant Gardner allele, some larger mRNA molecules

8. A 20-year-old Caucasian male with sensorineural deafness has a mother, grandmother, and other maternal relatives who are also affected. He has been counseled that his family's pattern fits autosomal dominant inheritance (eg, MIM*124900 among > 10 types), conferring a 50% risk for his offspring to be deaf with each pregnancy. His family has been involved with the deaf community and has resisted gene testing, but he and his wife are interested in preconception/prenatal diagnosis options. Which of the following statements accurately conveys DNA testing options for the man and his wife, focusing particularly on restriction fragment length polymorphism (RFLP) analysis?

a. The man and his wife could have RFLP analysis and determine fetal outcome by which paternal RFLP allele was inherited.
b. Survey of RFLPs for an allele cotransmitted with deafness in the man and his affected family members could provide a marker for deafness in his offspring.
c. Finding an RFLP-encoded protein could distinguish mutated and normal genes for deafness.
d. Survey of the man's DNA for mutations outside of the putative deafness gene would reveal a restriction site that reflected an amino acid coding change.
e. Restriction of the man's DNA would produce fragments of the same size but with differences in charge.

9. It is well known that DNA polymerases synthesize DNA only in the 5′ to 3′ direction. Yet, at the replication fork, both strands of parental DNA are being replicated with the synthesis of new DNA. An experiment examines incorporation of radio-labeled nucleotide triphosphates in unsynchronized cells, and finds a small amount of incorporated label in DNA fragments of small size. Which of the following statements explains why the experiment is compatible with new DNA from both strands being added in the 5′ to 3′ direction?

   a. A different DNA polymerase replicates the complementary DNA strand as a series of small fragments.

   b. A 3′ to 5′ DNA polymerase is active in cells with high rates of DNA replication.

   c. DNA synthesis on complementary strand produces small 5′ to 3′ fragments that are continuously ligated together.

   d. DNA replication switch strands every 100 nucleotides, a detail not resolved by microscopy.

   e. DNA synthesis on the complementary strand does not use RNA primers.

10. A newborn boy has a cleft lip and palate with severe limb defects. The hands emerge directly from the shoulders (phocomelia means literally "flipper" limb) and the legs consist of the roots of the thighs only. A medical student searches the Online Mendelian Inheritance in Man database and suggests the diagnosis of Roberts syndrome (MIM*268300), an autosomal recessive disorder associated with altered chromatin condensation. The attending postulates that the chromatin change may impair DNA replication, and discusses why mammalian genomes are 100 times the size of bacterial genomes yet are replicated in just a few minutes. Which of the following best explains this fact?

   a. Eukaryotic DNA polymerases are extraordinarily fast compared with prokaryotic polymerases.

   b. The higher temperature of mammalian cells allows for an exponentially higher replication rate.

   c. Hundreds of replication forks work simultaneously on each piece of mammalian genomic DNA.

   d. Histones and microRNAs complexed with bacterial DNA speed up the rate of DNA replication.

   e. The presence of histones in mammalian chromatin speeds up the rate of DNA replication.

11. A 24-year-old African-American female comes in for her first prenatal visit with an estimated gestational age of 9 weeks as confirmed by ultrasound. She had learning difficulties causing her to drop out of high school, and her family history led to a request for fragile X DNA analysis shown in the figure below. The test examines amplification of a 3 bp (triplet) CGG repeat adjacent to the fragile X mental retardation-1 (FMR-1) gene (MIM*309550) on the X chromosome by determining DNA fragment size after restriction cleavage and electrophoresis (Southern blot). Her analysis (lane 5) is shown after that of her father (lane 1), normal sister (lane 2), and her brothers with mental disability (lanes 3 and 4). Her mother also had mild mental disability and died in a motor vehicle accident. The bands of higher molecular weight (slower mobility by electrophoresis) derive from fragile X gene fragments that contain higher number of CGG repeats as read on the coding strand of the gene's 5'-untranslated region. A discrete upper band is seen in the patient's mother (lane 2), a more diffuse upper band in the patient (lane 5), and very diffuse, slowly moving bands in the patient's disabled brothers (lanes 3 and 4). Recalling that females can be carriers for X-linked conditions with one normal and one abnormal allele on their two X chromosomes, which of the following would be the best interpretation of the results?

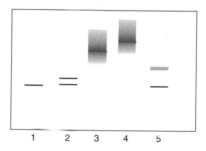

a. The patient has one fragile X gene with expanded triplet repeats and a 50% risk for a son with fragile X syndrome.
b. The patient has one fragile X gene with expanded triplet repeats and a 25% risk for a son with fragile X syndrome.
c. The patient has a restriction fragment length polymorphism within her fragile X genes with no increased risk for a child with fragile X syndrome.
d. The patient has one fragile X gene with expanded repeats that will produce a string of abnormal amino acids in fragile X protein; she has a 25% risk for a son with fragile X syndrome.
e. The patient has one fragile X gene with expanded triplet repeats and a 100% risk for a son with fragile X syndrome.

12. A 2-year-old child presents with poor weight gain, sparse hair, unusual face with sunken eyes, and skin that reddens markedly in sunlight. A diagnosis of Cockayne syndrome (MIM*216400) is considered and studies of DNA synthesis are undertaken. In vitro assay of labeled thymidine incorporation reveals decreased levels of DNA synthesis compared to controls, but normal-sized labeled DNA fragments. The addition of protein extract from normal cells gently heated to inactivate DNA polymerase restores DNA synthesis in Cockayne cells to normal. Which of the following enzymes used in DNA replication is most likely to be defective in Cockayne syndrome?

a. DNA-directed DNA polymerase
b. Unwinding proteins
c. DNA polymerase I
d. DNA-directed RNA polymerase
e. DNA ligase

13. A 20-year-old African-American male consults a physician because his father and a paternal aunt developed colon cancer in their mid-20s. Neither relative had multiple colonic polyps, so a diagnosis of hereditary nonpolyposis colon cancer (HNPCC-MIM*114500) is considered. The man's physician discusses testing for HNPCC, knowing that affected patients have genes with microsatellite instability; many gene regions containing abnormal, small loops of unpaired DNA. These DNA loops are the result of a mutation affecting which of the following?

a. Mismatch repair
b. Chain break repair
c. Base excision repair
d. Depurination repair
e. Nucleotide excision repair

14. A recombinant viral DNA containing a 300 bp human gene sequence is replicated in vitro using media containing bromodeoxyuridine triphosphate, completely saturating the DNA with bromodeoxyuridine residues. The bromo-substituted viral DNA is then switched to media with regular deoxyuridine triphosphate, and allowed to undergo two rounds of DNA replication. The human DNA fragment is then cleaved by restriction enzyme digestion and subjected to ultracentrifugation in cesium chloride under conditions that will separate bromo-substituted DNA duplexes, hybrid bromo-substituted/normal duplexes, and normal duplexes. Which of the results depicted in the figure below (with their interpretations) should be obtained?

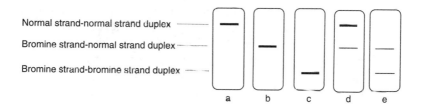

a. One DNA band of low density, meaning all DNA duplexes have two strands with normal uridine
b. One DNA band of intermediate density, meaning all DNA duplexes have one strand with uridine, one with bromouridine
c. One DNA band of high density, meaning all DNA duplexes have two strands with bromouridine
d. One DNA band of high density, one of intermediate density indicating the corresponding types of DNA duplexes
e. One DNA band of intermediate density, one of low density indicating the corresponding types of DNA duplexes

15. Sickle cell anemia (MIM*141900) is caused by a specific mutation in the gene for β-globin, one of the two globin proteins that complex with heme to form hemoglobin. The sickle cell anemia mutation is known to produce a single amino acid change, glutamic acid to valine, at position 6 of the β-globin peptide chain. Which of the following is the most likely mechanism for this mutation?

a. Crossing over
b. Two-base insertion
c. Three-base deletion
d. Single-base insertion
e. Single-base substitution (point mutation)

16. A newborn Caucasian girl is healthy with lightly colored eyes, hair, and skin that seem unremarkable. However, her parents are concerned because their first two children, a boy and a girl, have oculocutaneous albinism (MIM*203100) with pink irides, blond hair, and pale skin. Which of the following represents the best advice concerning the newborn child?

a. A one-eighth risk for albinism and skin cancer from DNA deletions
b. A one-eighth risk for albinism and skin cancer from DNA cross-linkage
c. A one-fourth risk for albinism and skin cancer from DNA point mutations
d. A one-fourth risk for albinism and skin cancer from DNA deletions
e. A one-fourth risk for albinism and skin cancer from DNA cross-linkage

17. A parent is correcting his child's photograph for red eye and notes one of the child's pupils reflects the flash as white rather than red. An ophthalmologist confirms the presence of a tumor in the back of the white-reflecting eye, telling the parents about the possibility of retinoblastoma (MIM* 180200). The parents return to their pediatrician, confused about the relation of retinoblastoma (*Rb*) and B-cell lymphoma (*bcl*) genes they saw on the Internet and the possibility their child's tumor is inherited. Which of the following is the most appropriate response?

a. Rb and bcl proteins are polymerases that prevent oncogenesis by stringent DNA repair; the parents are therefore carriers for autosomal recessive *Rb* deficiency with a one in four recurrence risk.

b. Rb protein binds transcription factors needed for cell division and bcl protein (cyclin D1) stimulates it; *Rb* is a tumor suppressor gene requiring homozygous mutations (two hits) that are likely sporadic in a child with unilateral tumor.

c. Rb and bcl proteins are DNA-binding factors that suppress promoters near oncogenes and act as tumor suppressors; the child represents a new, dominant-acting mutation and the parents have a minimal recurrence risk.

d. Rb protein stimulates cyclins specific for retinal tissue and bcl does the same for lymphatic cyclins; the child represents a new mutation with excess Rb activity.

e. Rb protein forms complexes with bcl protein that promotes cell division in rapidly proliferating tissues; the child represents a new mutation with excess Rb-bcl complex activity.

18. A 3-year-old boy offspring of first-cousin parents has a falloff in growth despite normal food intake. The child also has skin that is more darkly pigmented than his parents, and his skin also becomes bright red after sunlight exposure and leaves scars after healing. A skin biopsy is obtained and the cultured fibroblasts tested for xeroderma pigmentosum (XP-MIM*278700). The laboratory reports positive testing with assignment to complementation group A. Which of the following is the most likely information in this report?

a. The patient's fibroblasts had low amounts of thymine dimers after ultraviolet light exposure that were increased by fusion with other XP cell lines except those in complementation group A.

b. The patient's fibroblasts had low exogenous nucleotide-excision repair that could not be restored by fusion with any XP cell lines.

c. The patient's fibroblasts had low levels of RNA polymerase that were restored by fusion with XP cell lines except those from complementation group A.

d. The patient's fibroblast had low exogenous nucleotide-excision repair that was restored to normal levels by fusion with all XP cell lines except those in complementation group A.

e. The fibroblast had high amounts of thymine dimers after x-ray exposure that were increased by fusion with all XP cell lines.

19. Children with the Roberts syndrome (MIM*268300) of cleft palate and absence of one to all limbs have abnormal centromere structures visualized by routine chromosome studies. This observation highlights the complexity of animal DNA as compared to that of experimental models like *E coli* bacteria. Which of the following statements best describes the differences?

a. Animal nuclear DNA is discontinuous, with pieces (chromosomes) each of which are the same size as a bacterial genome.

b. Animal nuclear DNA has transcription factors that replace the histones and operons of bacterial DNAs.

c. Animal nuclear DNA is so large that it cannot be replicated semiconservatively.

d. Animal nuclear DNA is associated with many more histone and nonhistone proteins than bacterial DNA, producing a "second code" for genetic regulation.

e. Animal nuclear DNA is divided into nucleosomes that allow different transcription regulators to occupy specific nuclear compartments.

20. A large family has many individuals with colon cancer, affecting males and females in a manner compatible with autosomal dominant inheritance. The patients do not have multiple polyps as in Gardner syndrome or adenomatosis polyposis coli (APC-MIM*175100), so that colonoscopy screening has not been helpful. The family is thought most compatible with hereditary nonpolyposis colon cancer (HNPCC-MIM*114500), and the diagnosis is confirmed by skin biopsy and fibroblast studies. Which of the following best describes the diagnostic results?

a. Defect in mismatch repair with accumulation of nucleotide repeats by replication slippage.

b. Defect in double-strand break repair with accumulation of multiple small DNA fragments.

c. Defect in base-excision repair with accumulation of depurinated DNA.

d. Defect in nucleotide excision repair with accumulation of thymine dimers.

e. Defect in nucleotide excision repair with defects in an MSH protein that is homologous to an E coli mut gene.

21. A 21-year-old female has a history of frequent pneumonias and is hospitalized with fever, severe cough, low blood pressure, and bruises on her lower limbs that are interpreted as hemorrhage (purpura). *Streptococcus pneumoniae* is cultured from her blood stream and she improves after antibiotic therapy. She undergoes testing to evaluate white cell responsiveness to bacterial endotoxins that can be altered in the presence of mutated toll-like receptors (TLRs-MIM*603030). White cells from the patient and a control are isolated (buffy coat after centrifugation of heparinized blood) and incubated with endotoxin in the presence of tritiated thymidine to measure stimulation of DNA synthesis. DNA is isolated from the leucocyte samples and size-fractionated, yielding a large molecular weight fraction with slight differences and small molecular weight fractions with dramatically greater incorporation of tritiated thymidine in the control versus the patient. This result is interpreted as showing the patient has decreased leucocyte response to endotoxin, which is best explained by which of the following?

a. The large molecular weight fraction is mostly indicative of DNA repair while smaller DNA fragments reflect new and discontinuous DNA replication on both DNA strands.

b. The large molecular weight fraction arises from 3′ to 5′ DNA replication, while the smaller DNA fragments arise from 5′ to 3′ replication that reflects new DNA synthesis.

c. The large molecular weight fraction reflects continuous DNA replication on the leading (Watson) strand; this strand then serves as a template for new and discontinuous DNA synthesis on the lag (Crick) strand.

d. The small molecular weight fraction is a direct measure of DNA replication rather than repair, reflecting discontinuous 5′ to 3′ synthesis of DNA fragments on the lag strand using primase, RNA primers, and ligase.

e. The small molecular weight fraction is a direct measure of DNA replication rather than repair, reflecting newly synthesized Okazaki fragments directed by both DNA strands.

22. A 6-month-old Caucasian boy has been followed since birth because of extreme growth failure. His birth weight was 4 lb after a term 40-week uncomplicated pregnancy. Measures of tritiated thymidine incorporation by his stimulated white blood cells show a marked decrease compared to controls. Which of the following is the most likely interpretation of these results?

a. Homozygous nonsense mutation in the gene synthesizing the RNA primer used in DNA replication
b. Homozygous nonsense mutation in DNA polymerase
c. Homozygous mutation in helicase (rep protein) that continuously unwinds duplex DNA at the replication fork during synthesis
d. Homozygous mutation in an exonuclease used in excision repair
e. Homozygous mutation in DNA ligase that repeatedly joins the ends of DNA along the growing strand

23. A 13-year-old African-American adolescent notices decreased performance in basketball and drooping of his eyelids when tired. He complains to his pediatrician that his leg muscles seem smaller despite consistent weight training, and he has trouble keeping his balance with his eyes closed or when not concentrating. The physician suspects Kearns-Sayre syndrome (MIM*530000), and confirms the diagnosis by demonstrating a deletion of mitochondrial DNA in tissue obtained by muscle biopsy. Unique properties of mitochondrial DNA are best summarized as which of the following?

a. Circular, single-stranded, comprising 1% of cellular DNA with high mutation rates
b. Linear duplex DNA with a length similar to that of one nuclear chromosome, present as 50 to 100 copies per cell
c. Circular duplex DNA of about 16,000 bp that encodes unique tRNAs and several mitochondrial proteins
d. Circular, single-stranded DNA with low mutation rate that encodes a minority of mitochondrial peptides
e. Linear duplex DNA that encodes over 70 proteins of the respiratory chain and has a mutation rate 5 to 10 times higher than nuclear DNA

24. A 25-year-old adopted female uses a private detective to locate her birth hospital and likely biologic mother. She cannot see a family resemblance in this female and becomes concerned because this female had breast cancer at age 31 with several relatives having early-onset breast cancer. Upon questioning, the female recalls that she and her roommate in the hospital were both unwed, delivering on the same day and both giving up their babies for adoption. Which of the following would be the best option for the adopted female to pursue?

a. Compare blood leucocyte DNA for variable patterns of restriction fragments arising from tandemly repeated sequences (microsatellites) between the adoptee and her possible mother.

b. Compare fragment sizes of DNA copied from blood leucocytes using reverse transcriptase between the adoptee and her possible mother.

c. Compare blood leucocyte DNA fragment size distribution as analyzed by gel electrophoresis between the adoptee and her possible mother.

d. Compare HLA gene fragments obtained from blood leucocyte DNA between the adoptee and her mother.

e. Analyze blood leucocyte DNA for breast-ovarian cancer gene mutations (MIM*113705) in the adoptee and her prospective mother.

25. A 19-year-old female experiences recurrent respiratory infection and night sweats after becoming pregnant, attributing these symptoms to pregnancy until she notes a weight loss rather than expected weight gain. Obstetric evaluation reveals a positive test for tuberculosis and then a low white blood cell count. She admits to multiple sexual partners in the past, and an HIV antibody test is positive. Her doctor places her on a regimen of antituberculous drugs and recommends azidothymidine (AZT) therapy against her AIDS (MIM*609432) because it reduces maternal-to-child AIDS transmission by 30%. Which of the following describes the mechanism of action of AZT?

a. It inhibits viral protein synthesis.

b. It inhibits RNA synthesis.

c. It inhibits viral DNA polymerase.

d. It stimulates DNA provirus production.

e. It inhibits viral reverse transcriptase.

26. A 2-year-old girl is the product of a normal pregnancy and delivery and developed normally until age 12 months. After learning many words, crawling, and walking, she becomes progressively unsteady and stops walking, also refusing to speak. She begins wringing her hands frequently, has staring spells, and seems to be regressing in performance and memory. Her physician suspects a disorder called Rett syndrome (MIM*312750), and orders a diagnostic test that is based on increased DNA methylation around the *MECP* gene on the X chromosome. Which of the results below would be consistent with a positive diagnosis?

a. Increased expression of the MECP protein.
b. Increased size of *MECP* mRNA.
c. Loss of methylated sites as detected by methylation-sensitive restriction endonucleases.
d. Gain of methylated sites as detected by methylation-sensitive restriction endonucleases.
e. Amplification of triplet repeats surrounding the *MECP* gene promoter region.

27. A 6-month-old Hispanic girl has had six episodes of pneumonia, both viral and bacterial, and has spent only a few weeks outside of the hospital. Review of neonatal x-rays shows a very small thymus, and study of white cell markers suggests that both B (bursa-derived) and T (thymus-derived) cells are deficient. The autosomal recessive severe combined immune deficiency due to adenosine deaminase deficiency (ADA) (MIM*102700) is suspected and the physician-researcher team decides to try gene therapy as pioneered at other centers. Which of the following steps in performing gene therapy will be most challenging for the team?

a. Cloning of the ADA gene by digestion of human genomic and retroviral DNA with the appropriate restriction endonuclease and constructing a library of recombinant molecules.
b. Transformation of the child's bone marrow cells with DNA from a recombinant retrovirus that contains the ADA gene.
c. Engineering ADA gene insertion such that the retroviral ADA gene is replicated and regulated similarly to natural ADA genes.
d. Measuring ADA gene expression in transformed bone marrow cells to ensure sufficient immune function after transplant.
e. Suppression of the child's immune system so that transplanted bone marrow cells with recombinant ADA genes will not be rejected.

28. Nucleic acids extracted from normal and prostate cancer (MIM*176807) tissue are labeled with differently colored fluorescent probes and compared for their degree of hybridization to an array of DNA segments on a glass slide (DNA chip, technique known as comparative genomic hybridization— CGH—or microarray analysis). The DNA segments are chosen to represent the entire genome, and a segment from chromosome 2 gives a much stronger hybridization signal with the cancer tissue. This DNA segment is then used as a probe to characterize the nucleic acid that is more abundant in prostate cancer tissue. This nucleic acid is stable in acid, degraded by base, and migrates as a 30-base pair species in high or low salt by polyacrylamide gel electrophoresis. Which of the following statements best describes the nucleic acid that is more abundant in prostate cancer?

a. A 60 bp, double-stranded DNA fragment from chromosome 2
b. A 30 bp, single-stranded DNA fragment from chromosome 2
c. A 60 bp, double-stranded RNA fragment encoded by a gene on chromosome 2
d. A 30 bp single-stranded RNA encoded by a gene on chromosome 2
e. A 30 bp single-stranded RNA with a high degree of secondary structure, most likely a transfer RNA encoded by chromosome 2

29. Which of the following is the correct sequence of events in gene repair mechanisms in patients without a mutated repair process?

a. Nicking, excision, replacement, sealing, recognition
b. Nicking, recognition, excision, sealing, replacement
c. Nicking, sealing, recognition, excision, replacement
d. Recognition, nicking, excision, replacement, sealing
e. Sealing, recognition, nicking, excision, replacement

30. Which of the following indicates the correct sequence of chromosome constituents, going from smaller to larger?

a. Chromatin fibril, nucleosome, histone octamer, chromosome loop
b. Nucleosome, chromatin fibril, chromosome loop, histone octamer
c. Chromatin fibril, histone octamer, nucleosome, chromosome loop
d. Nucleosome, histone octamer, chromosome loop, chromosome fibril
e. Histone octamer, nucleosome, chromatin fibril, chromosome loop

31. A 2-year-old Caucasian girl presents with a 2-week history of fatigue, pallor, and recent chest pain localized to her sternum. Her physical examination is remarkable for general irritability, tenderness over her sternum, and a lemon-yellow hue to her skin. Blood counts show anemia with a hemoglobin of 5 g/dL (normal >12) and extreme leucocytosis (white blood cell count 130,000 cells/cubic millimeter with normal <12,000). A diagnosis of acute lymphocytic leukemia (MIM*187040) is made after further bone marrow studies, mandating a therapy protocol that includes radiation therapy of the central nervous system to destroy leukemic lymphoblasts. Which of the following describes the rationale for radiation therapy of certain cancers?

a. Cross-linking of DNA in rapidly growing cancer cells
b. Demethylation of DNA to prevent progression of precancerous cells
c. Cleavage of DNA double strands necessary for transcription in G phase
d. Disruption of DNA-RNA transcription complexes necessary for G phase
e. Disruption of purine rings in DNA crucial for S phase and rapidly growing cells

32. A 3-year-old Hispanic boy is evaluated because he says no words. He is being raised in a bilingual family, but he exhibits other behaviors during observation including poor eye contact, lining up of cars rather than imaginative play, and avoidance of touch or affection. The physician suggests a diagnosis of autism and recommends genetic testing including high resolution subtelomere FISH analysis that examines regions near the ends (telomeres) of each chromosome where aberrations are most common. Which of the following descriptions is accurate, perhaps accounting for subtelomere variability?

a. Unique replication of telomeric DNA involves a special polymerase called telomerase that uses a template RNA primer.
b. Unique replication of telomeric DNA involves telomeric oligonucleotides used on chromosome ends.
c. Standard replication of telomeres is possible because DNA polymerase has a special activity that cross-links DNA ends.
d. Standard replication of telomeres is possible because DNA polymerase has a subunit that facilitates binding to repetitive DNA.
e. Standard replication of telomeres is possible because DNA polymerase can reverse direction of replication at single-strand DNA termini.

33. A research study examines the nature of telomeres using DNA probes specific for the 6-nucleotide 5'-TTAGGG-3' repeats present in variable numbers at chromosome ends. The study includes children and adults with normal and abnormal development, including several patients with cancer (many genetic disorders cause both developmental disability and higher risks for cancer). Which of the following would be a likely result of this study?

a. Longer telomeres in older or disabled patients and in cancer tissues.
b. Shorter telomeres in younger patients and in cancer tissues, longer telomeres in some patients with developmental disabilities.
c. Shorter telomeres in older or disabled patients and in cancer tissues.
d. Longer telomeres in cancer tissue and single, specific telomere rearrangements in some patients with developmental disabilities.
e. Shorter telomeres in cancer tissue and single, specific telomere rearrangements in some patients' developmental disabilities.

34. A 9-month-old girl presents to hematology clinic after her 9-month checkup showed anemia. Her serum iron and transferring levels were normal, and her hemoglobin electrophoresis demonstrated an abnormal hemoglobin in addition to A and A2. Which of the following represents the most likely change at her β-globin locus and the genetic process that produced it? (Recall that the normal β-globin locus has the gene order Gγ-Aγ-Δ-β.)

a. Gγ-Aγ-deletion-β, gene conversion
b. Gγ-Aγ-β-deletion, gene conversion
c. Gγ-Aγ-fusion-Δ-β, unequal recombination
d. Gγ-Aγ-Δ-β fusion, unequal recombination
e. Gγ-Aγ-Δ-β-Gγ-Aγ-Δ-β, equal recombination

DNA Structure, Replication, and Repair

Answers

1. The answer is c. (*Lewis, pp 379-394. Murray, pp 388-405. Scriver, pp 11-18, 1257-1290.*) The figure accompanying this question shows DNA fragments displayed by Southern blotting (Dr Ed Southern developed the technique) with lanes 3 and 4 displaying single, diffuse bands derived from expanded DNA fragments from boys with fragile X syndrome. Males have one X chromosome and thus one DNA fragment per X chromosome gene (lane 4 for the patient, lane 3 for his affected brother, lane 1 for his unaffected brother) while women have two X chromosomes and two derived DNA fragments (lane 2 for the patient's normal sister, lane 5 for his carrier mother). The abnormally large DNA fragments (upper band in lane 5, single bands in lanes 3 and 4) are diffuse because abnormal fragile X alleles are unstable, with variable numbers of amplified triplet repeats among the different cells in one individual. Answers a (immunoblotting), d (Western blotting), or e (reverse transcription) are incorrect in suggesting the boy is unaffected, while Northern blotting in answer b examines RNA rather than DNA fragments.

For Southern blotting, the patient's genomic DNA (from blood, skin biopsy, amniocentesis, etc) is extracted, digested with the appropriate restriction enzymes, size-fractionated on agarose gels, blotted (transferred onto a membrane using capillary pressure), stabilized by heat/drying, hybridized with radioactive sequence-specific DNA probes, and exposed to x-ray film. Those fragments of size-fractionated DNA that are complementary to the probe are highlighted as dark bands on the autoradiogram. Boys with fragile X syndrome have over 500 to 1000 triplet repeats in a region proximal to the fragile X gene coding sequence, while normal males have repeat numbers of less than 60. In severely affected males with fragile X syndrome, amplifications are so great that restriction enzymes bracketing the triplet repeat region yield 500 to 2000 bp fragments that are easily distinguished from normal sizes of 15 to 60 bp (as illustrated in lanes 3 and 4 of the figure accompanying this question). Analogous blotting techniques were named as puns on the name of Southern, including "Northern" blotting to detect RNA molecules and "Western" blotting to detect proteins. Immunoblotting is one version of the "Western" blot technique where proteins are separated by electrophoresis and transferred to a membrane for probing with antibody to the proteins of interest. Reverse transcription of RNA into single, then double-stranded DNA, followed by polymerase chain reaction amplification (RT-PCR), is a more sensitive method for RNA measurement. RT-PCR could demonstrate altered levels of fragile X mRNA but would not measure triplet repeats because these are outside of the fragile X coding region.

Fragile X syndrome (MIM*309550) with amplified CGG repeats in the 5′ region upstream of the coding strand and Huntington chorea (MIM*143100) with similarly amplified CAG repeats exemplify a new category of genetic disease that involves triplet repeat instability. Fragile X syndrome is one of many disorders causing mental disability with autistic symptoms.

2. The answer is d. (*Murray, pp 302-305. Scriver, pp 677-704. Lewis, pp 172-174.*) DNA replication occurs in the 5′ to 3′ direction on both strands of DNA during the S phase of the cell cycle, as indicated in correct answer d. Measure of unscheduled DNA synthesis would not require cell synchrony as in answers a or c, DNA strands are not extended in the 3′ to 5′ direction (answer e), and purine bases are on the inside of the DNA duplex rather than outside as indicated in answer b.

DNA replication consists of five steps—unwinding by helicases, initiation of primase by short RNAs, 5′ to 3′ addition of deoxyribonucleotides via their triphosphates and DNA polymerase in elongation of the "leading" strand (discontinuously using Okazaki fragments for the "lag" strand), replacement of RNA primers with newly synthesized DNA, and sealing of gaps (on the lag strand) with DNA ligase. DNA repair occurs at all cell cycle phases, and among the types is excision repair that uses endonuclease to nick strands adjacent to thymine dimers, DNA polymerase to degrade and replace damaged nucleotides, ligase to restore integrity. All types of DNA synthesis will incorporate deoxyribonucleotide triphosphates rather than isolated bases or deoxyribose residues, and the new nucleotides are synthesized in the 5′ to 3′ direction using both strands of the DNA helix as templates.

3. The answer is a. (*Murray, pp 353-359. Scriver, pp 677-704. Lewis, pp 215-218.*) An individual homozygous for the ΔF508 cystic fibrosis mutation would have a 3 bp deletion beginning at nucleotide #1522 on both versions (alleles) of the cystic fibrosis gene, and such small changes are best detected by PCR followed by allele-specific-oligonucleotide (ASO) hybridization (answer a) or direct nucleotide sequencing. Note that the 3 bp genetic code predicts that amino acid #508 will correspond to nucleotides #1522 to 1524 of the coding sequence (excluding introns); this eliminates answers c and e. Homozygous individuals will have identical mutant alleles, meaning that molecular analyses would demonstrate a single size or band rather than two (normal and mutant) seen with a carrier (eliminating answers b, c, and d). Blotting techniques would not be sensitive enough to detect a 3 bp difference in DNA or RNA, and the effects on protein conformation could not be predicted. Acrylamide electrophoresis with direct visualization of DNA fragments could be performed as in answer e, but only one band corresponding to the two ΔF508 alleles (each 3 bp shorter than normal) would be detected.

4. The answer is c. (*Murray, pp 388-405. Lewis, pp 132-151. Scriver, pp 3-45.*) The result described in answer c is correct, emphasizing that the nucleotide change is a polymorphism associated with IDDM in Italian families, not a causative mutation and not necessarily associated with IDDM in other ethnic groups. PCR allows rapid amplification of target DNA sequences using heat-stable DNA polymerases and multiple denaturation, annealing, and extension cycles. Multiple PCR reactions coupled with DNA sequencing of amplified fragments has allowed systematic identification of single nucleotide polymorphisms (SNPs), occurring at an average 1 in every 600 nucleotides in the human genome. Genes that contribute to multifactorial diseases like diabetes mellitus, schizophrenia, and the like can be identified by scanning affected families with SNPs from all chromosome regions, using SNPs that cotransmit (are "associated") with the disease. The polymorphic HLA locus on chromosome 6 provided the first allele associations = linkage disequilibria, but the implicated genes near SNPs will not necessarily encode surface antigens as implied in answer e—they could influence insulin uptake, degradation, conformation, and the like.

5. The answer is d. (*Lewis, pp 248-261. Murray, pp 319-322.*) Chromosome deletion involves a breakage of DNA, with loss of the distal chromosome. The primary change in chronic myelogenous leukemia with chromosome 22 deletion would be a break in the chromosomal DNA that deletes certain sequences, joining DNA before the deletion point with telomeric sequences that foster chromosome replication (answer d). The other answers refer to changes in gene expression that could occur as a result of chromosome alteration, and do occur in various cancers—altered primary transcription (answer e), altered "second" code of epigenesis through histone modification (answer a), altered DNA methylation (answer b), or altered decoration patterns of small RNAs that influence chromatin transcription (answer c).

It is recognized now that all cancers involve genetic changes, even though few are hereditary. An early example was the discovery of a Philadelphia chromosome (terminally deleted chromosome 22) in chronic myeloid leukemia. In fact, most patients with the Philadelphia chromosome (22 deletion) actually have a chromosome 9:22 translocation that joins the Abelson ABL oncogene on chromosome 9 to a BCR (breakpoint cluster region) on chromosome 22. These discoveries follow a trend in cancer genetics where chromosomal abnormalities identify underlying cancer genes, in this case an ABL oncogene know from viral carcinogenesis and a BCR region known to be interrupted in other chronic myelogenous leukemias. Current research focuses on how altered expression of BCR-ABL gene products lead to chronic myelogenous leukemia.

6. The answer is e. (*Murray, pp 312-317. Scriver, pp 3-45. Lewis pp 127-128.*) DNA methylation occurs mainly at CpG dinucleotides that often cluster in at the upstream promoter regions of genes (CpG islands). Incorrect answers reflect double crossovers at meiosis that substitutes a normal allele for a mutant allele (gene conversion—answer a), reverse transcriptases copying intronless mRNA into complementary DNAs (cDNAs) that integrate into the genome as pseudogenes (answer c), gene rearrangement to unite variable, joining, and constant regions of immunoglobulin genes for expression of a unique antibody (answer d), or unequal crossing over between sister chromatids is thought to be an important mechanism for variation in copy number within gene clusters (answer b). Chromosomes subject to genomic imprinting may have different DNA methylation patterns on the homologue transmitted from mother versus that transmitted by father, producing balanced expression that is disrupted in disorders like Prader-Willi syndrome (MIM*176270).

7. The answer is b. (*Murray, pp 388-405. Lewis, pp 127-128. Scriver, pp 3-45.*) The DNA sequencing gel for the patient (figure below Question 7) indicates some bands at heavier density and others at lighter density, compatible with the autosomal Gardner syndrome/adenomatous polyposis coli (APC) alleles having identical sequence (homozygous) for the heavier bands and different sequences for the lighter bands (heterozygous). The gel can be read from top to bottom as CAG A/G GGT, where A/G represents comigrating DNA fragments of lighter density. The patient has one allele with CAGAGGT sequence (normal) and another with CAGGGGT (mutant), making her heterozygous (answer b, not d or e) and implying she is affected with Gardner syndrome and at increased risk for colon cancer. Interruption of a splice site for one copy of the gene will yield some larger mRNA molecules (answer b, not a or c) with failure of the intron to be removed.

DNA sequencing methodology primes DNA synthesis of key gene regions in the presence of the usual deoxynucleotides (dNTPs) plus low concentrations of a labeled deoxynucleotides that will terminate the synthesis (eg, a dideoxynucleotide (ddNTP) that has no free 3′ OH group for addition of the next nucleotide. Four reactions with A, C, T, and G ddNTPs are run, then applied to adjacent lanes on a gel to separate the labeled, synthesized strands by size. The sequence of the DNA is determined by reading the order of the terminated chains going up the gel.

8. The answer is b. (*Murray, pp 388-405. Scriver, pp 3-45. Lewis, pp 90-109.*) Restriction fragment length polymorphisms (RFLPs), now largely supplanted by single nucleotide polymorphisms (SNPs) detected by DNA sequencing, must be linked (located near) to putative disease genes by study of families with affected and unaffected members (answer b and not a, since the man's restriction fragments would not be linked with his deaf or normal alleles). The restriction site recognition sequence may vary among different individuals, yielding different DNA fragment sizes after cleavage (not different charges as in answer c or derived proteins as in answer c). Variable nucleotides that produce or eliminate restriction enzyme cleavage are often located outside of coding regions (not answer d). In order for an RFLP to cotransmit with normal or abnormal disease alleles, it must be within a few thousand base pairs of the disease gene. Even closely linked RFLPs or SNPs will require study of 10 or more family members to yield reliable probabilities for linkage and thus of disease diagnosis.

The method of RFLP analysis involves restriction of human DNA with endonucleases isolated from bacteria, producing an array of fragment sizes that can be separated by agarose or polyacrylamide electrophoresis. The differently sized DNA fragments migrate at speeds inversely proportional to their weights, and specific gene fragments can be detected amidst background DNA fragments after Southern transfer, hybridization with fluorescent or radiolabeled DNA probes, and visualization by fluorescence or autoradiography. Direct detection of the single nucleotide polymorphisms that alter restriction sites is now possible through DNA sequencing, now yielding a "Hap Map" of over 200 DNA markers that can rapidly locate genes for Mendelian or multifactorial diseases by determining which markers on which chromosome regions are coinherited with disease phenotypes.

9. The answer is c. *(Murray, pp 322-330. Scriver, pp 3-45. Lewis, pp 175-181.)* All DNA polymerases and repair enzymes can synthesize DNA only in the 5' to 3' direction, posing an apparent contradiction since the DNA strand (Crick) complementary to the coding strand (Watson strand) is oriented 3' to 5'. The Watson strand of DNA is synthesized continuously in the 5' to 3' direction while a different mechanism for replication on the Crick strand uses RNA primers (answer e is incorrect) and a distinctive enzyme (primase) to produce small Okazaki fragments (different DNA polymerases are not used as incorrectly suggested in answers a and b). Okazaki fragments of about 1000 nucleotides are synthesized in a 5' to 3' direction and then joined together by DNA ligase (DNA replication does not switch strands as suggested in answer e). Thus, while the overall direction of growth of the lagging strand that is made up of small fragments is in fact in the 3' to 5' direction, the actual polymerization of individual nucleotides is in the 5' to 3' direction.

10. The answer is c. *(Murray, pp 322-330. Scriver, pp 3-45. Lewis, 175-181.)* Despite the large size of mammalian genomes, DNA is replicated bidirectionally from multiple initiation sites and reduces copying times to minutes. Similar replication rates and cell temperatures among mammals and most bacteria (Archaea in ocean floor vents are exceptions) eliminate answers a and b, while the presence of histones and microRNAs in mammalian chromatin will slow replication and gene expression (incorrect answers d and e). Roberts syndrome (MIM*268300) exhibits altered chromosome condensation through special techniques for chromosome analysis, now defined by mutations in a gene stabilizing chromosome pairing during cell division. The resulting alteration in cell division likely impairs critical cell growth in embryonic regions like the palate and limbs.

The hundreds of initiation sites for DNA replication on chromosomes share a consensus sequence called an autonomous replication sequence (ARS). Thus, while the process of DNA replication in mammals is similar to that in bacteria, with DNA polymerases of similar optimal temperatures and speed, the many replication forks allow for a rapid synthesis of chromosomal DNA. Proteins such as histones, which are bound to mammalian chromosomes, inhibit DNA replication or transcription. Dissociation of the protein-DNA complex (chromatin) and unwinding of DNA supercoils (followed by chromatin reassembly) is part of the replication process.

11. The answer is b. *(Murray, pp 388-405. Lewis, pp 90-109. Scriver, pp 262-264.)* The female's upper band shown in lane 5 of the figure below Question 11 is derived from a fragile X gene fragment with amplified triplet repeats that makes her a carrier with a 25% risk for a son with fragile X syndrome (50% risk for a son × 50% risk for his inheriting her abnormal fragile X allele—answer b and not answer c suggesting an RFLP). Amplification above approximately 60 triplet repeats produces unstable DNA replication during meiosis as shown by the highly amplified bands in her brothers in lanes 3 and 4. The analysis implies that the female's deceased mother was also a fragile X carrier. The bands deriving from high numbers of repeats are diffuse because of variable DNA replication (not decreased as in answer a) and thus different sizes (differing numbers of repeats) in fragile X gene fragments from different cells of each individual. Location of these triplet repeat regions in the untranslated region would not produce a string of amino acids (note that CGG would encode proline) as implied by answer d.

12. The answer is b. *(Murray, pp 322-330. Scriver, pp 3-45. Lewis, pp 175-181.)* Before DNA replication can actually begin, unwinding protein must open segments along the DNA double helix. A defective unwinding protein (helicase) slows the overall rate of DNA synthesis, but does not alter the size of replicated DNA fragments. Defects in DNA synthesis or transcription may produce a phenotype of accelerated aging, as in Cockayne syndrome (MIM*216400 [usually defective in a transcription factor]). After unwinding, DNA-directed RNA polymerase (primase) catalyzes the synthesis of a complementary RNA primer of approximately 50 to 100 bases on each DNA strand. Then DNA-directed DNA polymerase III adds deoxyribonucleotides to the 3′ end of the primer RNA, which replicates a segment of DNA, the Okazaki fragment. DNA polymerase I then removes the primer RNA and adds deoxyribonucleotides to fill the gaps between adjacent Okazaki fragments. The fragments are finally joined together by DNA ligase to create a continuous DNA chain.

13. The answer is a. (*Murray, pp 388-405. Scriver, pp 769-784. Lewis, pp 355-377.*) One of the most common types of inherited cancers is non-polyposis colon cancer (HNPCC-MIM*114500). Most cases are associated with mutations of either of two genes that encode proteins critical in the surveillance of mismatches. Mismatches are due to copying errors leading to one- to five-base unmatched pieces of DNA. Two- to five-base-long unmatched bases form miniloops. Normally, specific proteins survey newly formed DNA between adenine methylated bases within a GATC sequence. Mismatches are removed and replaced. First, a GATC endonuclease nicks the faulty strand at a site complementary to GATC; then an exonuclease digests the strand from the GATC site beyond the mutation. Finally, the excised faulty DNA is replaced. In HNPCC, the unrecognized mismatches accumulate, leading to malignant growth of colon epithelium. The other forms of DNA repair are important for rectifying damage from ultraviolet light.

14. The answer is d. (*Murray, pp 322-330. Scriver, pp 3-45. Lewis, pp 175-181.*) The replication of double-stranded DNA is semiconservative, meaning that each strand separates and serves as a template for synthesis of a new complementary strand. Bromodeoxyuridine has a bromyl group at the fifth position of the pyrimidine ring, simulating the 5-methyl group of thymine and allowing it to replace thymidine in DNA (uridine is normally incorporated only into RNA). Incorporation of bases with the large bromine atom makes bromo-dU DNA strands more dense and separable from thymine-substituted DNA. The first round of replication of a bromodeoxyuridine (bromo-dU)-labeled DNA helix in a solution with normal dU will yield two daughter duplexes, each with one bromo-dU and one dU strand. The second round of replication will yield four daughter duplexes, two with one bromo-dU and one dU strand (intermediate density, middle of tube in the figure below Question 14) and two with both strands containing dU (low density, top of tube). Centrifugation to equilibrium in cesium chloride causes a density gradient to form in the centrifuge tube with banding of DNA duplex molecules at their corresponding density.

15. The answer is e. (*Murray, pp 353-359. Scriver, pp 3-45. Lewis, pp 188-194.*) A change from one DNA codon to another is required to cause a replacement of amino acids such as the valine to glutamic acid change in the β-globin peptide chain of hemoglobin S (MIM*141900). A single nucleotide substitution (point mutation) could effect such a codon change, and involves a thymine to adenine substitution at the second position of the codon 6. The other answers would not change one DNA/RNA codon and its translated amino acid. Equal exchange (crossing over) among homologous β-globin genes could exchange alleles, replacing normal alleles with mutant partners, or vice-versa (converting heterozygosity to homozygosity). Unequal crossing over could generate mutant alleles with duplicated or deficient nucleotides. One or two-base insertions would change the reading frame of the genetic code (frame-shift mutation) and produce a nonsense peptide or termination codon (chain-terminating mutation) after the point of insertion. Three-base deletions could also cause frame shifts if out of codon phase, or remove one codon and delete its corresponding amino acid from the peptide product.

16. The answer is e. (*Murray, pp 330-333. Scriver, pp 5587-5628. Lewis, pp 232-236.*) The normal parents having two hypopigmented children would fit the usual inheritance mechanism for oculocutaneous albinism (MIM*203100), an autosomal recessive disorder implying a one in four or 25% risk for their newborn to be affected with albinism (answer e, not a or b suggesting a one in eight risk). Decreased melanin synthesis in albinism increases the exposure of DNA in skin cells to ultraviolet rays from sunlight and leads to DNA cross-linkage (excluding answers c and d). Cross-linking occurs through the formation of thymine-thymine dimers. The DNA cross-links cause higher rates of mutation and skin cancer in albinism, mandating the wearing of protective clothing, sunglasses, and sunscreens by affected individuals. DNA deletions and point mutations are less common than DNA cross-links after sunlight exposure.

17. The answer is b. (*Scriver, pp 3-45. Murray, pp 446-458. Lewis, pp 355-377.*) DNA synthesis occurs only in the S phase of the cell cycle, a process regulated by numerous proteins called cyclins. A key cyclin (cyclin D) is phosphorylated as the cell commits from gap 1 (G1) quiescent phase to the S phase of DNA synthesis, and a cascade of secondary phosphorylations by cyclin-dependent kinases (CDK) activates cyclins, transcription factors, and the DNA synthesis machinery. The Rb protein, discovered as the product of the gene causing hereditary retinoblastoma, undergoes phosphorylation early in S phase and releases its inhibition (binding) of E2F transcription factor, promoting gene activation and DNA synthesis. *Rb*, like the genes for neurofibromatosis (neurofibromin) or breast cancer (BRCA1), acts as a tumor supressor gene requiring mutation of both Rb alleles to inactivate Rb protein and foster continuous E2F action and cell proliferation. Individuals with germ-line Rb mutations are more likely to incur a "second hit" in several retinal cells and present with retinoblastomas in both eyes. Individuals without germline Rb mutations are much less likely to incur two Rb mutations in the same retinal cell, having unilateral tumors if they occur at all. The bcl protein, discovered by its excess in B-cell lymphomas, was then identified as a stimulator of cell division called cyclin D1. *Bcl* is thus an oncogene, requiring one abnormal allele or "one hit" to be genetically activated in a cell and stimulate proliferation (oncogenesis). Several proteins of cancer-causing viruses (v-onc) have been adapted from putative cellular oncogenes (c-onc), while others inactivate the Rb protein and promote cell proliferation. Despite characterization of many tumor suppressor and oncogene proteins, the tissue specificity and variable ages of onset of different tumors speak for multifactorial, polygenic pathways to cancer.

18. The answer is d. (*Murray, pp 330-333. Scriver, pp 3-45. Lewis, pp 232-236.*) Xeroderma pigmentosum is caused by defects in excision repair, a mechanism involving several different enzymes and thus several different genes. Cells from XP patients should have lower nucleotide-excision repair activity and higher amounts of thymine dimers. Since the individual enzymes contributing to excision repair cannot be assayed, patients must be grouped by complementation testing—fusing patient cells with other XP cell lines to see which complement or correct the defective excision repair and high levels of thymine dimers—the question states that the patient falls into complementation group A and implies all XP cells except those from group A should rectify abnormalities in the patient's cells (answer d). Incorrect answers postulate either low thymine dimers (answer a), low RNA polymerase that is not an excision-repair enzyme (answer c), or correction by all XP cell lines (answers b and e).

Xeroderma pigmentosum (XP-MIM*278700) is an autosomal recessive disorder with enhanced DNA damage from ultraviolet irradiation, manifest by photosensitivity (reddening of skin and eyes from sunlight), pigmentation, blistering and scarring, and a 1000-fold greater risk for skin cancer. Autosomal recessive inheritance implies an enzyme deficiency (heterozygous carriers will be normal with 50% enzyme levels), and the deficient enzyme is part of a complex mediating excision repair. A UV-specific exonuclease nicks the dimer on its 5′ side, DNA polymerase I replicates the damaged sequence, the damaged piece is hydrolyzed by the 5′ to 3′ exonuclease activity of DNA polymerase I, and DNA ligase joins the patched and original DNA. Cultured skin cells (fibroblasts) from patients with XP are deficient in nucleotide excision repair, and fusion with cells from different XP patients could restore excision-repair activity (complement the repair deficiency). Systematic testing of various XP fibroblast lines demonstrated there were seven groups of XP cells, implying seven different enzymes involved in the process, each susceptible to mutations that would produce the disease.

19. The answer is d. (*Murray, pp 322-330. Scriver, pp 3-45. Lewis, pp 175-181.*) Like bacterial DNA, eukaryotic DNA is replicated in a semiconservative manner. However, in contrast to most bacterial DNA, which is circular in structure, nuclear chromosomal DNA is a single, uninterrupted molecule that is linear and unbranched. A eukaryotic chromosome contains a strand of DNA at least 100 times as large as the DNA molecules found in prokaryotes. The animal DNA is thousands of times as long as its nuclear diameter, and is condensed with proteins to form chromatin. Chromatin consists of fundamental 146 bp DNA-histone octamer units called nucleosomes, with many nucleosomes per gene. The chromatin histones can be modified covalently through attachment of acetyl, methyl, phosphate, or ubiquitin groups and the DNA bases can be variously opened to nucleoplasm by nonhistone proteins and subjected to methylation or other modifications. Chromatin modifications and protein interactions produce tremendous variation in DNA structure, visualized by karyotyping (centromeres, satellites, etc) and in DNA expression, visualized by "puffs" of transcription in the fruit fly or by imprinted (DNA methylation) regions in mammals. The chromatin interactions comprise a "second code" for gene regulation that, with vastly more genes and gene families, far transcends the simple operon models of bacteria. The significance of many animal DNA variations, like the premature centromere condensation in Roberts syndrome, is not yet understood.

20. The answer is a. *(Murray, pp 330-333. Scriver, pp 3-45. Lewis, pp 232-236.)* Hereditary nonpolyposis colon cancer (HNPCC-MIM*114500) is caused by defects in *hMLH1* or *hMSH2* genes that cause faulty mismatch repair. Mismatch repair corrects errors in newly synthesized DNA that arise from abnormal base-pairing or slippage at the replication fork that introduces point mutations or small nucleotide repeats (microsatellites). The mismatch repair apparatus, first characterized as *Mut S*, *Mut C*, and *Mut H* proteins in *E coli*, match newly synthesized DNA strands with their templates relative to adenine-methylated GATC sequence sites. New strands have unmethylated GATC sites, and mismatched sequences are excised by exonuclease and restored correctly by polymerase and ligase. Human *hMLH* genes are homologous to *E coli mut* genes, but the way in which accumulated point mutations and microsatellites in colon cell DNA lead to cancer is not yet clear. It is known that accumulation of abnormal DNA inhibits the cell cycle, so perhaps the continuous demand for high-turnover intestinal cells drives some colon cells to aberrant and unregulated pathways of proliferation.

21. The answer is d. *(Murray, pp 322-330. Lewis, pp 175-181. Scriver, pp 3-45.)* DNA polymerase moves along the DNA in one direction and synthesizes new DNA from both antiparallel strands at one replication fork. Since DNA is always synthesized 5' to 3', one of the strands (the leading strand) is synthesized continuously, whereas the other (the lagging strand) is synthesized in short stretches called Okazaki fragments that are made only during DNA replication (as implied by correct answer d). Answers a and e are incorrect because they posit discontinuous synthesis on both strands, b is incorrect because it posits 3' to 5' synthesis, and c is incorrect because it violates semiconservative DNA replication.

Discontinuous synthesis on the lag strand requires an RNA primer because DNA polymerase I, the major enzyme for DNA replication, can only add bases to an existing strand in the presence of template strand. A unique enzyme called primase synthesizes the short RNA molecules required to prime synthesis of Okazaki fragments and a ligase joins these fragments to elongate the lagging strand. Initiation of DNA replication occurs at specific sites with easily unwound AT-rich sequences characterized as autonomously replicating sequences (ARS) or origin recognition complexes (ORC) in *E. coli*. Formation and procession of the replication fork requires helicases for DNA unwinding, SSBs (single-strand binding proteins) to prevent premature reannealing, and DNA polymerase I for chain elongation.

22. The answer is d. (*Murray, pp 322-330. Scriver, pp 3-45. Lewis, pp 175-181.*) Homozygous mutations in DNA repair enzymes can lead to primordial dwarfism (short stature beginning with intrauterine growth retardation and low birth weight) or predispose to cancers as with hereditary nonpolyposis colon cancer (HNPCC-MIM*114500). Other answers involve mutations in key DNA replication components and would be incompatible with life, presenting as an early embryonic death that might not be recognized as a pregnancy. DNA replication involves continuous synthesis in the 5′ to 3′ direction from the leading strand and discontinuous DNA synthesis, also in the 5′ to 3′ direction, by DNA polymerase III on the lagging strand. RNA primers, primase enzyme, and DNA ligase are used repeatedly to make and join Okazaki DNA fragments along the growing lagging strand. Mutation of both alleles for the major DNA polymerase, DNA polymerase III, the gene synthesizing RNA primer, primase, or the special replication DNA ligase would make DNA replication and cell division impossible and be genetically lethal to the embryo.

23. The answer is c. (*Murray, pp 317-319. Scriver, pp 2415-2512. Lewis, pp 98-100.*) Mitochondrial DNA is similar to bacterial DNA in structure as a circular, double-stranded molecule of 16,569 bp (eliminates answers a and d positing single-stranded DNA, b and e positing linear DNA). Present in 500 to 1000 copies per cell, it comprises 1% of cellular DNA and encodes 13 peptides of the respiratory chain compared to 54 encoded by nuclear DNA. Mitochondrial DNA encodes unique ribosomal and transfer RNAs, has some unique coding properties (UGA stop codon read as tryptophan), and exhibits a 5- to 10-fold higher mutation rate than nuclear DNA. This fragility contributes to a dozen mitochondrial DNA diseases that range from optic atrophy to Kearns-Sayre syndrome (MIM*530000), not to be confused with similar disorders caused by mutation of nuclear-encoded peptides that are imported into mitochondria. Sperm heads contain few mitochondria, so mitochondrial DNA diseases often exhibit maternal inheritance due to contribution of zygote mitochondria from oocyte cytoplasm. Mitochondrial DNA mutations may arise during oogenesis, causing appearance of new disease, and may affect only a portion of the cell's mitochondria, producing mutant-normal mitochondrial mixtures (heteroplasmy).

Proportions of mutant mitochondria can differ with age and among tissues, accounting for worsening symptoms, variable ages of onset, and variable symptoms in disorders such as Kearns-Sayre syndrome.

24. The answer is a. (*Murray, pp 388-405. Scriver, pp 3-45. Lewis, pp 399-402.*) Restriction fragment length polymorphisms (RFLPs) arising from variable numbers of tandem repeats (VNTRs) are visualized by Southern blotting, yielding patterns called DNA fingerprints. If the restriction patterns from several VNTRs are used as in answer a, then differences between prospective parent and child can exclude parentage or support it (nonexclusion) at a probability equal to the number of RFLPs examined and the frequencies of the DNA fragment sizes in that population. Visualization of specific RFLP patterns using appropriate DNA probes after Southern blotting is required, since the gross distribution of DNA sizes (incorrect answer c), including that made by reverse transcriptase (incorrect answer b) will be similar in all individuals. Specific analysis of a gene encoding the highly variable HLA cell surface proteins would only provide one RFLP/gene variant for comparison (incorrect answer d), and the female would be at only 50% risk to inherit a breast-ovarian cancer gene (BRCA1 or 2-MIM*113705) from her mother even if the female were her biological mother and did have such a mutant allele (incorrect answer e).

DNA fingerprinting involves (1) isolation of DNA from parent/child or forensic specimens using blood, skin, or semen; (2) PCR amplification and radioactive labeling of DNA from variable regions in each sample; (3) separation of the variable DNA fragments by gel electrophoresis; and (4) comparison of the DNA fragment patterns among samples. Since numbers of arrays of repeats of 2, 3, or 4 bp (microsatellites) may vary from 5 to 100 at a particular chromosome locus, particular alleles may occur in less than 1% of the population. As a result, analysis of three loci, each with two alleles, can produce odds as high as $(100)^6$ that the pattern matches a putative father or suspect as compared to a random person from the general population.

25. The answer is e. (*Murray, pp 322-330. Scriver, pp 3-45. Lewis, pp 175-181.*) The AIDS treatment drug azidothymidine (AZT) inhibits viral reverse transcriptase that is essential for replication of the human immunodeficiency virus (as in answer e). AZT does not inhibit DNA polymerase, RNA polymerase, or protein synthesis (incorrect answers a-d). Reverse transcriptase is an RNA-directed DNA polymerase that synthesizes the HIV-DNA provirus, which in turn synthesizes new viral RNA. Since AZT (zidovudine) was approved in 1987, nonnucleoside reverse transcriptase inhibitors (eg, nevirapine) and viral protease inhibitors (eg, ritonavir) were developed that allow very effective combination therapies that provide long life spans and low fetal transmission rates for AIDS patients.

26. The answer is d. *(Murray, pp 312-317. Lewis, pp 172-174. Scriver, pp 3-45.)* The DNA of eucaryotes is associated with histone and nonhistone proteins and small RNAs. The DNA and its associated components are subject to chemical modifications that can alter gene expression, a process known as epigenesis or the "second code" to distinguish it from the primary code by which DNA codons are converted to protein amino acids. DNA methylation is an important mode of epigenesis that usually operates to shut genes down (inactivation). Diseases that involve methylation changes in a specific gene, like those of the *MECP* gene in Rett syndrome, are amenable to DNA diagnosis by demonstrating altered DNA methylation patterns. Primers are used to amplify characterized *MECP* gene fragments using the polymerase chain reaction, and their size distribution after methylation-sensitive endonuclease cleavage is determined by gel electrophoresis. Increased DNA methylation will modify cytosines within the gene sequence that are not normally methylated, causing insensitivity to endonuclease cleavage and larger fragment sizes on the appropriate size-separating gel.

27. The answer is c. *(Murray, pp 388-405. Scriver, pp 3-45. Lewis, pp 379-394.)* Restriction of vector (viral or plasmid) DNA and mammalian DNA with the same endonuclease produces cohesive ends that may be joined together with DNA ligase and produce recombinant DNA molecules. Mammalian genes can first be isolated using bacterial vectors (identified in recombinant populations—libraries—using the relevant radioactive DNA probe). The recombinant vector is replicated (cloned), the gene fragment purified, and mammalian cells transformed (DNA absorbed directly into the cell) or transfected (recombined with the DNA of a retrovirus with infection) to study properties of the inserted gene. One type of therapy expresses recombinant genes at high levels in bacterial or animal cells, purifies their protein products, and administers them to deficient patients as with human growth hormone or enzyme therapy. When administration of gene products cannot enter or be delivered to the deficient cells, then the gene itself must be delivered into these cells to accomplish expression of the defective gene (gene replacement or gene therapy). All of the listed steps are now routine (incorrect answers a, b, d, and e) except insertion of the replacement gene such that it is replicated and expressed like the natural gene (correct answer c). While bone marrow transplant still has significant mortality of approximately 10% due to lethal infections of graft-versus-host reaction after immune suppression, this patient with immune deficiency would require lower doses of suppressive drugs. Continuing challenges of gene therapy include abnormal expression of the inserted retroviral vectors as well as the inserted human gene, as evidenced by deaths in some gene replacement recipients and later leukemias in others.

28. The answer is d. (*Murray, pp 285-291.*) DNA is composed of 2'-deoxyribose sugars while RNA is composed of ribose sugars. The 2' and 3' hydroxyls of ribose allow alkaline release of one proton and initiation of phosphate cleavage by oxide, making RNA unstable at basic pH and less stable in general than DNA. The lability of the prostate cancer nucleic acid in base and its similar electrophoretic migration in high or low salt suggests it is a single-stranded RNA with little secondary structure (correct answer d). DNA species would be stable in base (incorrect answers a and b), and high salt would dissociate hydrogen bonds in double-stranded or highly coiled RNAs, reducing their apparent molecular weight estimated by migration on gel electrophoresis (incorrect answers c and e). Comparative genomic hybridization or microarray analysis provides a rapid method for defining nucleic acid excess or deficiency in patient samples, revealing subtle extra or missing chromosome segments in the patient's genomic DNA (high resolution chromosome analysis) or abnormally abundant/deficient RNAs in cancer tissues. DNA "chips" composed of 40 to 100,000 segments arrayed on a glass slide are hybridized with fluorescently-labeled patient and control samples, and a machine graphs the relative hybridization signals for each DNA segment, ordered by their chromosome location. DNA samples from patients with autism or related disabilities are revealing novel microdeletions and microduplications in these disorders while RNA samples from cancer tissues are revealing tumor-specific hybridization patterns (RNA profiles) or particular microRNA markers (implied by this question) that forecast tumor type, prognosis, and optimum therapy.

29. The answer is d. *(Murray, pp 322-330. Scriver, pp 3-45. Lewis, pp 232-236.)* In all of the forms of DNA repair in normal cells, a common sequence of events occurs:

1. The single or multiple base abnormality is surveyed and detected by a specific protein or proteins.
2. The DNA is nicked on one side of the damaged DNA.
3. A specific enzyme excises the damaged portion (steps 2 and 3 can be combined if an exonuclease cuts on both sides of the damaged DNA).
4. The damaged portion of the strand is replaced by resynthesis catalyzed by DNA polymerase I.
5. A ligase seals the final gap.

With some variability, these general principles apply in nucleotide excision repair (segments of about 30 nucleotides), base excision repair of single bases, and mismatch repair of copying errors (1-5 bases).

30. The answer is e. *(Murray, pp 312-317. Lewis, pp 172-174. Scriver, pp 3-45.)* DNA does not exist naked in eucaryotic cells but as a complex with histones and nonhistone proteins. The four core histones are present as the dimers H2A-H2B and H3-H4, and these dimers in turn pair to produce a histone octamer. The histone octamer associates with DNA and histone H1 to form nucleosomes—arrayed like beads on a string to form a chromatin fibril of 30 nm width. Each histone octamer complexes with 146 base pairs of coiled (superhelical) DNA, and each of the core histones or histone H1 is susceptible to chemical modification by acetylation, methylation, phosphorylation, ribosylation, or ubiquination. Phosphorylation of histone H1 causes chromatin condensation, and the 10 nm fibril can condense to form successive 30 nm fibrils, chromosome loops or domains, and finally the highly condensed metaphase chromosomes that are analyzed in human cytogenetics. Chromatin upstream of active genes is typically less condensed, forming hypersensitive sites to nuclease. The modification of histones, along with methylation of DNA and changes in chromosome condensation, comprises a "second code" for regulation of gene expression. These changes are often distinguished as "epigenetic" in contrast to genetic changes in the primary code of DNA to RNA to protein.

31. The answer is e. (*Murray, pp 322-330. Scriver, pp 3-45. Lewis, pp 355-377.*) Chemo- and radiotherapies target deregulated and/or rapidly growing cancer cells that have more active DNA replication (S phase) and transcription compared to quiescent cells in G or stationary phase. Radiation damages cellular DNA by opening purine rings and rupturing phosphodiester bonds, not by other actions suggested by incorrect answers a to d. Chemical agents such as formaldehyde can cross-link DNA, and inhibitors of DNA methylation, such as methotrexate (an inhibitor of folic acid), were the first anticancer drugs. Experimental gene therapies for cancer include the inhibition of oncogene expression and the enhancement of tumor suppressor gene activity. These therapies target particular DNA-RNA transcription complexes or signal transduction cascades that are active in cancer cells.

32. The answer is a. (*Murray, pp 322-330. Scriver, pp 3-45. Lewis, pp 355-377.*) A special DNA polymerase called telomerase is responsible for replication of the telomeric DNA. This enzyme contains an RNA molecule that guides the synthesis of complementary DNA and therefore is an RNA-dependent DNA polymerase like reverse transcriptase. Incorrect answers c to e do not recognize that the multiple TTAGGG repeats extending for several kilobases plus other unique characteristics of chromosome ends (telomeres) require a special replication enzyme. Incorrect answer b postulates oligonucleotide rather than RNA templates for the telomerase.

33. The answer is c. (*Murray, pp 322-330. Lewis, pp 172-174. Scriver, pp 3-45.*) Special DNA structures at the end of chromosomes, called telomeres, consist of repetitive DNAs including a particular 6-base pair repeat (5'-TTAGGG-3') at each chromosome terminus. The number of 6-base pair repeats is normally in the thousands, but has been noted to shorten in tumor tissues and in normal tissues as a function of aging. Multicolor, fluorescent DNA probes to regions adjacent to telomeric repeats detect subtle deletions (missing signal) or duplications (extra signal) that are more common in these regions (subtelomere fluorescent in situ hybridization [FISH]). The described research study uses probes to the 6-bp repeats rather than the adjacent regions, and thus will show fewer repeats (shorter telomeres) in older patients and cancer tissues (incorrect answers a and d) without revealing rearrangement of adjacent DNA in select patients with disabilities (incorrect answers b and e). Subtelomere FISH studies, now being supplanted by microarray analysis, can reveal subtle chromosome aberrations in 3% to 6% of individuals with developmental disabilities who have a normal routine karyotype.

34. The answer is d. (*Murray, pp 319-322. Lewis, pp 219-232. Scriver, pp 3-45.*) Gene recombination during chromosome synapsis at the first and second meiotic divisions produces unique genetic constitutions in each gamete and derived conception. In the first meiotic division, the chromosomes are tetraploid and recombination occurs mostly between sister chromatids of the same chromosome. In the second meiotic division, recombination may occur between chromosome homologues. Recombination is normally "equal," meaning that the crossover of DNA strands is at the same base pair on each chromosome arm and produces no excess or deficient DNA. Among chromosome regions with repetitive DNAs, including gene families like the globins that are similar in sequence, it is common to have "unequal" crossovers with mismatched pairing. The child with anemia proved to have hemoglobin Lepore (MIM*141900), produced by unequal recombination between a Δ-globin gene on one chromatid and a β-globin gene on the other. The child therefore had normal fetal hemoglobin produced from α- and γ-globin genes, but produced an abnormal hemoglobin due to $\Delta\beta$-globin gene fusion on one chromosome. The reciprocal anti-Lepore recombination would be lost at meiosis II, and the child would have a normal β-globin locus on the chromosome 11 received from the other parent. This produces a mild to moderate anemia once the switch occurs from fetal to adult hemoglobin at 3 to 6 months.

Gene Expression and Regulation

Questions

35. A 6-year-old boy of Scandinavian descent presents with recurrent vomiting, fatigue, and weight loss. Physical examination reveals scleral icterus (yellow whites of eyes) and tenderness over the right upper quadrant of the abdomen. Laboratory studies reveal elevated levels of serum glutamic oxaloacetic transaminase (AST—reflecting liver or heart cell death) and bilirubin (reflecting icterus or jaundice) but no hepatitis A or B viral antigens. A diagnosis of nonviral hepatitis is made and a family history reveals the father and his sister suffer from early-onset emphysema and that the paternal grandmother died from this illness. A suspected diagnosis of α_1 antitrypsin (AAT-MIM*104700) deficiency is confirmed by finding the child has only the Z form of AAT on protein electrophoresis, confirmed by DNA sequencing showing homozygous AAG sequences at the 342nd codon (expected to encode lysine) rather than normal GAG (expected to encode glutamine). Which of the following statements about the "genetic code" explain this molecular diagnosis?

a. There are 64 codons, each of which can encode several different amino acids.
b. There are 64 possible combinations of 3 nucleotides, each combination specifying a specific amino acid or serving as a termination signal.
c. There are 16 possible combinations of 2 nucleotides, allowing the first two nucleotides of each codon to specify unique amino acids and rendering the third nucleotide as irrelevant (degenerate).
d. Information is stored as sets of trinucleotide repeats called codons, accounting for the evolution of complex genes from simpler ones.
e. The 5' to 3' sequence of 3-base pair codons within genes is exactly matched by the amino to carboxy sequence of amino acids within the translated protein.

36. A 25-year-old male presents for evaluation of declining athletic performance and fatigue. Physical examination shows mild tachycardia and a palpable spleen, followed by blood counts revealing low hemoglobin (11.7 g/dL) and rounded red blood cells with dense centers on blood smear. A diagnosis of spherocytosis (MIM*182900) is made and DNA analysis for mutations in the causative ankyrin gene performed so prenatal or early neonatal diagnosis would be possible for future generations. This mutation is best detected by which of the following?

a. Isolation of DNA from red blood cells followed by polymerase chain reaction (PCR) amplification and restriction enzyme digestion.

b. Isolation of DNA from blood leukocytes followed by Southern blot analysis to detect ankyrin gene exon sizes.

c. Isolation of DNA from blood leukocytes followed by DNA sequencing of ankyrin gene introns.

d. Isolation of DNA from blood leukocytes followed by complete gene sequencing or polymerase chain reaction (PCR) amplification/allele-specific oligonucleotide (ASO) hybridization.

e. Western blot analysis of red blood cell extracts.

37. A 3-year-old Caucasian boy has grown along the third percentile for age despite his parents being tall. He also has required treatment for chronic asthma, and his pediatrician notes unusual curvature of his knees and wrists typical of rickets. Testing confirms rickets by x-ray and deficiency of vitamin D, a fat-soluble vitamin that can become deficient with inadequate sunlight or intestinal malabsorption. The latter possibility, together with the asthma and growth delay, suggests a diagnosis of cystic fibrosis (MIM*219700). DNA testing is now very accurate, examining over 100 possible mutations including the 3 bp deletion that removes a codon for phenylalanine (ΔF508). The DNA sequence shown below is the sense strand from a coding region known to be a mutational "hot spot" for a gene. It encodes amino acids 21 to 25. Given the genetic and amino acid codes CCC = proline (P), GCC = alanine (A), TTC = phenylalanine (F), and TAG = stop codon, which of the following sequences is a frameshift mutation that causes termination of the encoded protein 5'-CCC-CCT-AGG-TTC-AGG-3'?

a. -CCA-CCT-AGG-TTC-AGG-

b. -GCC-CCT-AGG-TTC-AGG-

c. -CCA-CCC-TAG-GTT-CAG-

d. -CCC-CTA-GGT-TCA-GG-

e. -CCC-CCT-AGG-AGG-

38. A 5-year-old Caucasian girl returns from a mushroom hunt in Northern Michigan and begins vomiting, then shows tremors, extreme anxiety, and finally disorientation—not recognizing her parents. She is taken to the emergency room where jaundice and delirium are noted and followed by liver function tests showing elevated ammonia, liver enzymes, and bilirubin. A toxicologist is called, who suggests poisoning from *Amanita phalloides*, a mushroom containing the toxin α-amanitin that inhibits RNA polymerase II. The child's liver failure is most likely due to which of the following?

a. Inhibition of tRNA and protein synthesis
b. Inhibition of mRNA synthesis
c. Inhibition of small RNA synthesis
d. Inhibition of ribosomal RNA synthesis
e. Inhibition of mitochondrial RNA synthesis

39. A 9-month-old Italian American boy presents with tachypnea and respiratory distress. His physical examination reveals a large spleen and his blood counts reveal severe anemia with targeted red blood cells on smear. A diagnosis of β-thalassemia (MIM*141900) is suggested and analysis of gene structure and expression is begun. As shown in the diagram below Question 40, the β-globin gene contains three exons that encode a protein of 150 amino acids, separated by introns of 150 and 750 bp. The β-globin messenger RNA (mRNA) has 5′- and 3′-untranslated regions of 50 nucleotides. Measure of β-globin gene expression in the child would normally recognize a mature β-globin messenger RNA of which of the following sizes?

a. 1450 bp
b. 700 bp
c 550 bp
d. 300 bp
e. 450 bp

40. A "factor" is studied that stimulates a gene controlling differentiation of human immune stem cells into B-cells that fight bacterial infection. Some diseases like Bruton agammaglobulinemia (MIM*300300) involve an inability to produce B-cells. The factor can hybridize to DNA, is hydrolyzed by alkali treatment, and migrates as a 2 to 30 bp species on electrophoresis. The differentiation gene is not stimulated by the factor if a 10 bp promoter element near the initiation site for transcription is removed. Which of the following factors is most likely?

a. A transfer RNA that recognizes a codon within the promoter element
b. An mRNA that is translated to produce a stimulatory transcription factor
c. A small RNA that binds the promoter and enhances transcription
d. A transposon that recognizes the promoter element and inserts to activate the gene
e. An RNA catalyst that is essential for mRNA splicing

Questions 41 to 48. Refer to the figure below for these questions.

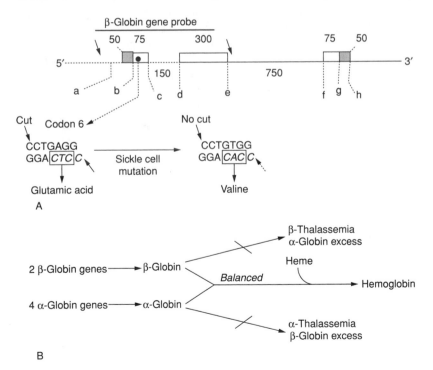

41. A 3-year-old boy immigrant from Somalia presents for evaluation of priapism (prolonged and painful erection). The parents report through a translator that he has an illness well known in their family and that several cousins are affected. The illness causes fatigue, poor growth, and bone pain, and the physician suspects sickle cell anemia (MIM*603903). Sickle red cells are observed on peripheral smear, and the physician suggests confirmation by DNA diagnosis so the couple can consider preimplantation/prenatal diagnosis with future pregnancies.

The β-globin gene is diagrammed in the upper portion (A) of the figure, consisting of untranslated RNA regions (gray boxes), three exons (clear boxes), and two introns (lines between exons). DNA diagnosis for sickle cell anemia was facilitated by finding that a cleavage site for restriction endonuclease (MstII) included the sixth codon of β-globin gene exon 1 (solid circle in first exon). When this codon is mutated to cause the glutamate to valine amino acid change in sickle cell anemia, the MstII site is ablated. MstII sites in normal β-globin genes are shown as solid arrows in the upper part of the figure, yielding gene fragments of 165 bp (5′ MstII site to that in the glutamate codon) and 515 bp (MstII site in glutamate codon to the 3′ MstII site). Recall that the β-globin gene is on chromosome 16, and that both copies are mutated (homozygous) in individuals with sickle cell anemia. Analysis of β-globin gene structure and expression in an individual with sickle cell anemia would yield which of the following results? (Southern blotting is performed using MstII endonuclease cleavage and hybridization with the β-globin gene probe shown in the figure.)

a. MstII DNA cleavage segment of 515 and 165 bp by Southern blot, nucleic acid segment of ~550 bp by Northern blot, abnormal protein by hemoglobin electrophoresis

b. MstII DNA cleavage segments of 515 and 165 bp by Southern blot, no nucleic acid segment detected by Northern blot, abnormal protein by hemoglobin electrophoresis

c. MstII DNA cleavage segments of 515 and 165 bp by Southern blot, nucleic acid segment of ~1400 bp by Northern blot, abnormal protein by hemoglobin electrophoresis

d. MstII DNA cleavage segment of 680 bp by Southern blot, nucleic acid segment of ~550 bp by Northern blot, abnormal protein by hemoglobin electrophoresis

e. MstII DNA cleavage segments of 680, 515, and 165 bp by Southern blot, nucleic acid segment of ~550 bp by Northern blot, abnormal protein by hemoglobin electrophoresis

42. An 18-month-old Caucasian boy of Italian ancestry is evaluated for "failure to thrive"—his height and weight have leveled off and have gone from the 50th to the 3rd percentiles for age. Parental neglect is suspected and he is hospitalized for calorie counts and daily weights to see if normal feeding results in weight gain. Upon physical admission, a medical student notes he is pale with brownish-yellow pigmentation to his skin, and that his face seems unusual. Because of these observations, laboratory testing is initiated before the dietary treatment is completed and reveals a low hemoglobin (5 g/dL with normals of 12-14 for age) and target cells on smear that suggest a diagnosis of β-thalassemia (MIM*141900). Molecular studies show a mutation just upstream (5′) to the transcription initiation site of both β-globin alleles (point a in the figure below Question 40). In homozygous individuals, this mutation decreased the amount of β-globin mRNA and subsequent β-globin protein and hemoglobin, producing anemia. Which of the following best describes this mutation?

a. It affects a promoter sequence that codes for RNA polymerase, lowering β-globin mRNA levels.

b. It affects a promoter sequence and the rate at which RNA polymerase II initiates transcription, lowering β-globin mRNA levels.

c. It affects the termination site of an upstream gene, increasing β-globin mRNA levels.

d. It alters a sequence encoding a subunit of RNA polymerase II (the sigma factor), increasing α-globin mRNA levels.

e. It affects a promoter sequence and the rate at which RNA polymerase II terminates transcription, increasing α-globin mRNA levels.

43. A 24-year-old African American mountain climber in excellent physical condition suffers shortness of breath and low oxygen (hypoxia) at high altitude in Nepal. After transport to base camp and oxygen treatment, a family history reveals that his mother has sickle cell anemia (MIM*603903). With reference to the upper portion (A) of the figure below Question 40, laboratory studies of his β-globin gene structure and expression would be expected to show which of the following results? (Note that the same MstII restriction and β-globin probe in the figure is used for Southern blotting.)

a. MstII DNA cleavage segment of 515 and 165 bp by Southern blot, RNA segment of ~550 and 700 bp by Northern blot, normal and abnormal proteins by hemoglobin electrophoresis

b. MstII DNA cleavage segments of 680, 515, and 165 bp by Southern blot, RNA segment of ~550 and 700 bp by Northern blot, normal and abnormal proteins by hemoglobin electrophoresis

c. MstII DNA cleavage segments of 515 and 165 bp by Southern blot, RNA segment of ~1400 bp by Northern blot, single abnormal protein by hemoglobin electrophoresis

d. MstII DNA cleavage segment of 680 bp by Southern blot, RNA segment of ~700 bp by Northern blot, single normal protein band by hemoglobin electrophoresis

e. MstII DNA cleavage segments of 680, 515, and 165 bp by Southern blot, RNA segment of ~1400 and 700 bp by Northern blot, single abnormal protein by hemoglobin electrophoresis

44. An 8-year-old African American girl presents with severe anemia despite several years treatment with iron supplementation. A blood smear is examined carefully and reveals both target cells suggestive of β-thalassemia (MIM*141900) and sickle cells suggestive of sickle cell anemia (MIM*603903). Referring again to the figure below Question 40, molecular analysis demonstrates a mutation at the promoter site (point a in the figure) on one β-globin gene and a sickle cell mutation on the other. Which of the following laboratory results would be expected in such an individual, using the same MstII restriction and β-globin probe for Southern blotting described previously?

a. MstII DNA cleavage segment of 515 and 165 bp by Southern blot, normal amounts of ~700 bp RNA segment by Northern blot, normal and abnormal proteins by hemoglobin electrophoresis

b. MstII DNA cleavage segments of 680, 515, and 165 bp by Southern blot, decreased amounts of ~550 and 700 bp RNA segment by Northern blot, normal and abnormal proteins by hemoglobin electrophoresis

c. MstII DNA cleavage segments of 680, 515, and 165 bp by Southern blot, decreased amounts of a ~550 and 700 bp RNA segment by Northern blot, mostly abnormal protein by hemoglobin electrophoresis

d. MstII DNA cleavage segment of 680 bp by Southern blot, normal amounts of a ~550 and 700 bp RNA segment by Northern blot, mostly normal protein band by hemoglobin electrophoresis

e. MstII DNA cleavage segments of 680, 515, and 165 bp by Southern blot, lower amounts of 550 and 700 bp DNA segment by Northern blot, mostly normal protein by hemoglobin electrophoresis

45. A population study in a rural area of Greece examines several patients with anemia revealed a homozygous mutation in a sequence 5'-TATAAAA-3' at the 5' end of the β-globin gene (site a in the figure below Question 40). This sequence has been found at the 5' boundary of other eukaryotic genes, and is quite similar to a consensus sequence observed in prokaryotes. Which of the following best describes the significance of this mutation?

a. Likely β-thalassemia due to disruption of RNA polymerase III binding

b. Likely hemoglobinopathy like sickle cell anemia due to promoter disruption

c. Likely β-thalassemia due to disruption of transcription termination

d. Major binding site of RNA polymerase I

e. Likely β-thalassemia due to disruption of transcription initiation by RNA polymerase II

46. A 2-year-old Caucasian from a Greek community in Chicago presents with severe anemia, targeted red blood cells on peripheral smear, skin pallor, jaundice, and growth failure. Molecular analysis demonstrates a homozygous mutation in the β-globin gene at the junction of exon 1 and intron 1 (site c in the figure below Question 40). Which of the following best describes the nature and clinical consequence of this mutation?

a. Altered splice donor site, absent mRNA by Northern blotting, β-globin protein deficiency presenting as α-thalassemia

b. Altered splice acceptor site, altered mRNA size by Northern blotting, β-globin protein deficiency presenting as β-thalassemia

c. Altered splice donor site, altered mRNA size by Northern blotting, β-globin protein deficiency presenting as β-thalassemia

d. Altered promoter site, altered mRNA size by Northern blotting, β-globin protein deficiency presenting as β-thalassemia

e. Altered promoter site, deficient β-globin mRNA by Northern blotting, β-globin protein deficiency presenting as α-thalassemia

47. A 22-year-old male is found to have a hemoglobin of 11.5 during his army induction physical and his red cell indices include a mean corpuscular volume (MCV) of 79 (mean 90 femtoliters, 80 is −2 SD). The microcytosis and anemia first suggest iron deficiency, but ferritin levels (reflection of total body iron) are normal. A diagnosis of hemoglobin H disease (MIM*141800) is considered, recalling that the α-globin genes are similar in structure to the β-globin genes diagrammed in the figure below Question 40 but are present in duplicate copies on each chromosome 16 in humans. Which of the following α-globin mutations would be compatible with moderate anemia of the type seen in hemoglobin H disease α-globin genes?

a. Heterozygous point mutation within the TATA box of one α-globin gene

b. Homozygous point mutation within the TATA box of one α-globin gene

c. Homozygous mutation deleting both α-globin gene copies

d. Heterozygous mutation deleting both α-globin gene copies paired with a heterozygous mutation with the TATA box of one α-globin gene

e. Homozygous frameshift mutation within the coding sequence of the 5′ α-globin gene

48. A population survey of a Northern Italian population reveals a variety of mutations in the β-globin gene. It is known that eucaryotic mRNAs undergo several forms of posttranscriptional processing, and that some forms of thalassemia are due to incorrect processing of the α- and β-globin mRNAs. Referring to the β-globin gene structure shown in the figure below Question 40, which of the following homozygous mutations would most likely present as altered hemoglobin (hemoglobinopathy) but not as a β-thalassemia?

a. Mutations changing the consensus AGGUAAGU splice donor sequence at exon-intron junctions
b. Missense mutations in exon 2
c. Mutations changing the AAUAA recognition sequence at the terminus (3′-end) of the gene
d. Mutations altering TATA or CAAT boxes
e. Mutations changing the consensus UACUAAC-30bp-CAGG splice acceptor sequence at intron-exon junctions

49. A 3-week-old Caucasian girl has returned for follow-up after her initial newborn metabolic screen showed elevated levels of phenylalanine, causing concern for phenylketonuria (PKU-MIM*261600). The second screen performed at age 2 weeks showed a phenylalanine level of 30 mg/dL with upper limits of normal being 6 mg/dL. Molecular characterization demonstrated a single-base change GT to AT at an intron-exon junction in both of her phenylalanine hydroxylase (PAH) alleles, and an unusually large PAH mRNA. Which of the following most accurately describes these test results?

a. The PAH mutation has disrupted RNA catalysis, producing a PKU carrier.
b. The PAH mutation has disrupted RNA self-splicing and caused PKU.
c. The PAH mutation has disrupted spliceosome activity and caused PKU.
d. The PAH mutation has disrupted action of RNA polymerase and caused PKU.
e. The PAH mutation has disrupted RNA helicase, producing a PKU carrier.

50. Antibiotics that selectively inhibit bacterial growth exploit differences between bacterial and mammalian cells. Design of a drug that would selectively inhibit bacterial RNA synthesis would target which of the following?

a. Spliceosome components
b. 3′ ends of tRNA unprotected by caps
c. 3′ ends of mRNA unprotected by caps
d. 5′ ends of mRNA unprotected by caps
e. Poly(A) addition to the 5′ end

51. A 36-year-old female elects to have amniocentesis with her third pregnancy because of "advanced" maternal age—her family history and that of her 38-year-old husband are normal. The fetal chromosomes show a normal number of 46 but one chromosome 21 has a large satellite region. The couple is called back for parental chromosomes and is extremely anxious that their fetus may have Down syndrome. The same enlarged satellite is seen on one chromosome 21 of the father, and silver staining shows this amplified DNA to be part of the nucleolar organizing region (NOR). The counselor explains that these NOR regions are seen on chromosomes 13 and 15 and 21 and 22 (acrocentric chromosomes) and are transcriptionally active in the nucleolus. The molecules associated with these NOR would most likely be which of the following?

a. Messenger RNA used to synthesize histone proteins
b. Small silencing RNA (siRNA)
c. Poly(A) RNA
d. Ribosomal RNA
e. Transfer RNA

52. Which one of the following statements best describes the synthesis of mammalian messenger RNA (mRNA)?

a. There is colinearity of the RNA nucleotides transcribed from a gene and the amino acids encoded by each nucleotide.
b. Each mRNA often encodes several different proteins.
c. Several different genes may produce identical mRNA molecules.
d. The RNA sequence transcribed from a gene is virtually identical to the mRNA that exits from nucleus to cytoplasm.
e. Mammalian mRNA undergoes minimal modification during its maturation.

53. A 22-year-old single Ashkenazi Jewish female has a strong family history of breast cancer, with her mother, maternal aunt, and grandmother all having breast cancer before menopause. She understands that the family likely exhibits autosomal dominant inheritance for predisposition to breast cancer due to mutations in the *BRCA* tumor suppressor genes; a pathologic BRCA mutation causes an ~80% lifetime risk for breast and 45% risk for ovarian cancer . Her mother undergoes testing and a mutation in the *BRCA1* gene (MIM*113705) is found, potentially defining her daughter's cancer risks. Which of the following maternal test results and consequent lifetime cancer risks for daughter are most accurate?

a. Homozygous mutation in the BRCA1 TATA box, 80% cancer risk for daughter
b. Heterozygous mutation in the BRCA1 TATA box, 80% cancer risk for daughter
c. Heterozygous mutation in the BRCA1 coding sequence changing the third nucleotide in a codon for glycine, 80% cancer risk in daughter
d. Heterozygous frameshift mutation in the BRCA1 coding sequence, 40% cancer risk for daughter
e. Homozygous frameshift mutation in the BRCA1 coding sequence, 80% cancer risk for daughter

54. An 18-year-old Ashkenazi Jewish female had developed worsening balance and coordination (ataxia) with declining vision at night. She also had chronic diarrhea that had been attributed to irritable bowel syndrome but was recognized as fat malabsorption from gastroenterology studies. A diagnosis of autosomal recessive abetalipoproteinemia (MIM*200100) was considered and analysis of apolipoprotein B (*apoB*) gene expression was initiated. Northern blots of the patient's duodenal biopsy tissue showed an apoB mRNA of expected size while Western blots demonstrated an apoB peptide that was smaller than that characterized in control liver tissue. A nonsense, chain-terminating mutation was thought likely until the same small peptide was found in intestinal biopsies of controls. Which of the following interpretations is most likely?

a. ApoB mRNA undergoes alternative splicing in intestine; the patient has a heterozygous *apoB* gene deletion.

b. An exon of the *apoB* gene is deleted in intestine; the patient has homozygous *apoB* gene deletion.

c. Intestinal apoB mRNA undergoes a codon alteration that causes termination of translation and a smaller peptide; the patient may have homozygous apoB missense mutation.

d. Polyadenylation of apoB mRNA is deficient in intestine; the patient has heterozygous apoB mutation affecting transcription termination.

e. Transcription of apoB mRNA occurs from a different promoter in intestine; the patient has heterozygous apoB mutation deleting this promoter.

55. A 35-year-old African American male has noted deteriorating skills in activities like golf and tennis, lately noting difficulties with handwriting. Evaluation reveals poor tandem walking and finger to nose coordination, and a peripheral smear shows shrunken and spiny red blood cells called acanthocytes. Serum lipoprotein electrophoresis shows very low density (VLDL) and low density (LDL) lipoproteins, suggesting a diagnosis of abetalipoproteinemia (MIM*200100). Which of the following is the best method to demonstrate yield of different apolipoprotein B (apoB) protein sizes through RNA editing?

a   Western blot using apoB DNA as probe

b. Northern blot using antibody to apoB protein as probe

c. Southern blot using the proximal *apoB* gene segment as probe

d. Western blot using apoB cDNA as probe

e. Western blot using antibody to the amino-terminal portion of apoB protein

56. A 26-year-old male medical student contracts a skin infection from an elderly patient and notes an expanding circular red lesion on his thigh at dinner that night. He places a warm washrag on the lesion at bedtime and awakens in early morning feeling hot with shortness of breath. After reluctantly going to the health clinic, he faints during the registration process and awakens in the intensive care unit. An infectious disease specialist tells him he has methicillin-resistant *Staphylococcus aureus* with toxic shock syndrome (low blood pressure) and adult respiratory distress syndrome (swelling of alveolar membranes with hypoxemia). The attending wishes to use a new antibiotic that acts on the earliest step of protein synthesis. Which of the following steps would most likely be targeted?

a. Peptide bond formation
b. Loading of the small ribosomal subunit with initiation factors, messenger RNA, and initiation aminoacyl-tRNA
c. Sliding of the ribosome three bases forward to read a new codon
d. Binding of the small ribosomal subunit to the large ribosomal subunit
e. Elongation factors deliver aminoacyl-tRNA to the A site of the small ribosomal subunit

57. A 15-year-old Caucasian adolescent of Scandinavian descent has suffered from mild liver disease thought related to receiving parenteral nutrition as a premature infant. Recently she has developed shortness of breath and has decreased oxygen saturation measured at rest. Emphysema is suspected that with liver disease suggests α_1-antitrypsin (AAT) deficiency (MIM*107400), confirmed by protein electrophoresis that shows only mutant protein. Given that normal AAT blocks serum proteases, which of the following is the most likely mechanism for AAT disease?

a. Disruption of signal peptide function with accumulation of AAT protein in the Golgi apparatus
b. Disruption of signal peptide function with increased amounts of AAT in plasma
c. Disruption of AAT protease function
d. Decreased targeting of AAT mRNA to smooth ER ribosomes
e. Increased targeting of AAT mRNA to rough ER ribosomes

58. A couple request genetic counseling because their first child had severe β-thalassemia (MIM*141900) and expired at age 1 year from graft-versus-host reaction after bone marrow transplant. DNA analysis of the child demonstrated a promoter mutation on one copy of the β-globin gene and a mutation in the middle of exon 2 on the other copy. What is the most likely type of mutation in exon 2 that would lead to β-thalassemia (ie, decreased production of β-globin peptide from both β-globin gene copies) and what is the couple's recurrence risk for their next child to be affected?

a. Deletion of 3 bp, 50%
b. Insertion of 1 bp, 25%
c. Insertion of 3 bp, 25%
d. Missense mutation, 25%
e. Silent mutation, virtually zero recurrence risk

59. A 21-year-old Hispanic female presents for evaluation of recurring kidney stones, leg pain, and blanching of her hands with the cold (Raynaud phenomenon). Her prior care was in Mexico and records of prior stone episodes (urolithiasis) or the nature of the stones are not available. Laboratory testing shows elevated blood urea nitrogen (BUN) and creatinine suggesting chronic renal disease, and urinary excretion of oxalic acid is greatly elevated. A diagnosis of primary oxalosis or hyperoxaluria (MIM*259900) is suggested, known to be caused by abnormal location of alanine-glyoxylate aminotransferase enzyme in the endoplasmic reticulum (ER) rather than the peroxisome. Patients can be treated by liver transplant to restore a source of peroxisomal enzyme, but a less invasive cure could be achieved by engineering one mutant allele so its product enzyme was not targeted to the ER. This alteration would be achieved by which of the following strategies?

a. Cleaving the enzyme's carboxy-terminal segment
b. Changing RNA splicing to include an extra exon in the mRNA
c. Adding a proteolytic cleavage site near the protein terminus
d. Changing the enzyme's protein processing to produce a smaller peptide
e. Altering the enzyme's amino-terminal sequence

60. How many high-energy phosphate-bond equivalents are utilized in the process of activation of amino acids for protein synthesis?

a. Zero
b. One
c. Two
d. Three
e. Four

61. The hydrolytic step leading to the release of a polypeptide chain from a ribosome is catalyzed by which of the following?

a. Dissociation of ribosomes
b. Peptidyl transferase
c. Release factors
d. Stop codons
e. UAA

62. The sequence of the template DNA strand is 5'-GATATCCATTAGT-GAC-3'. What is the sequence of the RNA produced?

a. 5'-CAGUGAUUACCUAUAG-3'
b. 5'-CTATAGGTAATCACTG-3'
c. 5'-CUAUAGGUAAUCACUG-3'
d. 5'-GTCACTAATGGATATC-3'
e. 5'-GUCACUAAUGGAUAUC-3'

63. Which of the following statements about ribosomes is true?

a. They are composed of RNA, DNA, and protein.
b. They are composed of three subunits of unequal size.
c. They are bound together so tightly they cannot dissociate under physiologic conditions.
d. They are found both free in the cytoplasm and bound to membranes.
e. They are an integral part of transcription.

64. Guanosine triphosphate (GTP) is required by which of the following steps in protein synthesis?

a. Aminoacyl-tRNA synthetase activation of amino acids
b. Attachment of ribosomes to endoplasmic reticulum
c. Translocation of tRNA-nascent protein complex from A to P sites
d. Attachment of mRNA to ribosomes
e. Attachment of signal recognition protein to ribosomes

65. A 50-year-old African American male develops cough and fever for 3 days while attending a convention, then returns to his home city for medical evaluation. Chest x-rays reveal diffuse (interstitial) pneumonia and the male's poor oxygen saturation and severe cough mandates hospitalization. His physician calls a hospital in the convention town and hears that over a dozen conventioneers received ER treatment for similar symptoms. The physician suspects mycoplasma or pertussis infection similar to Legionnaires disease and prescribes erythromycin. Erythromycin, azithromycin (Zithromax), and clarithromycin (Biaxin). They are macrolide antibiotics that inhibit protein synthesis in certain bacteria by doing which of the following?

a. Inhibiting translocation by binding to 50S ribosomal subunits
b. Acting as an analogue of mRNA
c. Causing premature chain termination
d. Inhibiting initiation
e. Mimicking mRNA binding

66. An immigrant family from rural Mexico brings their 3-month-old son to the emergency room because of whistling inspiration (stridor) and high fever. The child's physician is perplexed because the throat examination shows a gray membrane almost occluding the larynx. A senior physician recognizes diphtheria, now rare in immunized populations. The child is intubated, antitoxin is administered, and antibiotic therapy is initiated. Diphtheria toxin is often lethal in unimmunized persons because it does which of the following?

a. Inhibits initiation of protein synthesis by preventing the binding of GTP to the 40S ribosomal subunit
b. Binds to the signal recognition particle receptor on the cytoplasmic face of the endoplasmic reticulum receptor
c. Shuts off signal peptidase
d. Blocks elongation of proteins by inactivating elongation factor 2 (EF-2 or translocase)
e. Causes deletions of amino acid by speeding up the movement of peptidyl-tRNA from the A site to the P site

67. Aminoacyl-tRNA synthetases must be capable of recognizing which of the following?

a. A specific tRNA and a specific amino acid
b. A specific rRNA and a specific amino acid
c. A specific tRNA and the 40S ribosomal subunit
d. A specific amino acid and the 40S ribosomal subunit
e. A specific amino acid and the 60S ribosomal subunit

68. Ribosomes similar to those of bacteria are found in which of the following?

a. Cardiac muscle cytoplasm
b. Liver endoplasmic reticulum
c. Neuronal cytoplasm
d. Pancreatic mitochondria
e. Plant nuclei

69. Endogenous insulin is ineffective in type II diabetes mellitus (MIM*222100), leading to high blood glucose levels (hyperglycemia) with gradual effects on blood vessels in eye, kidney, and skin. Pregnant women with diabetes mellitus present high glucose loads to their fetus; this stimulates production of fetal insulin (hyperinsulinemia) and causes rapid fetal growth with large birth weight (macrosomia). The stimulation of fetal growth by insulin may be correlated with its effect on gene expression, which is which of the following?

a. Stimulation of mRNA production by enhancing 5′ capping
b. Acceleration of protein synthesis by phosphorylating initiation inhibitors
c. Acceleration of protein synthesis by phosphorylating the 40S ribosomal subunit
d. Acceleration of protein synthesis by phosphorylating proteinase K
e. Stimulation of mRNA production by enhancing RNA splicing

70. Which of the following eukaryotic promoter/regulatory elements has the most variable position with respect to the start site of transcription?

a. Downstream promoter element (DPE)
b. Enhancer
c. Initiator sequence
d. Operator
e. TATA box

71. Which of the following is required for certain types of eucaryotic protein synthesis but not for prokaryotic protein synthesis?

a. GTP
b. Messenger RNA
c. Ribosomal RNA
d. Peptidyl transferase
e. Signal recognition particle

72. A 72-year-old Caucasian male experiences progressive shortness of breath and is diagnosed with emphysema. He had smoked up to one pack per day of cigarettes until 5 years ago. Family history reveals that his father, two paternal uncles, and his father's mother all died of emphysema, and a diagnosis of α_1-antitrypsin deficiency (AAT-MIM*107400) is suspected. He is found to have decreased amounts and abnormal mobility of AAT protein in his serum when analyzed by serum protein electrophoresis. Liver biopsy discloses mild scarring (cirrhosis) and demonstrates microscopic inclusions due to an engorged endoplasmic reticulum. Which of the following is the most likely explanation for these findings?

a. Defective transport from hepatic ER to the plasma
b. A mutation affecting the N-terminal methionine and blocking initiation of protein synthesis
c. A mutation affecting the signal sequence
d. Defective structure of the signal recognition particles
e. Defective energy metabolism causing deficiency of GTP

73. A 6-month-old Caucasian boy has had chronic yeast diaper rash and four episodes of pneumonia, two with positive blood cultures for Group A streptococcus. Knowing that Group A strep infections are rare in infants and that the patient likely has defective B-cells that fight bacteria and defective T-cells that fight viruses and fungi, his physician thinks a diagnosis of severe combined immune deficiency (SCID) due to adenosine deaminase (ADA) deficiency (MIM*102700) is likely. Which of the following treatment options would permanently cure the patient?

a. Germ-line gene therapy to replace one *ADA* gene copy
b. Germ-line gene therapy to replace both *ADA* gene copies
c. Somatic cell gene therapy to replace one *ADA* gene copy in circulating lymphocytes
d. Somatic cell gene therapy to replace both *ADA* gene copies in circulating lymphocytes
e. Somatic cell gene therapy to replace one *ADA* gene copy in bone marrow lymphoblasts

74. A major obstacle to gene therapy involves the difficulty of homologous gene replacement. Which of the following strategies best addresses this issue?

a.   A recombinant vector contains complementary DNA sequences that will facilitate site-specific recombination.
b.   A recombinant vector expresses antisense nucleotides that will hybridize with the targeted mRNA.
c.   A recombinant vector replaces inessential viral genes with a functional human gene.
d.   A recombinant vector transfects patient cells, which are returned to the patient.
e.   A recombinant vector contains DNA sequences that target its expressed protein to lysosomes.

75. A 26-year-old black African American suffers vision loss after hitting his head while playing handball. Ophthalmologic evaluation reveals detachment of the retina that seems unusual for such mild trauma, and further medical history notes the male has lax joints, tall and thin build, and chronic joint pain after exercise. The family history is further revealing in that several individuals have had arthritis and detached retina. The symptoms and history suggest a diagnosis of Stickler syndrome (MIM*108300), a collagen disease that results in lax joints, arthritis, and retinal detachments. The locus for Stickler syndrome has been mapped near that for type II collagen on chromosome 12, and mutations in the *COL2A1* gene have been described in Stickler syndrome. The family became interested in molecular diagnosis to distinguish normal from mildly affected individuals. Which of the following results would be expected in an individual with a promoter mutation at one *COL2A1* gene locus?

a.   Western blotting detects no type II collagen chains.
b.   Southern blotting using intronic restriction sites yields normal restriction fragment sizes.
c.   Reverse transcriptase-polymerase chain reaction (RT-PCR) detects one-half normal amounts of COL2A1 mRNA in affected individuals.
d.   Fluorescent in situ hybridization (FISH) analysis using a COL2A1 probe detects signals on only one chromosome 12.
e.   DNA sequencing reveals a single nucleotide difference between homologous COL2A1 exons.

76. Gyrate atrophy (MIM*258870) is a rare autosomal recessive genetic disorder caused by a deficiency of ornithine aminotransferase. Affected individuals experience progressive chorioretinal degeneration with vision and neurologic defects. The gene for ornithine aminotransferase has been cloned, its structure has been determined, and mutations in affected individuals have been extensively studied. Which of the following mutations best fits with test results showing normal Southern blots with probes from all ornithine aminotransferase exons but absent enzymatic activity?

a. Duplication of entire gene
b. Two-kb deletion in coding region of gene
c. Two-kb insertion in coding region of gene
d. Deletion of entire gene
e. Missense mutation

77. A 5-year-old Egyptian boy receives a sulfonamide antibiotic as prophylaxis for recurrent urinary tract infections. Although he was previously healthy and well nourished, he becomes progressively ill and presents to your office with pallor and irritability. A blood count shows that he is severely anemic with jaundice due to hemolysis of red blood cells. Which of the following is the simplest test for diagnosis?

a. Northern blotting of red blood cell mRNA
b. Enzyme assay of red blood cell hemolysate
c. Western blotting of red blood cell hemolysates
d. Amplification of red blood cell DNA and hybridization with allele-specific oligonucleotides (PCR-ASOs)
e. Southern blot analysis for gene deletions

78. A 1-year-old Caucasian girl who has been treated for scoliosis and club foot is noted to be developmentally delayed with no walking and no speech. Examination reveals increased subcutaneous tissue in her face that causes a coarse appearance, enlarged liver and spleen, scoliosis with a posterior spinal prominence called a gibbus, and increased body hair (hirsutism). A diagnosis of Hurler syndrome (MIM*252800) is considered, and analysis of her white blood cells shows the characteristic deficiency of L-iduronidase. Exogenous L-iduronidase can be taken up by deficient cells via a targeting signal that directs the enzyme to its normal lysosomal location. Which of the following therapeutic strategies is the most realistic and efficient mode of therapy?

a. Germ-line gene therapy
b. Heterologous bone marrow transplant
c. Infection with a disabled adenovirus vector that carries the L-iduronidase gene
d. Injection with L-iduronidase purified from human liver
e. Autologous bone marrow transplant after transfection with a virus carrying the L-iduronidase gene

79. It is now recognized that all cancers involve genetic changes, even though few are hereditary. An early example was the discovery of a Philadelphia chromosome (terminal deletion of chromosome 22) in leucocytes from patients with chronic myeloid leukemia (MIM*608232). Later work demonstrated that the deleted material was in fact translocated to the terminus of chromosome 9, being an example of a balanced translocation between 9 and 22. Of the following results, which would be most diagnostic of the 9;22 translocation in chronic myeloid leukemia?

a. All chromosome 22 genes show increased incorporation of labeled acetate into histones of chromatin regions.
b. A particular gene near the terminus of chromosome 22 shows altered DNA restriction endonuclease patterns.
c. The pattern of small RNA "decoration" along leukemic chromatin is changed.
d. Increased transcription of mRNA from genes near the terminus for chromosome 9.
e. Decreased transcription of mRNA from all loci on the chromosome 22 long arm.

80. A 14-year-old Caucasian adolescent of Ashkenazi Jewish descent is evaluated for fatigue and aching legs at night that had been attributed to "growing pains." Examination revealed a palpable spleen (splenomegaly because the spleen is not normally palpated at this age). His white blood cells showed the typical foamy appearance of cytoplasm due to lipid accumulation in Gaucher disease (MIM*231000). Gaucher disease was considered and blood obtained for DNA testing, examining the gene for glucocerebrosidase enzyme that when deficient causes accumulation of complex lipids in white cells, brain, liver, and spleen. A homozygous glucocerebrosidase gene mutation was found that changed the mRNA sequence of codon 93 from UAC to the UAA depicted in the table below. Which of the following best describes this result?

88	89	90	91	92	93	94
GUC	GAC	CAG	UAC	GGC	UAA	CCG

a. Missense mutation that may interfere with glucocerebrosidase function and could be diagnostic of Gaucher disease
b. Silent mutation that should not interfere with glucocerebrosidase function and is not diagnostic of Gaucher disease
c. Nonsense mutation that produces a truncated, nonfunctional glucocerebrosidase polypeptide and is diagnostic of Gaucher disease
d. Suppressor mutation that interferes with glucocerebrosidase mRNA transcription and is diagnostic of Gaucher disease
e. Frameshift mutation that produces a nonfunctional glucocerebrosidase and is diagnostic of Gaucher disease

81. A 3-month-old Caucasian boy fails to grow and has very low muscle tone with strange "kinky" hair. A diagnosis of Menkes kinky hair syndrome (MIM*309400) is made by showing deficient copper in fibroblasts. A likely candidate gene encoding an ATP-dependent copper transporter protein is known, and antibodies to this protein are available. Experimental analysis of the patient's fibroblast DNA is performed to see if a pathologic mutation can be found, thus confirming the copper transport gene as the cause of Menkes disease. The table below shows a partial DNA sequence from the transporter coding strand as amplified by PCR; the amplified sequence is from a region where a TATA box has been located.

Normal	3'-ATT-ATT-TAC-AAA-ATA-5'
Patient	3'-ATT-ATT-GAC-ATA-ATA-5'

Which of the following experimental results would be most compatible with a pathologic mutation in the transporter gene

a. Usual band of usual intensity on Northern and Western blots
b. Absent bands on Northern and Western blots
c. Usual band plus a second band of lower size on Northern, usual band on Western
d. Usual band on Northern, band of unusual size and reduced intensity on Western blot
e. Two unusual bands on Northern blot, usual bands on Western blot

82. Lipoproteins transport lipids from intestine and liver where they are absorbed and metabolized to peripheral tissues via the bloodstream. They contain core proteins (apo proteins) that bind various types of lipid, thus producing lipoprotein complexes of varying densities—very low density lipoproteins (VLDL), low density lipoproteins (LDL), and high density lipoproteins (HDL) after plasma lipoprotein electrophoresis. A disorder called abetalipoproteinemia (MIM*200100) was distinguished by its deficiency of the bands for very low density lipoproteins (VLDL) and low density lipoproteins (LDL) after plasma electrophoresis. Affected patients have ataxia (wide gait, incoordination), retinopathy (retinal degeneration with blindness), and myopathy (muscle weakness). VLDL and LDL contain the same apoB core protein, their different densities produced by association with different lipids, and apoB became good candidate for mutation in the disorder. Initial characterization of the *apoB* gene together with its mRNA and protein products demonstrated identical mRNA sizes in all tissues. Western blotting using antibody specific for the amino-terminus of apoB protein showed a 100-kDa species in liver and a 48-kDa species in intestine, as did antibody specific for the C-terminus of the 48-kDa intestinal protein. Molecular study of a patient with abetalipoproteinemia showed normal mRNA sizes, but 100-kDa peptide species were identified in both liver and intestine using the amino- or carboxy-terminus antibody probes. Which of the following processes is most likely deficient in this patient with apobetalipoproteinemia?

a. RNA splicing
b. DNA amplification
c. Transcription initiation
d. Transcription factor phosphorylation
e. RNA editing

83. During the analyses described in Question 82, another patient with abetalipoproteinemia was found to have negligible amounts of apoB protein in either liver or intestine. Analysis of the patient's DNA and RNA would most likely yield which of the following results?

a. Substitution of the last base of a codon near the middle of the first apoB exon
b. Insertion of two bases near the apoB amino-terminus
c. Transversion producing a nonsense mutation within the first apoB intron
d. Transition affecting the 30th base of the first apoB intron
e. Base substitution changing glycine for alanine near the apoB carboxyl-terminus

84. Cancers may be caused by mutations in two types of genes, those that affect cell proliferation (oncogenes, tumor suppressor genes) and those that control rates of mutation (caretaker genes—ie, those altering DNA repair). A child develops a wide gait and is found to have different leg lengths. On examination, one leg is larger (hemihypertrophy) and a mass is found in the lower abdomen. Surgery reveals a Wilms tumor (MIM*194070), and the *IGF2* (insulin-like growth factor 2) gene is known to be specifically overexpressed in Wilms tumor. Restriction analysis of the child's tumor DNA showed that both IGF2 alleles were undermethylated. It is known that normal adult tissues have one methylated and one undermethylated IGF2 allele, while the single IGF2 allele in sperm DNA is always undermethylated. The results are best summarized as which of the following?

a. A loss of imprinting (LOI) mutation that increased tumor IGF2 expression and identifies *IGF2* as a caretaker gene
b. A loss of imprinting (LOI) mutation that increased tumor IGF2 expression and identifies *IGF2* as an oncogene
c. A loss of imprinting (LOI) mutation that increased tumor IGF2 expression and identifies it as a tumor suppressor gene
d. A loss of imprinting (LOI) mutation that increased tumor IGF2 expression and causes Wilms tumor in females only
e. A loss of imprinting (LOI) mutation that increased tumor IGF2 expression and causes Wilms tumor in males only

85. Part of the triplet genetic code involving mRNA codon triplets that start with U is shown below. Using the portion of the genetic code shown, which of the following mutations in the 3′ to 5′ DNA template segments corresponds to a nonsense mutation?

5′ End (Nucleotide 1)	Middle		3′ End (Nucleotide 2)	(Nucleotide 3)
	U	C	A	G	
	Phe	ser	tyr	cys	U
	Phe	ser	tyr	cys	C
U	Leu	ser	stop	stop	A
	Leu	ser	stop	stop	G

a. ACGACGACG to ACAAACACG
b. AGGAATATG to AGGAATATT
c. AGAATAACA to AAAATAACA
d. AAAATGAGC to AAAATAAGC
e. AACAACAAC to AACAAGAAC

86. An abdominal mass is palpated during a well visit for a 15-month-old African American boy with a normal past medical history. Urinalysis demonstrates blood cells and other cells of unusual morphology, suggesting a diagnosis of Wilms tumor (MIM*194070). The physicians suspected erosion of surrounding kidney with invasion of the renal pelvis, causing tumor cells to be excreted in urine. Because a version of the *p57* gene is known to be silenced preferentially in Wilms tumor, analysis of *p57* gene methylation and expression was performed on the urine tumor cells with the results shown below (normal cells-N, tumor cells-T). Which of the following best summarizes these results?

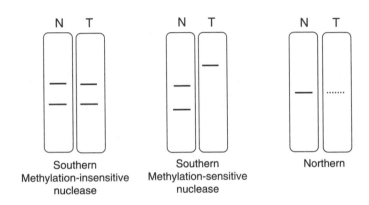

a. Bi-allelic *p57* gene methylation and with normal *p57* gene expression making a diagnosis of Wilms tumor unlikely
b. Bi-allelic *p57* gene methylation and with increased *p57* gene expression making a diagnosis of Wilms tumor unlikely
c. Bi-allelic *p57* gene methylation and with decreased *p57* gene expression supporting the diagnosis of Wilms tumor
d. Undermethylation of both p57 alleles with increased *p57* gene expression supporting the diagnosis of Wilms tumor
e. Methylation of one p57 allele with increased *p57* gene expression supporting the diagnosis of Wilms tumor

87. The lactose operon is negatively controlled by the lactose repressor and positively controlled by which of the following?

a. Increased concentrations of glucose and cyclic AMP (cAMP)
b. Decreased concentrations of glucose and cAMP
c. Increased concentrations of glucose, decreased concentration of cAMP
d. Decreased concentrations of glucose, increased concentration of cAMP
e. Increased concentrations of glucose and adenosine triphosphate (ATP)

88. Which of the following regulators are said to act in "cis"?

a. The lac repressor and the lac operator
b. The lac operator and mammalian transcription factors
c. The lac operator and mammalian enhancers
d. Mammalian transcription factors and enhancers
e. The lac repressor and mammalian transcription factors

89. A severe birth defect syndrome called retinoic acid embryopathy (MIM*243440) is caused by medications such as isotretinoin (Accutane) when taken by pregnant women for treatment of acne. Retinoic acid and steroid hormones are group I signals that cross the cell membrane to interact with cytosolic or nuclear receptors. Which of the structural domains of such receptors would interact with retinoic acid?

a. Response elements
b. Antirepressor domains
c. Transcription-activating domains
d. Ligand-binding domains
e. DNA-binding domains

90. The proopiomelanocortin (POMC-MIM*176830) gene encodes several regulatory proteins that affect pituitary function. Children with severe brain defects like holoprosencephaly (MIM*157170) often have abnormalities in the hypothalamic-pituitary axis. In different brain regions, proteins encoded by this gene have different carboxy-terminal peptides. Which of the following best explains the regulatory mechanism?

a. POMC transcription is regulated by different factors in different brain regions.
b. POMC translation elongation is regulated by different factors in different brain regions.
c. POMC transcription has different enhancers in different brain regions.
d. POMC protein undergoes different protein processing in different brain regions.
e. POMC protein forms different allosteric complexes in different brain regions.

91. A 3-year-old Chinese boy has severe anemia with prominence of the forehead (frontal bossing) and cheeks. The red cell hemoglobin concentration is dramatically decreased, and it contains only β-globin chains with virtual deficiency of α-globin chains. Which of the following mechanisms is the most likely explanation?

a. A transcription factor regulating the α-globin gene is mutated.
b. A regulatory sequence element has been mutated adjacent to an α-globin gene.
c. A transcription factor regulating the β-globin gene is mutated.
d. A transcription factor regulating the α- and β-globin genes is deficient.
e. A deletion has occurred surrounding an α-globin gene.

92. A mutation that results in a valine replacement for glutamic acid at position 6 of the β chain of hemoglobin S hinders normal hemoglobin function and results in sickle cell anemia (MIM*602903) when the patient is homozygous for this mutation. This is an example of which of the following types of mutation?

a. Deletion
b. Frameshift
c. Insertion
d. Missense
e. Nonsense

93. Two boys with mental disability are found to have mutations in a gene on the X chromosome that has no homology with globin genes. Both are also noted to have deficiency of α-globin synthesis, causing imbalance of globin chains and the severe anemia and skeletal changes of α-thalassemia plus mental retardation (MIM*301040). Which of the following is the best explanation for their phenotype?

a. The mutation disrupted an enhancer for an α-globin pseudogene.
b. The mutation disrupted an X-encoded transcription factor that regulates the α-globin loci.
c. There is a second mutation that disrupts an enhancer near the α-globin gene.
d. There is a DNA rearrangement that joins the mutated X-chromosome gene with an α-globin gene.
e. There is a second mutation that disrupts the promoter of an α-globin gene.

94. A 50-year-old Caucasian male presents with a markedly enlarged tonsil and recurrent infections with serum immunoglobulin deficiency. He has enlarged lymph nodes along his neck. Chromosome analysis demonstrates a translocation between the immunoglobulin heavy-chain locus on chromosome 14 and an unidentified gene on chromosome 8. Which of the following is the most likely cause of his phenotype?

a. The translocation has deleted constant chain exons on chromosome 14 and prevented heavy-chain class switching.
b. The translocation has deleted the interval containing diversity (D) and joining (J) regions.
c. The translocation has activated a tumor-promoting gene on chromosome 8.
d. The translocation has deleted the heavy-chain constant chain Cμ so that virgin B-cells cannot produce IgM on their membranes.
e. The translocation has deleted an immunoglobulin transcription factor gene on chromosome 8.

Gene Expression and Regulation

Answers

35. The answer is b. *(Murray, pp 353-359. Scriver, pp 3-45. Lewis, pp 188-194.)* The "genetic code" uses 64 possible combinations of three-nucleotide "words" (codons) each specifying one of 20 amino acids or three stop signals that catalyze translational termination when present in the transcribed messenger RNA (answer b correct, answers a, c, d incorrect). Single nucleotide changes in genes (point mutations) can thus change the codon in transcribed mRNA and produce single amino acid changes in the translated protein. It follows that the genetic code must be degenerate, with different codons specifying the same amino acid. Amino acid changes in proteins implied by altered enzyme activity or altered electrophoretic migration (eg, the abnormal Z form of AAT) can now be predicted by DNA sequencing of the encoding gene to demonstrate specific altered codons (eg, the GAG to AAG change in the *AAT* gene that changed the 342nd amino acid from lysine to glutamine. Mutations are best described by reference to amino acid position since the linear correspondence of codons in DNA and of amino acids in protein domains is interrupted by the presence of introns in DNA (answer e is incorrect). The genetic code is universal in the sense that codon-amino acid relationships are the same in all organisms.

36. The answer is d. *(Murray, pp 388-405. Scriver, pp 3-45. Lewis, pp 219-232.)* Spherocytosis (MIM*182900), like other single gene or Mendelian disorders, is subject to DNA diagnosis by demonstrating an altered nucleotide sequence within or around the causative gene. This process is simpler and less expensive if common mutations like that for sickle cell anemia have been previously characterized, allowing PCR amplification of that specific gene region and using sequence-specific oligonucleotides to determine the presence of normal or mutated DNA sequence.

The equivalence of DNA in most tissues (with the exception of red blood cells that extrude their nucleus—incorrect answer a) makes DNA diagnosis a powerful technique that is independent of gene or protein expression. Analysis of exon sizes or intron (noncoding) DNA sequences within a gene would be insensitive, detecting only DNA insertions/deletions for the former and possibly mutations altering splicing in the latter (incorrect answers b, c) Western blotting is a technique that uses antibodies to highlight the size and amount of mutant protein in cell extracts; it is less sensitive and specific than DNA diagnosis (incorrect answer e). The sensitivity of DNA diagnosis is also lowered when several genes can cause the same disease phenotype, as is the case with spherocytosis.

37. The answer is c. (*Murray, pp 353-359. Scriver, pp 3-45. Lewis, pp 188-194.*) Insertion (correct answer c) or deletion (incorrect answer d) because no termination codon generated of nucleotides shifts the reading frame unless the change is a multiple of three (incorrect answer e). Frameshifts may create unintended stop codons as in correct answer c. Point mutations resulting in nucleotide or amino acid substitutions are conveniently named by their position in the protein, that is, $P_{21}A$ (choice b). The protein change $P_{21}A$ could also be denoted by the corresponding change in the DNA reading frame, that is, $C_{63}A$. Note that the single base substitution of $C_{65}A$ for incorrect answer a does not result in an amino acid change. Deletions may be prefixed by the letter delta, as with ΔF_{25} (incorrect answer e).

38. The answer is b. (*Murray, pp 336-346. Scriver, pp 3-45. Lewis, pp 188-194.*) Three RNA polymerases are responsible for RNA transcription in mammalian cells, RNA polymerase I for ribosomal RNA, RNA polymerase II for messenger RNA, and RNA polymerase III for transfer and small RNAs (5s, μRNAs). Mammalian RNA polymerase II is highly sensitive to the mushroom toxin α-amanitin, and thus synthesis of mRNA (correct answer b) rather than other RNA species (incorrect answers a, c-e) will be inhibited by α-amanitin (even experienced mushroom gatherers can confuse the toxic *Amanita* species with edible varieties). Inhibition of RNA polymerase II-catalyzed HnRNA/mRNA transcription seems to have the most dramatic effects in liver, perhaps because of its active role in protein synthesis. The liver damage caused by α-amanitin ingestion cannot be treated, requiring regeneration in milder ingestions and transplant in severe ones.

39. The answer is c. (*Murray, pp 346-351. Scriver, pp 3-45. Lewis, pp 215-218.*) The size of the primary β-globin RNA transcript will include the 5'- and 3'-untranslated regions (50 plus 50 bp) and the exons encoding protein domains (450 amino acids requires 150 coding bp), producing a processed (mature) mRNA of 550 bp (correct answer c). Introns (900 bp) would be included in the 1450 bp primary or HnRNA (answer a incorrect). RNA processing removes the 150 and 750 bp introns, yielding a mature mRNA of 550 bp (excluding answers b, d, e that incorrectly include an intron or exclude untranslated regions that remain in the mRNA). Any mutation that reduces β-globin relative to α-globin (β-thalassemia) reduces hemoglobin ($\alpha_2\beta_2$) synthesis. Severe forms lead to extramedullary hematopoiesis in liver in an attempt at compensation (causing liver enlargement or hepatomegaly).

Exons are the coding portions of genes and consist of trinucleotide codons that guide the placement of specific amino acids into protein. Introns are the noncoding portions of genes that may function in evolution to provide "shuffling" of exons to produce new proteins. The primary RNA transcript contains both exons and introns, but the latter are removed by RNA splicing. The 5′ (upstream) and 3′ (downstream) untranslated RNA regions remain in the mature RNA and are thought to regulate RNA transport or translation. A polyA tail is added to the primary transcript after transcription, which facilitates transport and processing from the nucleus. The discovery of introns complicated Mendel's idea of the gene as the smallest hereditary unit; a modern definition might be the colinear sequence of exons, introns, and adjacent regulatory sequences that accomplish protein expression.

40. The answer is c. (*Murray, pp 346-351. Scriver, 3-45. Lewis, pp 206-212.*) The small size and alkaline lability of the factor suggests it is a small RNA (correct answer c) rather than mRNA (>100 to thousands of bp—incorrect answer b) or tRNA (75-90 bp—incorrect answer a). Some simple RNAs can self-catalyze their own splicing, but such mechanisms are less important during the complex processing of mammalian mRNAs (incorrect answer e). A transposon is a mobile DNA element that usually inhibits gene expression (incorrect answer d).

Small RNAs ranging from 21 to 30 nucleotides in length are now recognized in all eucaryotes and include more than 1000 species in humans. Small RNAs may stimulate genes (μRNAs) or silence them (interfering or siRNAs), influencing gene transcription by binding to chromatin or DNA sequence elements. Regulation by small RNAs is complex since many have double-stranded or hairpin regions that are cleaved and activated by specific nucleases like *Dicer, Drosha,* or *Pasha* in flies. Small RNAs have been implicated in regulating the conversion of mouse hematopoietic stem cells to B-cells. Silencing or interfering RNAs have become an important tool for genetic analysis, allowing specific knockout of genes in animals or in vitro systems to define their effects.

41. The answer is d. *(Murray, pp 353-359. Scriver, pp 4571-4636. Lewis, pp 188-194.)* Recognition of the 7-bp CCTGAGG site that includes the codon for glutamate by MstII restriction endonuclease provided a simple DNA test, since the sickle cell mutation ablates this middle site and yields a 680 bp fragment after Southern blotting and hybridization with the DNA segment illustrated in the figure. Normal globin alleles will retain the middle MstII site and yield 515 bp and 165 bp fragments after restriction, electrophoretic size-separation, capillary transfer to a nitrocellulose membrane, and hybridization to the indicated probe (Southern blotting named after Ed Southern). Northern blotting, a pun on Southern's name, is an analogous technique for detection of RNA fragments through transfer and hybridization. A nucleic acid species of about 550 bp representing β-globin mRNA (discussed in Question 39; incorrect answers b, c) would be expected upon Northern blotting of tissue extracts from normal or sickle cell individuals since the mutation should not change transcription or RNA processing. Both β-globin alleles would be mutated in a person with sickle cell anemia, ablating the MstII site on both alleles and yielding only the 680 MstII restriction fragment (incorrect answers a, e).

The single nucleotide transition from A to T on the sense strand in codon six of the β-globin gene causes the amino acid substitution glutamic acid to valine in the encoded β-globin protein. The valine lacks the negative charge of the glutamic acid carboxyl group, changing the shape of the β-globin protein and its subsequent complex with α-globin protein and heme to form hemoglobin. Correlation of this DNA change with its effect on hemoglobin and its resulting clinical symptoms earned Linus Pauling a Nobel Prize and initiated the era of molecular medicine. The lack of a negative charge and change in protein conformation also produced altered mobility of the hemoglobin, uniquely visualized by hemoglobin electrophoresis because of its red color.

42. The answer is b. *(Murray, pp 336-346. Scriver, pp 3-45. Lewis, 188-194.)* Promoter sites are initiation sites for transcription that are located just upstream (5′) of the transcription unit (site a in the figure for the β-globin gene). Alterations of promoter DNA sequences or the enhancer/controller regions that surround them will decrease RNA polymerase binding and transcription of the downstream gene. In this case, the decrease in β-globin mRNA and thus of β-globin protein levels disrupts the β-globin/α-globin chain balance in hemoglobin and prevents normal hemoglobin synthesis. Upstream promoter sequences bind rather than code for RNA polymerase (incorrect answers a, d) and do not influence transcription termination (incorrect answers c, e). The severe hemoglobin deficiency (anemia) in β-thalassemia causes pale skin (pallor) and prevents effective tissue oxygenation and growth. Hemoglobin-deficient red blood cells are destroyed more quickly, causing increased bilirubin and yellow skin (jaundice). The red cell deficiency causes continuous bone marrow cell proliferation, thickening of marrow spaces, and thus prominence of the forehead and cheeks.

RNA transcription starts when RNA polymerase binds to the promoter, unwinds the closed promoter complex, and forms the open promoter complex with unwound template DNA. RNA synthesis begins with a pppA or pppG at the 5′ terminus and continues in the 5′ to 3′ direction. The nascent, single-stranded RNA (heterogenous or HnRNA) is terminated (a process linked to transcription that when disrupted is another cause of β-thalassemia-MIM*141900). DNA sequence elements achieve specificity of transcription in eucaryotes, providing promoter/enhancer sites or encoding transcription factors that form a multiprotein RNA polymerase II aggregate. Mammalian transcription is more complex and variable than in bacteria where special subunits of RNA polymerase (eg, sigma factor) regulate specificity of transcription.

43. The answer is b. (*Murray, pp 353-359. Scriver, pp 4571-4636. Lewis, pp 206-212.*) The offspring of a female with sickle cell anemia (MIM*603903) must receive one of her abnormal β-globin alleles and be a heterozygote or carrier known as sickle cell trait. Those with sickle trait will have one β-globin gene with a sickle mutation that ablates the sixth codon MstII site, yielding a 680 bp fragment by Southern blot in addition to the 515 and 165 bp fragments yielded by the normal β-globin gene (eliminating incorrect answers a, c, and d). RNA transcription and processing will not be affected, yielding a β-globin mRNA of about 550 bp (eliminating incorrect answer e). The sickle hemoglobin will have a different charge and conformation due to its glutamic acid to valine substitution, migrating differently by electrophoresis and yielding a second, abnormal hemoglobin band in addition to that of normal hemoglobin.

Approximately 1 in 12 African Americans will have sickle trait, justifying its inclusion in American neonatal screening protocols. Caucasians, especially those of Mediterranean origin, can also be affected. Individuals with sickle trait will be asymptomatic under normal conditions, but may show symptoms under conditions of low oxygen tension (high altitudes, diving, etc) due to the lower oxygen-binding capacity of their red blood cells (half normal, half sickle cell hemoglobin).

44. The answer is c. (*Murray, pp 336-346. Scriver, pp 4571-4636. Lewis, pp 206-212.*) A mutation affecting the transcription initiation or promoter site of the β-globin gene will decrease transcription of that allele and diminish the amount of ~550 bp β-globin mRNA detected by Northern blot (eliminating incorrect answers a, d). The β-globin mRNA produced will be mostly that encoding sickle globin, appearing as abnormal β-globin protein on hemoglobin electrophoresis (incorrect answers b, d, e). The promoter mutation on one β-globin allele will not affect the 515 and 165 bp MstII cleavage fragments detected by Southern blotting, but the sickle cell mutation on the other allele will ablate the MstII site at the sixth codon and produce an additional 680 bp fragment. Because both β-thalassemia and sickle cell anemia are common in Mediterranean populations, compound heterozygotes with both mutations, known colloquially as "sickle-thal," are fairly common. Their symptoms will be as severe as those of sickle cell homozygotes, including anemia, strokes, and pain crises due to vascular occlusion from sickled red blood cells.

45. The answer is e. (*Murray, pp 336-346. Scriver, pp 4571-4636. Lewis, pp 188-194.*) The mutated sequence is that for a TATA box, thus disrupting binding by transcription factor IID and initiation of transcription by RNA polymerase II (incorrect answers a, c, d). Mutations that interfere with β-globin mRNA synthesis or disrupt encoding of β-globin protein (eg, frameshift, nonsense mutations in the exon sequences) will produce β-globin chain deficiency, imbalance of globin chains, and β-thalassemia (correct answer e—severe and chronic anemia due to hemoglobin deficiency). Amino acid substitutions in the globin coding sequence would cause hemoglobinopathies—altered hemoglobin structure or binding properties as with sickle cell anemia (incorrect answer b).

The initiation of eukaryotic mRNA transcription involves the binding of transcription factor TFIID to a TATA box upstream of virtually all eukaryotic genes. The TATA box occurs about 25 nucleotides upstream from the gene and initiates a sequence of binding involving TFIID, TFIIA, TFIIB, RNA polymerase II, and TFIIE. The TATA box is similar to a 10-sequence promoter box found in prokaryotes, and is recognized by a TATA box-binding protein within TFIID.

46. The answer is c. (*Murray, pp 336-346. Scriver, pp 4571-4636. Lewis, pp 188-194.*) Site c at the first exon-intron junction of the β-globin gene (figure below Question 40) is a likely splice donor site, lying at the upstream border of the intron; alteration would prevent excision of intronic sequences from β-globin mRNA, increasing its size and interfering with β-globin protein translation (incorrect answers a, b, d, e). Mediterranean peoples have increased frequency of hemoglobinopathies and thalassemias (literally, sea anemias) due to migration from Africa where they conferred resistance to malaria. Decrease of β-globin protein production rather than alteration of its amino acid sequence produces imbalance of α-/β-chain synthesis and β-thalassemia (incorrect answers a, e).

The primary RNA transcript produced by RNA polymerase is a heterogenous RNA containing introns and exons. RNA processing then occurs as the newly transcribed RNA is transported from nucleus to cytoplasm, and includes RNA splicing to remove intronic sequences in the transcript, methyl capping of the 5′ end, and polyadenylation (addition of 50-200 adenylate residues) to the 3′ end. RNA splicing is catalyzed by a spliceosome, using consensus donor sites at the proximal exon-intron junction and consensus acceptor sites at the distal intron-exon junction. Mutation of splice donor or acceptor sequences will disrupt normal splicing, yielding an aberrant mRNA that contains intronic sequences (if not degraded, a larger size by Northern blot). Decreased amounts of normal mRNA and production of an aberrant protein due to translation of nonsense intronic sequences will decrease the amounts of normal β-globin protein and produce β-thalassemia. Mutations at splice sites will not affect promoter sites or transcription initiation, producing a different category of β-thalassemia that is due to aberrant RNA processing.

47. The answer is d. (*Murray, pp 353-359. Scriver, pp 4571-4636. Lewis, pp 219-232.*) Two α-globin genes are present in tandem within the human α-globin gene cluster on chromosome 16. Mutations affecting 1, 2, 3, or all 4 α-globin genes are thus possible, causing α-thalassemia trait when one or both α-globin genes on the same chromosome homologue are mutated—this leaves two normal α-globin genes on the other homologue that can produce sufficient amounts of α-globin (incorrect answer a). Homozygous mutations affecting the first or second α-globin gene on both chromosome homologues also produce α-thalassemia trait, since one active α-globin gene remains on each homologue (incorrect answers a, b, e). Mutations in all four α-globin genes that severely impact α-globin expression (eg, gene deletions, frameshift or nonsense mutations) produce severe α-thalassemia with fetal demise from tissue edema (fetal hydrops) or chronic, lethal anemia during childhood (incorrect answer c). Severe α-thalassemia is associated with hemoglobin Bart, made from four γ-chains when fetal hemoglobin ($\alpha_2 \gamma_2$) cannot be synthesized due to severe α-globin deficiency. Mutations affecting 3 of the 4 α-globin genes produce hemoglobin H disease, named for the formation of hemoglobin containing four β-globin chains (hemoglobin H) on account of α-globin deficiency.

The α-globin and β globin gene clusters on chromosomes 11 and 16, respectively consist of major and minor globin genes in tandem. Individual globin genes are highly similar to one another, suggesting that their clusters evolved by unequal crossing over to generate duplicate genes with later divergence of function. Both clusters have globin genes that are expressed during embryonic or fetal life, exemplified by the switch from fetal γ-globin to adult β-globin expression in the β-globin cluster at age 6 months of infancy. The β-globin mutations that decrease β-globin mRNA can be heterozygous (β-thalassemia trait) or homozygous (β-thalassemia), but the corresponding α-globin mutations can be present in 1, 2, 3, or 4 α-globin genes. Only patients with mutations in 3 or 4 α-globin genes will have significant α-thalassemia.

48. The answer is b. (*Murray, pp 336-346. Scriver, pp 4571-4636. Lewis, pp 188-194.*) Mutations changing the β-globin amino acid sequence will likely present as hemoglobinopathies while those that decrease β-globin mRNA synthesis will likely cause β-thalassemia. Mutations can decrease mRNA amounts by interfering with sequence elements (promoters, enhancers—incorrect answer d) that promote gene transcription or sequence elements (consensus splice donor and acceptor sites, consensus polyadenylation sites—incorrect answers a, c, e) that interfere with mRNA processing.

Eukaryotic mRNAs are polyadenylated at the 3' end to protect it from exonuclease attack. The polyadenylation signal AAUAA is found 10 to 30 bp upstream of the polyadenylation site. Homozygous mutations affecting the β-globin gene polyadenylation signal can reduce β-globin mRNA synthesis by 95% to 97%, producing β-thalassemia. Single-base substitutions within exons should not change mRNA transcription or processing, but may produce amino acid changes (missense mutations) and yield an aberrant protein with defective function (eg, a hemoglobinopathy).

49. The answer is c. (*Murray, pp 346-351. Scriver, pp 3-45. Lewis, pp 206-212.*) The splicing of messenger RNA is carried out by spliceosomes—complexes of small ribonucleoprotein particles (snRNPs) and messenger RNA precursor. The presence of the GT to AT mutation in both PAH alleles, together with the larger (incompletely spliced) mRNA precursor, indicates a homozygote affected with PKU. Self-splicing by RNA catalysis (ribozymes) occurs in simpler organisms and some ribosomal RNA precursors but not in spliceosome-mediated processing of mammalian mRNAs (incorrect answers a, b). Spliceosomes use snRNPs to recognize the 5' splice site and the 3' splice site followed by excision of the intronic RNA; RNA polymerase or helicase are not involved because it is the RNA within the spliceosome that catalyzes intron excision (incorrect answers d, e).

The indicated splicing mutation was the first molecular change demonstrated in PKU, a necessary step in diagnosis because PAH enzyme activity cannot be measured in blood leucocytes or in cultured fibroblasts. Although use of phenylalanine-deficient formula provides excellent therapy for PKU patients like the mentioned child, severe forms of PKU reflecting defective biopterin cofactor binding make prenatal diagnosis desirable.

50. The answer is d. (*Murray, pp 346-351. Scriver, pp 3-45. Lewis, 206-212.*) The primary transcripts of all eukaryotic mRNAs are capped at the 5' ends as opposed to prokaryotic RNAs or eukaryotic tRNAs and rRNAs (incorrect answers b, c). Spliceosomes accomplish RNA splicing and excision of intronic sequences from mammalian mRNA (incorrect answer a), and poly(A) is added to the 3' end (incorrect answer e). The cap is composed of 7-methylguanylate attached by a pyrophosphate linkage to the 5' end. The cap protects the 5' ends of mRNAs from nucleases and phosphatases and is essential for the recognition of eukaryotic mRNAs in the protein-synthesizing system.

51. The answer is d. (*Murray, pp 346-351. Scriver, pp 3-45. Lewis, 243-248.*) The nucleolus, an organelle unique to eukaryotic cells, is the site where RNA polymerase I transcribes the multiple, tandemly repeated genes for ribosomal RNAs to give 45S primary transcripts that form the 28S and 18S ribosomal RNAs. The ribosomal RNA (rRNA) gene clusters can undergo amplification through unequal crossing over, accounting for individual variability in the size of these clusters, located at the ends of the five pairs of acrocentric chromosomes (numbers 13-15, 21-22). These variably sized clusters form stalks and "satellites" on the acrocentric chromosomes when visualized at metaphase by karyotyping, and their associated rRNA gives a distinctive dark color when incubated with silver stain. The rRNA gene clusters (rDNA) associate within nucleoli at interphase and comprise nucleolar organizing regions (NOR) on chromosomes visualized at metaphase.

Enzymatic modification and cleavage remove spacer regions to yield 28S, 18S, and 5.8S ribosomal RNA. The 5S subunit is synthesized by RNA polymerase III in the nucleoplasm rather than in the nucleolus. Ribosomal proteins combine with the ribosomal subunits to assemble into a 60S subunit containing the 5S, 5.8S, and 28S RNAs and a 40S subunit containing the 18S RNA. Combined, the two subunits produce a functional eukaryotic ribosome with a sedimentation coefficient of 80S. Messenger RNAs are synthesized by RNA polymerase II in the nucleoplasm, while 5S, tRNA, and small RNAs are synthesized by RNA polymerase III in the cytoplasm.

52. The answer is c. (*Murray, pp 346-351. Scriver, pp 3-45. Lewis, 206-212.*) Although precursor heterogenous RNA may undergo alternative processing to encode several different proteins, mature mRNAs are highly processed (incorrect answers d, e) to encode one specific protein (incorrect answer b). A collinear 3-nucleotide to amino acid code is employed (incorrect answer a).

About 30% of the DNA of humans and other mammals consists of repeated sequences. Repetitive DNA includes numerous families of genes like those for histones. Some families of repeated genes make identical mRNA molecules, suggesting that their multiple gene copies are needed to make adequate amounts of protein. Although many genes in bacteria produce a polycistronic mRNA that encodes several different peptides, all mRNAs in mammals encode a single peptide and are monocistronic. In addition, RNA is initially transcribed from protein-encoding genes as larger molecules called heterogenous nuclear RNA (hnRNA). These immature hnRNA molecules must be spliced to remove introns and chemically modified with 5' caps and 3'-poly(A) sequences before reaching the cytoplasm as functional mRNA. The initial hnRNA transcript is colinear with its encoded protein within exons but not within introns. Mature mRNAs also have 5'- and 3'-untranslated regions that are not colinear with the encoded peptide.

53. The answer is d. (*Murray, pp 336-346. Scriver, pp 3-45. Lewis, pp 355-377.*) Tumor suppressor genes like *BRCA1* and 2 require expression of both alleles to inhibit cell growth and transformation to malignancy. A pathologic BRCA1 mutation would be expected to affect one of the two alleles (incorrect answers a, e) and severely impact protein expression or function (incorrect answer c—"wobble" in the nucleotide code allows for differences in the third position of codons to encode the same amino acid). Mutations affecting the RNA polymerase-transcription factor IID binding site (TATA box) or frameshifts that garble the amino acid code would be pathologic, that is, would cause disease rather than representing harmless DNA variation (polymorphism). Since pathologic mutations for tumor suppressors will be heterozygous (homozygosity would be extremely rare), daughter has a 50% chance to inherit the mutant allele with its 80% lifetime risk for breast cancer. This would give a joint probability of 50% to inherit the mutation and 80% lifetime cancer risk if she did = 40% risk for breast cancer (and 22.5% risk for ovarian cancer). If a BRCA1 mutation were found in the mother that was likely to be pathologic (cause her breast cancer), the daughter could have the DNA test and elect prophylactic mastectomy and oophorectomy if positive. Young women can either plan marriage and child-bearing before surgery or have eggs frozen for future use.

54. The answer is c. (*Murray, pp 346-351. Scriver, pp 2717-2752. Lewis, pp 206-212.*) Though unanticipated, the apoB mRNA was found to undergo RNA editing wherein a cytidine deaminase in intestine changed a CAA codon to UAA. The UAA is a termination codon and caused a truncated 48-kDa apoB mRNA peptide to be synthesized in intestine compared to the full-length 100 kb peptide synthesized in liver. The other explanations (alternative splicing, exon deletion, polyadenylation, different promoter) would not produce mRNA of similar size and abundance (incorrect answers a, b, d, e). In addition, the autosomal recessive inheritance of abetalipoproteinemia (MIM*200100) requires homozygous or compound heterozygous (both alleles with different mutations) mutation to produce disease. A homozygous missense mutation changing the amino acid sequence and function of the apoB protein could be diagnostic (correct answer c), best demonstrated by DNA sequencing studies.

55. The answer is e. *(Murray, pp 388-405. Scriver, pp 2717-2752. Lewis, pp 380-388.)* Northern blotting to detect RNA and Western blotting to detect protein were named as puns on the name of Ed Southern who developed his cognate method for electrophoretic separation and hybridization probe detection of DNA segments. Changes in protein size due to RNA editing (two forms of mRNA from the same gene) would be detected by Western blotting (incorrect answers b, c). Specific antibodies to apoB protein are needed to visualize the protein after Western blotting (incorrect answers a, d). Specific antibodies are usually raised by injection into rabbits and purification of antibody from rabbit serum. Antibodies are labeled with radioactive iodine or fluorescent dyes, then floated over the Western blot membrane to bind and identify specific peptides. Antibody to the amino-terminus region of apoB protein is needed to identify.

56. The answer is b. *(Murray, pp 359-368. Scriver, pp 3-45. Lewis, pp 188-194.)* Despite the more complex initiation factors loading the small ribosomal subunit (correct answer b), protein synthesis in prokaryotes and eukaryotes is quite similar. The ribosomal subunits are odd numbers 30S and 50S in prokaryotes, even numbers 40S and 60S in eukaryotes. At the start of translation, initiation factors, mRNA, and initiation aminoacyl-tRNA bind to the dissociated small ribosomal subunit (answers a, c-e thus incorrect). Only after the small ribosomal subunit is primed with mRNA and initiation aminoacyl-tRNA does the large ribosomal subunit bind to it. Once this happens, elongation factors bring the first aminoacyl-tRNA of the nascent protein to the A site. This is the step inhibited by tetracycline. Then peptidyl transferase forges a peptide bond between the initiation amino acid and the first amino acid of the forming peptide. The now uncharged initiation tRNA leaves the P site and the peptidyl-tRNA from the A site moves to the now vacant P site with the two amino acids attached. The ribosome advances three bases to read the next codon and the process repeats. Macrolide antibiotics (eg, azithromycin, Zithromax, and erythromycin) bind to the bacterial 50S ribosome and inhibit this translocation step. When the stop signal is reached after the complete polypeptide has been synthesized, releasing factors bind to the stop signal, causing peptidyl transferase to hydrolyze the bond that joins the polypeptide at the A site to the tRNA. Factors prevent the reassociation of ribosomal subunits in the absence of new initiation complex.

57. The answer is a. *(Murray, pp 359-368. Scriver, pp 3-45. Lewis, pp 188-194.)* Protein synthesis occurs in the cytoplasm, on groups of free ribosomes called polysomes, and on ribosomes associated with membranes, termed the rough endoplasmic reticulum. However, proteins destined for secretion have a signal peptide targeting their ribosomes to the endoplasmic reticulum and the synthesized protein is extruded into the ER lumen. Normal AAT synthesis would involve signal peptide targeting to the ER, secretion from ER lumen to plasma membrane and the blood stream, and subsequent inhibition of damaging serum proteases (incorrect answer c). Mutations causing AAT deficiency could disrupt signal peptide function and rough ER targeting with decreased serum AAT levels (incorrect answers b, d, e).

58. The answer is b. *(Lewis, pp 215-218. Murray, pp 353-359. Scriver, pp 4571-4636.)* The insertion or deletion of nucleotides other than multiples of three will change the reading frame by which the linear nucleotides of RNA parsed three at a time (codons) into the linear amino acids of protein (eliminates answers a, c). Substitution with a different nucleotide will usually produce missense (change in amino acid) or silent (no change in amino acid) that have milder effects on protein function (incorrect answers d, e—rare substitutions could produce a terminating codon and truncated protein). The inserted base pair or similar nonsense mutation would have to be present in both β-globin alleles of the deceased child in order to cause disease, and thus both parents (assuming correct paternity) would be heterozygotes or carriers. The next child of carrier parents would have a $1/4$ or 25% chance to be affected ($1/2$ chance for the abnormal allele in each parental gamete) and could be given the option of preimplantation/prenatal diagnosis (the 25% risk eliminates answers a, e).

A shift in the reading frame by one or two positions will change the sense of ensuing nucleotides, causing all subsequent codons to be read out of frame to produce a completely different (nonsense) amino acid sequences. Often the shift in frame will introduce a stop codon after the frameshift and produce a truncated protein. Whether the amino acid sequence is garbled or truncated, a frameshift mutation will disrupt production of normal protein. In the case of frameshift mutations in the β-globin gene, production of β-globin protein will be reduced as with transcription or RNA processing mutations, causing another form of β-thalassemia when both β-globin gene copies are ineffective. Missense mutations may produce a protein with variant structure and function (eg, as in a hemoglobinopathy) while silent mutations will have no effect on protein structure/function and may be called polymorphisms (harmless genetic variations).

59. The answer is e. *(Murray, pp 359-368. Scriver, pp 3219-3256. Lewis, pp 215-218.)* An amino-terminal sequence of about 70 amino acids (signal or leader sequence) causes secretory proteins and their polysomes to become associated with the endoplasmic reticulum; cotranslational insertion then directs the protein to the ER lumen and, ultimately, the plasma membrane. Amino-terminal signal sequences also direct proteins to the mitochondria or peroxisomes, explaining why a mutation affecting the signal sequence could cause reroute a peroxisomal protein to the ER (answers a-d thus incorrect).

An important and practical result of genetic engineering is the use of recombinant DNA techniques to produce mRNAs that yield chimeric proteins (ie, composites of peptides). When DNA encoding an amino-terminal signal sequence is inserted upstream of the α-globin gene, the usual cytosolic α-globin becomes a secretory protein and is translocated into the lumen of endoplasmic reticulum. The signal sequence thus contains all the information needed to direct the translocation of protein across endoplasmic reticulum. Biologically important proteins like insulin or growth hormone can thus be engineered for secretion and manufactured in cell culture. Gene therapies that appropriately target and express replacement or repositioned proteins are not yet practical, but enzyme therapies for disorders like Hunter syndrome (MIM*309900) use natural mannose-6-phosphate signals to target infused enzyme from blood to intracellular lysosomes.

60. The answer is c. *(Murray, pp 359-368. Scriver, pp 3-45. Lewis, pp 188-194.)* ATP is required for the esterification of amino acids to their corresponding tRNAs. This reaction is catalyzed by the class of enzymes known as aminoacyl-tRNA synthetases. Each one of these enzymes is specific for one tRNA and its corresponding amino acid:

$$\text{amino acid} + \text{tRNA} + \text{ATP} \rightarrow \text{aminoacyl-tRNA} + \text{AMP} + \text{PP}_i$$

As with most ATP hydrolysis reactions that release pyrophosphate, pyrophosphatase quickly hydrolyzes the product to Pi, which makes the reaction essentially irreversible. Since ATP is hydrolyzed to AMP and PPi during the reaction, the equivalent of two high-energy phosphate bonds is utilized.

61. The answer is b. (*Murray, pp 359-368. Scriver, pp 3-45. Lewis, pp 188-194.*) During the course of protein synthesis on a ribosome, peptidyl transferase catalyzes the formation of peptide bonds. However, when a stop codon such as UAA, UGA, or UAG is reached, aminoacyl-tRNA does not bind to the A site of a ribosome. One of the proteins, known as a release factor, binds to the specific trinucleotide sequence present. This binding of the release factor activates peptidyl transferase to hydrolyze the bond between the polypeptide and the tRNA occupying the P site. Thus, instead of forming a peptide bond, peptidyl transferase catalyzes the hydrolytic step that leads to the release of newly synthesized proteins. Following release of the polypeptide, the ribosome dissociates into its major subunits.

62. The answer is e. (*Murray, pp 336-346. Scriver, pp 3-45. Lewis, pp 188-194.*) The template strand refers to the DNA strand that is transcribed into RNA. As for DNA, RNA is synthesized in the 5′ to 3′ direction, so the template strand shown in the question should be rewritten in the 3′ to 5′ direction (eg, 3′-CAGTGA . . ., giving a 5′ to 3′ RNA transcript of 5′-GUCACU . . ., correct answer e). The DNA complementary to the template strand is known as the coding strand and will have the same sequence as the RNA transcript, except that U replaces T in RNA. This coding strand sequence is used for DNA sequence databases so potential genes can be identified by coding sequences that would yield stretches of amino acids and thus encode proteins. Incorrect answers b and d show DNA sequences without U, while incorrect answers a and c have the wrong sequence orientation.

63. The answer is d. (*Murray, pp 359-368. Scriver, pp 3-45. Lewis, pp 188-194.*) The two subunits of ribosomes are composed of proteins and rRNA. Ribosomes are found in the cytoplasm, in mitochondria, and bound to the endoplasmic reticulum. Transcription refers to the synthesis of RNA complementary to a DNA template and has nothing immediately to do with ribosomes.

64. The answer is c. (*Murray, pp 359-368. Scriver, pp 3-45. Lewis, pp 188-194.*) Two molecules of GTP are used in the formation of each peptide bond on the ribosome. In the elongation cycle, binding of aminoacyl-tRNA delivered by EF-2 to the A site requires hydrolysis of one GTP. Peptide bond formation then occurs. Translocation of the nascent peptide chain on tRNA to the P site requires hydrolysis of a second GTP. The activation of amino acids with aminoacyl-tRNA synthetase requires hydrolysis of ATP to AMP plus PPi.

65. The answer is a. (*Murray, pp 359-368. Scriver, pp 3-45. Lewis, pp 188-194.*) Virulent strains of bacteria such as *Mycoplasma pneumoniae*, various *Legionella* species, and *Bordetella pertussis* that cause severe, life-threatening respiratory tract infections can often be successfully treated with erythromycin. The mechanism of action of erythromycin is to specifically bind the 50S subunit of bacterial ribosomes (answers b-e incorrect). Under normal conditions, after mRNA attaches to the initiation site of the 30S subunit, the 50S subunit binds to the 30S complex and forms the 70S complex that allows protein chain elongation to go forward. Elongation is prevented in the presence of erythromycin.

66. The answer is d. (*Murray, pp 359-368. Scriver, pp 3-45. Lewis, pp 188-194.*) The gene that produces the deadly toxin of *Corynebacterium diphtheriae* comes from a lysogenic phage that grows in the bacteria. Prior to immunization, diphtheria was a frequent cause of death in children. The protein toxin produced by this bacterium inhibits protein synthesis by ADP-ribosylation of elongation factor 2 (EF-2 or translocase). Diphtheria toxin is a single protein composed of two portions (A and B). The B portion enables the A portion to translocate across a cell membrane into the cytoplasm. The A portion catalyzes the transfer of the adenosine diphosphate ribose unit of NAD1 to a nitrogen atom of the diphthamide ring of EF-2, thereby blocking translocation. Diphthamide is an unusual amino acid residue of EF-2.

67. The answer is a. (*Murray, pp 359-368. Scriver, pp 3-45. Lewis, pp 188-194.*) Aminoacyl-tRNA synthetases are responsible for charging a tRNA with the appropriate amino acid for translation. Charging a tRNA is a two-step reaction. In the first step, the enzyme forms an aminoacyl-AMP enzyme complex in a reaction that requires one ATP. In the second step, the activated amino acid is attached to the appropriate tRNA and the enzyme and AMP are released.

68. The answer is d. (*Murray, pp 359-368. Scriver, pp 3-45. Lewis, pp 188-194.*) Prokaryotic ribosomes have a sedimentation coefficient of 70S and are composed of 50S and 30S subunits (odd numbers). Eukaryotic cytoplasmic ribosomes, either free or bound to the endoplasmic reticulum, are larger—60S and 40S subunits that associate to an 80S ribosome (even numbers). Nuclear ribosomes are attached to the endoplasmic reticulum of the nuclear membrane. Ribosomes in chloroplasts and mitochondria of eucaryotic cells are more similar to prokaryotic ribosomes than to eukaryotic cytosolic ribosomes. Like bacterial ribosomes, chloroplast and mitochondrial ribosomes use a formylated tRNA and are sensitive to bacterial protein synthesis inhibitors. Antibiotics that target bacterial protein synthesis may interfere with human mitochondrial function at high doses.

69. The answer is b. (*Murray, pp 359-368. Lewis, pp 188-194. Scriver, pp 1471-1488.*) The initiation of protein synthesis is a multistep process that includes several protein factors—eIF-4E and eIF-4G proteins that bind the mRNA cap, eIF-4A and eIF-4B proteins that bind to the 5′ end of mRNA and reduce its secondary structure. The eIF-3 proteins bind to the prior factors, linking them to the 40S ribosomal subunit and scanning for suitable AUG codons that will initiate peptide bond formation. This is usually the 5′-most AUG, but others may be selected by virtue of Kozak consensus sequences that surround it (GCC-AUG-UGG). Other protein factors regulate the rate of protein synthesis initiation by acting on eIF-4E, including those such as BP1 that bind and inactivate eIF-4E unless it is phosphorylated. Insulin and other growth factors act to phosphorylate BP-1 at several sites, releasing eIF-4E and stimulating initiation and protein synthesis. Though stimulation of protein synthesis by insulin is one plausible factor in increased fetal growth, other factors undoubtedly contribute to this complex process.

Once the EF factors, 40S subunit, and relaxed mRNA are associated (as a 43S preinitiation complex), it binds the 60S ribosomal subunit and its peptidyl transferase that is a component of the 28S rRNA—an example of a ribozyme. In translation, the P site of the ribosome is occupied by the peptidyl-tRNA, which has the growing peptide chain attached. The appropriate aminoacyl-tRNA enters the A site and the carboxyl group of the peptidyl tRNA undergoes nucleophilic attack by the α-amino group of the aminoacyl-tRNA, as catalyzed by peptidyl transferase. The peptide chain is transferred to the tRNA in the A site, which is subsequently displaced to the P site, freeing the A site to bind the next charged tRNA.

70. The answer is b. (*Murray, pp 336-346. Scriver, pp 3-45. Lewis, pp 188-194.*) Eukaryotic promoters are much more complex than bacterial promoters. The most common bacterial promoter elements are the −10 and −35 sequences, which are the recognition sites for RNA polymerase binding. In addition, bacterial promoters may have operators (repressor binding sites) and activator binding sites. Eukaryotic promoters have a core region that may contain a TATA box (which is bound by TBP, the TATA binding protein), an initiator sequence, and downstream promoter elements. Many promoters lack one or more of these elements. In addition, eukaryotic promoters have upstream elements such as GC boxes and CCAAT boxes that bind specific transcription factors (Sp1 and CTF, respectively). Enhancers are elements that increase or enhance the rate of transcription initiation from a promoter. Enhancers can be upstream or downstream of the transcription start site and can exert their effect from hundreds or thousands of bases away. In addition, enhancers are orientation-independent (ie, whether their recognition sequence is on the Watson or Crick strand).

71. The answer is e. (*Murray, pp 359-368. Scriver, pp 3-45. Lewis, pp 403-410.*) Signal recognition particles (SRPs) recognize the signal sequence on the N-terminal end of proteins destined for the lumen of the endoplasmic reticulum (ER). SRP binding arrests translation and an SRP receptor facilitates import of the nascent protein into the ER lumen. A signal peptidase removes the signal sequence from the protein, which may remain in the membrane or be routed for secretion. Common to both eukaryotic and prokaryotic protein synthesis is the requirement for ATP to activate amino acids. The activated aminoacyl-tRNAs then interact with ribosomes carrying mRNA. Peptidyl transferase catalyzes the formation of peptide bonds between the free amino group of activated aminoacyl-tRNA on the A site of the ribosome and the esterified carboxyl group of the peptidyl-rRNA on the P site; the liberated rRNA remains on the P site.

72. The answer is a. (*Murray, pp 359-368, 498-513. Scriver, pp 5559-5628. Lewis, pp 403-410.*) The decreased amount of AAT protein, its abnormal mobility, and the engorgement of liver ER suggest a mutant AAT that is inefficiently transported from the ER to plasma. Since other plasma protein abnormalities were not mentioned, general deficiencies of protein synthesis arising from defective energy metabolism or defective signal recognition particles are unlikely. A mutation affecting the N-terminal methionine of AAT or its signal sequence should drastically decrease its synthesis and import to the ER lumen. This would not explain the engorgement of liver ER. The usual binding of the signal recognition particle to the signal sequence of AAT, followed by import into the ER lumen, seems intact. An altered amino acid necessary for signal peptidase cleavage of the signal sequence of AAT might be invoked, but a general deficiency of the signal peptidase should disrupt many secreted proteins and be an embryonic lethal mutation. AAT deficiency (MIM*107400) is a well-characterized autosomal dominant disease with common ZZ, SZ, and SS genotypes that can cause childhood liver disease and adult emphysema. The Z and S mutations alter AAT conformation and interfere with its secretion from ER to plasma. Lack of AAT protection from proteases in lung is thought to cause the thinning of alveolar walls and dysfunctional "air sacs" of emphysema.

73. The answer is e. (*Murray, pp 359-368. Scriver, pp 175-192. Lewis, pp 403-410.*) For autosomal recessive disorders, only one of the two defective alleles must be replaced or supplemented to allow normal enzyme function (incorrect answers b, c). Somatic gene therapy to correct stem cells such as bone marrow would provide a continuous source of ADA enzyme and curative therapy; germ-line therapy would target his spermatogonia and thus future offspring (incorrect answers a, b, c).

Gene therapy refers to a group of techniques by which gene structure or expression is altered to ameliorate a disease. Because of ethical and practical difficulties, germ-line therapy involving alterations of genes in primordial germ cells is not being explored in humans. Although germ-line genetic engineering is being performed in animals with the goals of improved breeding or agricultural yield, it alters the characteristics of offspring rather than the treated individuals. Somatic cell gene therapy is targeted to an affected tissue or group of tissues in the individual and is most effective if stem cells such as bone marrow can be treated. Somatic cell gene therapy offers the hope of replacing damaged tissue without the rejection problems of transplantation. For autosomal recessive disorders, only one of the two defective alleles must be replaced or supplemented.

74. The answer is a. (*Murray, pp 388-405. Scriver, pp 175-192. Lewis, pp 403-410.*) Challenges for gene therapy include the construction of recombinant viral genomes that can propagate the replacement gene (gene constructs or vectors), delivery of the altered gene to the appropriate tissues (gene targeting), and recombination at the appropriate locus so that replacement of the defective gene is achieved (site-specific recombination). The latter step positions DNA sequences in the vector so that the replacement gene pairs and recombines precisely with homologous DNA in the native gene. Ex vivo transfection (introduction of vector DNA into patient cells outside the body) is an ideal method for gene targeting if the engineered cells can repopulate the tissue/organ in question. Transfection of bone marrow stem cells with a functional adenosine deaminase gene, followed by bone marrow transplantation back to the patient, has been successful in restoring immunity to children with severe deficiency. Even when tissue targeting and precise gene replacement are feasible, mimicking the appropriate patterns of gene expression can be a substantial barrier to gene therapy. Injection of deficient enzymes into plasma (enzyme therapy) has been successful in disorders such as non-neurologic Gaucher disease (MIM*231000)— storage of lipids in the spleen and bone—and takes advantage of cellular pathways that target enzymes to lysosomes.

75. The answer is c. (*Murray, pp 388-405. Scriver, pp 175-192. Lewis, pp 219-232.*) After the locus responsible for a genetic disease is mapped to a particular chromosome region, "candidate" genes can be examined for molecular abnormalities in affected individuals. The connective tissue abnormalities in Stickler syndrome (MIM*108300) make the COL2A1 collagen locus an attractive candidate for disease mutations, prompting analysis of COL2A1 gene structure and expression. Western blotting detects gene alterations that interfere with protein expression, while use of the reverse transcriptase-polymerase chain reaction (RT-PCR) detects alterations in mRNA levels. Each analysis should detect one-half the respective amounts of COL2A1 protein or mRNA in the case of a promoter mutation that abolishes transcription of one COL2A1 allele. Southern blotting detects nucleotide changes that alter DNA restriction sites, but this is relatively insensitive unless large portions of the gene are deleted.

Fluorescent in situ hybridization (FISH) analysis using DNA probes from the COL2A1 locus is a sensitive method for detecting deletions of the entire locus, and DNA sequencing of the entire gene provides the gold standard for detecting any alteration in the regulatory or coding sequences. Nucleotide sequence changes are still subject to interpretation, since they may represent polymorphisms that do not alter gene function. Population studies and/or in vitro studies of gene expression are often needed to discriminate DNA polymorphisms from mutations that disrupt gene function. For any autosomal locus, the interpretation of molecular analyses is complicated by the presence of two homologous copies of the gene.

76. The answer is e. (*Murray, pp 353-359. Scriver, pp 1857-1896. Lewis, pp 188-194.*) Missense mutations, which cause the substitution of one amino acid for another, may significantly alter the function of the resultant protein without altering the size of DNA restriction fragments detected by Southern blotting. In this case, Northern blot results would most likely also be normal. Single-base changes may also result in nonsense mutations. Large insertions or deletions in the exon or coding regions of the gene alter the Southern blot pattern and usually ablate the activity of one gene copy. In the case of an autosomal locus like that for ornithine aminotransferase, the homologous allele remains active and gives 50% enzyme activity (heterozygote or carrier range with a normal phenotype). Similar effects on enzyme activity would be predicted from complete gene deletions at one locus, while duplication might produce 150% or 50% of normal enzyme activity depending on the status of promoter sites.

77. The answer is b. (*Murray, pp 359-368. Scriver, pp 4517-4554. Lewis, pp 215-218.*) Red cell hemolysis after drug exposure suggests a red cell enzyme defect, most easily confirmed by enzyme assay to demonstrate deficient activity. A likely diagnosis here is glucose-6-phosphate dehydrogenase (G6PD) deficiency (MIM*305900), probably the most common genetic disease (it affects 400 million people worldwide). Tropical African and Mediterranean peoples exhibit the highest prevalence because the disease, like sickle cell trait, confers resistance to malaria. DNA analysis is available to demonstrate particular alleles, but simple enzyme assay is sufficient for diagnosis. More than 400 types of abnormal G6PD alleles have been described, meaning that most affected individuals are compound heterozygotes. The phenotype of jaundice and red blood cell hemolysis with anemia is triggered by a variety of infections and drugs, including a dietary substance in fava beans. Sulfonamide and related antibiotics as well as anti-malarial drugs are notorious for inducing hemolysis in G6PD-deficient individuals. G6PD deficiency exhibits X-linked recessive inheritance, explaining why male offspring but not the parents become ill when exposed to antimalarials.

78. The answer is b. (*Murray, pp 388-405. Scriver, pp 3421-3452. Lewis, pp 403-410.*) All of the modes of therapy are theoretically possible, and enzyme therapy (ie, injection of purified enzyme) has been successful in several lysosomal deficiencies, particularly those in which the central nervous system is not affected (ie, non-neurologic Gaucher disease [MIM*231000]). Unfortunately, antibodies frequently develop to the injected enzyme and limit the term of successful enzyme delivery. Heterol-ogous bone marrow transplant, preferably from a related donor, offers the most realistic and effective therapy since the graft provides a permanent source of enzyme. Bone marrow transplants do have a 10% mortality, how-ever, and the enzyme diffuses poorly into the central nervous system. Somatic gene therapy (ie, delivery of enzyme to somatic cells via viral vec-tors or transfected tissue) is now possible; however, targeting of the gene product to appropriate tissues and organelles is still a problem. Transfected autologous bone marrow transplant (ie, marrow from the patient) has been used in a few cases of adenosine deaminase deficiency, an immune disorder affecting lymphocytes. Germ-line gene therapy requires the insertion of functional genes into gametes or blastomeres of early embryos prior to birth. The potential for embryonic damage, lack of knowledge regarding developmental gene control, and ethical controversies regarding selective breeding or embryo experimentation make germ-line therapy unrealistic at present.

79. The answer is e. (*Murray, pp 359-368. Scriver, pp 3-45. Lewis, pp 127-128.*) Because chromosomes are large chains of DNA comprising several thousand genes (links of chain), even small deletions will remove tens to hundreds of genes. Deletions involving the autosomes (chromosomes 1-22) will reduce genes within the deletion from diploid to haploid dosage, decreasing the amount of mRNA produced from these genes (answer e). The other answers concern changes in epigenesis—histone acetylation, DNA methylation, small RNA decoration—or a change in gene sequence that may not occur if the deletion cuts between genes. Changes in epigenesis undoubtedly occur with chromosome rearrangements (eg, translocations, duplicated segments, interstitial deletions between chromosome ends) that make new links between noncontiguous chromosome segments. Epigenetic changes likely contribute to the diverse phenotypic effects of trisomies, where an extra dose of normal chromosomal DNA sequence is added to cells (eg, trisomy 21 causing Down syndrome).

80. The answer is c. (*Murray, pp 353-359. Scriver, pp 3635-3643. Lewis, pp 188-194.*) The replacement of the codon UAC with UAA would be a nonsense mutation since UAC encodes tyrosine and UAA is a "stop" signal (see HY Facts Table 4). Missense mutations substitute one amino acid for another, silent mutations do not change the amino acid code, suppressor mutations are rare changes in tRNA that allow normal reading of a stop codon, and frameshift mutations insert or delete a nucleotide so as to change the reading frame (incorrect answers a, b, d, e).

Nonsense or terminating codons in mRNA signal the ribosome to stop translation. Mutation of an internal codon to a termination codon results in a shortened peptide that in the case of enzymes would not function as a catalyst. Homozygous nonsense mutation affecting both glucocerebrosidase alleles would result in no enzyme produced and no ability for the cells to break down stored lipids.

81. The answer is d. (*Murray, pp 353-359. Scriver, pp 3-45. Lewis, pp 188-194.*) The change in the patient's DNA coding strand sequence from TAC to GAC would change AUG to CUG in mRNA, substituting the amino acid leucine for methionine but also changing a likely AUG translation initiation signal since this AUG is near a TATA signal mediating transcription initiation. The mutation would logically affect the conformation of the translated protein and alter its mobility on electrophoresis while also ablating an AUG translation signal and reducing the amount of protein detected on Western blot (correct answer d, incorrect answers a-c and e). Transcription of mRNA should not be affected, also making answers b, c, e that suggest an abnormal signal by Northern blotting incorrect.

Note that RNA is transcribed 5' to 3' from the coding strand of DNA that is 3' to 5'; it is the 5' to 3' complement of this coding strand that is represented in genome databases so the gene sequence can be easily visualized in terms of its product RNA. When researchers examine a cloned DNA sequence for potential coding activity, they must consider reads from both complimentary strands to see if either gives a sensible peptide translation. Sequences encoding RNA can come from either DNA strand, indicating the asymmetry of leading and lagging strand during DNA replication is not preserved for transcription. Another facet of the patient's mutation is its change from T (thymine, a pyrimidine) to G (guanine, a purine). This is a transversion with change in base class rather than a transition that substitutes one purine or pyrimidine for another. Transversions will usually have more severe consequences than transitions, and both will be less severe than frameshift or nonsense mutations that garble or truncate the protein product.

82. The answer is e. (*Murray, pp 346-351. Lewis, pp 188-194. Scriver, pp 2717-2721.*) The *apoB* gene, which encodes apolipoprotein B, is transcribed in the liver normally and the mRNA is translated into a 100-kDa protein (apoB100). In the intestine, however, the apoB mRNA is edited by the enzyme cysteine deaminase, which alters a CAA codon (encoding a glutamine) to UAA (a stop codon). This change results in synthesis of a 48-kDa form of apolipoprotein B (apoB48) that lacks the carboxy-terminal end. The apoB100 and apoB48 proteins serve different functions in the liver and the intestine. A mutation that ablates apoB mRNA editing and its resulting apoB48 protein product in intestine could interfere with lipid absorption and production of VLDL and LDL in plasma. Other answers besides e indicate processes that would affect mRNA transcription, not protein size.

Although RNA editing is not widespread, there are a growing number of other examples. Alternative RNA splicing is a much more common means of generating alternative forms of a protein. In splicing, intron sequences are removed and exon (protein coding) sequences are joined together. Use of alternative splice sites can include or exclude certain exons, resulting in different primary sequence, conformation, and size of a protein. RNA splicing will usually preserve the carboxy-terminal exon since it is needed for mRNA polyadenylation and its transport from nucleus to cytoplasm.

83. The answer is b. (*Murray, pp 353-359. Scriver, pp 2717-2721. Lewis, pp 188-194.*) The structures of glycine and alanine are quite similar, with the —H side group of glycine being replaced with the —CH_3 side group of alanine. Consequently, a mutation causing such a change, particularly near the carboxy-terminus is unlikely to produce a dysfunctional protein. Similarly, the third position of mRNA codons is least crucial for amino acid coding due to "wobble"—similar or identical amino acids are often produced regardless of the third codon nucleotide (see HY Facts Table 4). In contrast, a mutation inserting two bases into DNA and mRNA will change the reading frame of translation, producing a truncated (misread termination codon) or garbled amino acid sequence with apoB dysfunction. Introns are spliced out of RNA and do not encode segments of the protein product unless splicing is defective; intronic mutations should therefore not disrupt protein function unless they affect the splice sites near exon-intron junctions.

84. The answer is b. (*Murray, pp 359-368. Scriver, pp 525-537. Lewis, pp 127-128.*) The undermethylation of IGF2 alleles in sperm as compared to methylated and undermethylated alleles in diploid adult tissues suggests that the gene is imprinted. During germ cell formation, certain chromosome regions are patterned differently or "imprinted" in males versus females, producing different levels of maternal versus paternal allele expression in tissues of the resulting embryos and adults. These imprinting patterns are associated with DNA methylation at key CpG dinucleotide sites, up- or down-regulating allele transcription and expression. Biparental origin of alleles in diploid tissues is thus necessary for normal levels of gene expression, a balance disrupted by uniparental disomy (both copies of a chromosome and its alleles from one parent) or loss of imprinting (LOI) of one allele. Imprinted genes are often growth factors, perhaps arising to regulate embryo-fetal growth but persisting in diploid tissues as potential sources of cell proliferation and tumors. The specific increased IGF2 expression in Wilms tumor suggests it is a potential regulator of cell proliferation rather than rates of mutation. The fact that one allele can increase expression and cause a tumor suggests *IGF2* is an oncogene rather than a tumor suppressor that must have both alleles inactivated to produce a tumor.

85. The answer is b. (*Murray, pp 353-359. Scriver, pp 3-45. Lewis, pp 188-194.*) The following mutations were shown in the DNA changes:

a. Missense (Cys to Leu)
b. Nonsense (Tyr to stop)
c. Missense (Ser to Phe)
d. Harmless (Tyr to Tyr)
e. Missense (Leu to Phe)

Most of the mutations shown result in a missense effect, with a different amino acid being incorporated into the same site in a protein. This may or may not have an effect depending on its location. Some single-base mutations are harmless because of the degeneracy of the genetic code, whereby more than one triplet code exists for all amino acids except tryptophan and methionine. Choice a contains two mutations, one degenerate and the other missense.

DNA coding: 3'-ACGACGACG-5' to 3'-ACAAACACG-5'
mRNA: 5'-UGCUGCUGC-3' to 5'-UGUUUGUGC-3
Protein: Cys-Cys-Cys to Cys-Leu-Cys

Nonsense mutations occur when the reading of the normal termination signal is changed. This can occur by mutation to a stop signal as in choice b, by deletions near a stop codon, or by insertions.

86. The answer is c. (*Murray, pp 359-368. Scriver, pp 525-537. Lewis, pp 127-128.*) Southern analysis using methylation-sensitive or insensitive endonuclease restriction in the first two panels of the figure suggests both p57 alleles in the tumor are methylated. Only the larger fragment is detected in the patient sample when restricted with methylation-sensitive endonuclease (second panel). The accompanying Northern blot shows markedly decreased amounts of p57 mRNA, supporting a connection between p57 allele methylation and silencing of expression. The maternal allele of p57 is undermethylated and expressed in normal tissues, and its loss of imprinting (methylation) is one of the few situations where epigenetic silencing appears to be the sole carcinogenic event.

87. The answer is d. (*Murray, pp 359-368. Scriver, pp 3-45.*) Several operons in *Escherichia coli*, including the lac operon, are subject to catabolite repression. In the presence of glucose, there is decreased manufacture of cyclic AMP (cAMP) by adenylate cyclase. Low glucose levels increase production of cAMP, which binds to the catabolite activator protein (CAP). The cAMP-CAP complex binds to the promoters of several responsive operons at catabolite activator protein (CAP) binding sites, greatly enhancing transcription of operon RNA. This positive control stimulates use of more exotic metabolites when glucose is not available and conserves energy when glucose is plentiful. High levels of glucose lower cAMP levels and direct metabolism toward constitutive glucose pathways such as glycolysis.

88. The answer is c. (*Murray, pp 336-346. Scriver, pp 3-45. Lewis, pp 188-194.*) Certain regulatory elements act on genes on the same chromosome ("cis"), while others can regulate genes on the opposite chromosome ("trans"). The terminology makes analogy to carbon-carbon double bonds, where two modifying groups may both be above or below the bond (cis) or opposite it (trans). Cis regulatory elements like the lac operator and promoter or mammalian enhancers are usually DNA sequences (regulatory sequences) adjoining or within the regulated gene. Transregulatory elements like the lac repressor protein or mammalian transcription factors are usually diffusible proteins (regulatory factors) that can interact with adjoining target genes or with target genes on other chromosomes. Classification of bacterial elements as cis or trans requires mating experiments where portions of a second chromosome are introduced by transduction (with bacteriophage) or conjugation (with other bacteria). The distinction between cis and trans is fundamental for understanding how regulators work.

89. The answer is d. (*Murray, pp 359-368. Scriver, pp 3-45. Lewis, pp 188-194.*) Mammalian regulatory factors are much more diverse than those of bacteria, possessing several types of structural domains. Activators of transcription, such as steroid hormones, may enter the cell and bind to regulatory factors at specific sites called ligand-binding domains; these intracellular "receptors" are analogous to G protein-linked membrane receptors that extend into the extracellular space. Response elements are not regulatory factors but DNA sequences near the transcription site for certain types of genes (eg, steroid-responsive and heat shock-responsive genes). Regulatory factors interact with specific DNA sequences through their DNA-binding domains and with other regulatory factors through transcription-activating domains. Some regulatory factors have antirepressor domains that counteract the inhibitory effects of chromatin proteins (histones and nonhistones).

90. The answer is d. (*Murray, pp 359-368, Scriver, pp 3-45. Lewis, pp 202-213.*) The *POMC* gene provides a mammalian example in which several proteins are derived from the same RNA transcript. Unlike the polycistronic mRNA of the bacterial lactose operon, mammalian cells generate several mRNAs or proteins from the same gene by variable protein processing or by alternative splicing. Variable protein processing preserves the peptide products of some gene regions but degrades those from others. Alternative splicing would often produce proteins composed of different exon combinations with the same terminal exon and carboxy-terminal peptide, but could remove the terminal exon in some proteins and produce different C-terminal peptides. Different transcription factors or enhancers in different brain regions could regulate the total amounts of *POMC* gene transcript but not the types of protein produced. Elongation of protein synthesis involves GTP cleavage but is not differentially regulated in mammalian tissues.

91. The answer is a. (*Murray, pp 359-368. Scriver, pp 4571-4636. Lewis, pp 206-212.*) Imbalance of globin chain synthesis occurs in the thalassemias. Deficiency of α-globin chains (α-thalassemia—MIM*141900) is common in Asian populations and may be associated with abnormal hemoglobins composed of four β-globin chains (hemoglobin H) or (in fetuses and newborns) of four γ-globin chains (hemoglobin Bart). Mutation in a transcription factor necessary for expression of α-globin could ablate α-globin expression, since the same factor could act in trans on all four copies of the α-globin genes (two α-globin loci). Mutation of a regulatory sequence element that acts in cis would inactivate only one α-globin gene, leaving others to produce α-globin in reduced amounts (mild α-thalassemia). Deletions of one α-globin would produce a similar mild phenotype, and deficiencies of transcription factors regulating α- and β-globin genes would not produce chain imbalance.

92. The answer is d. (*Murray, pp 353-359. Scriver, pp 4571-4636. Lewis, pp 206-212.*) Missense mutations are those in which a single-base change (point mutation) results in a codon that encodes for a different amino acid residue. The effects of these types of mutations can range from very minor or even undetectable to major, depending on the importance of the altered residue to protein folding and function. Nonsense mutations are also point mutations in which the affected codon is altered to a stop (nonsense) codon, resulting in a truncated protein. Frameshift mutations are due to one or two base pair insertions or deletions such that the reading frame is altered. These mutations generally lead to truncated proteins as well, since in most protein coding regions the unused reading frames contain numerous stop codons.

93. The answer is b. (*Murray, pp 336-346. Scriver, pp 3-45. Lewis, pp 188-194.*) The boys have an X-linked recessive condition called α-thalassemia/

mental retardation or ATR-X syndrome (MIM*301040). The X-encoded gene has an unknown function in the brain as well as being a factor that regulates α-globin gene transcription. In order to affect all four α-globin genes, the X-encoded gene must produce a transacting factor; second mutations altering enhancers or promoters would be cis-acting and affect only one α-globin gene. Pseudogenes are functionless gene copies, so altered expression would not influence α-globin chain synthesis.

94. The answer is c. (*Murray, pp 566-582. Scriver, pp 645-664. Lewis, pp 333-354.*) This case is an example of Burkitt lymphoma, which may affect the tonsils or other lymphoid tissues. The translocation places the *myc* oncogene on chromosome 8 downstream of the very active heavy-chain locus on chromosome 14, activating *myc* gene expression in B-cells and their derivatives. The translocation is likely an aberrant form of the normal DNA rearrangements that generate unique heavy-chain genes in each B-cell. The translocation joins one chromosome 8 to one chromosome 14, leaving their homologues unaffected. The cause for the phenotype must therefore be transacting, since cis-acting effects would pertain only to the translocated loci and not affect the homologous untranslocated loci. Activation of a tumor-promoting gene (oncogene) on chromosome 8 could produce an enlarged tonsil, while underactivity of immunoglobulin production due to one-half expression could decrease immune function but would not completely ablate the processes in choices a, b, d, and e. At the genetic level, transacting events are autosomal dominant in that one of the two homologous loci is abnormal and produces a phenotype. Mutations of cis-acting events must disrupt both homologous loci to produce phenotypes, making them autosomal recessive at the genetic level.

Acid-Base Equilibria, Amino Acids, and Protein Structure

Questions

95. A 2-day-old African American boy becomes lethargic and uninterested in breast-feeding. Physical examination reveals hypotonia (low muscle tone), muscle twitching that suggests seizures, and tachypnea (rapid breathing). The child has a normal heartbeat and breath sounds with no indication of cardiorespiratory disease. Initial blood chemistry values include normal glucose, sodium, potassium, chloride, and bicarbonate (HCO_3^-) levels; initial blood gas values reveal a pH of 7.53, partial pressure of oxygen (PCO_2) normal at 103 mm Hg, and partial pressure of carbon dioxide (PCO_2) decreased at 27 mm Hg. Which of the following treatment strategies is most appropriate?

a. Administer alkali to treat metabolic acidosis.
b. Administer alkali to treat respiratory acidosis.
c. Decrease the respiratory rate to treat metabolic acidosis.
d. Decrease the respiratory rate to treat respiratory alkalosis.
e. Administer acid to treat metabolic alkalosis.

96. A 2-day-old Caucasian boy develops tachypnea and cyanosis with a blood pH of 7.1. A serum bicarbonate (HCO_3^-) is measured as 12 mM, but the partial pressures of oxygen (PO_2) and carbon dioxide (PCO_2) are not yet available. Recall the pK_a of 6.1 for carbonic acid (reflecting the HCO_3^-/CO_2 equilibrium in blood) and the fact that the blood CO_2 concentration is equal to the PCO_2 in mm Hg (normal value = 40 mm Hg) multiplied by 0.03. Which of the following treatment strategies is most appropriate?

a. Administer oxygen to improve tissue perfusion and decrease metabolic acidosis.
b. Administer oxygen to decrease respiratory acidosis.
c. Increase the respiratory rate to treat respiratory acidosis.
d. Decrease the respiratory rate to treat respiratory acidosis.
e. Administer medicines to decrease renal hydrogen ion excretion.

97. A 72-year-old African American male with diabetes mellitus (MIM*222100) is evaluated in the emergency room because of lethargy, disorientation, and long, deep breaths (Kussmaul respirations) that often compensate for acidosis. Initial chemistries on venous blood demonstrate high glucose at 380 mg/dL (normal up to 120) and a pH of 7.3. Recalling the normal bicarbonate (22-28 mM) and PCO_2 (33-45 mm Hg) values, which of the following additional test results is consistent with the man's pH and breathing pattern?

a. A bicarbonate of 5 mM and PCO_2 of 10 mm Hg
b. A bicarbonate of 15 mM and PCO_2 of 30 mm Hg
c. A bicarbonate of 15 mM and PCO_2 of 40 mm Hg
d. A bicarbonate of 20 mM and PCO_2 of 45 mm Hg
e. A bicarbonate of 25 mM and PCO_2 of 50 mm Hg

98. A 1-year-old Caucasian girl has had frequent wet diapers and seems to always want her bottle or cup. Her pediatrician is concerned about her growth at her 1-year well visit and notes that she had two prior hospitalizations for dehydration. The pediatrician suspects nephrogenic diabetes insipidus (MIM*125800) and orders serum electrolytes that show concentrations of sodium at 155 mEq/L (normal 133-146) and chloride at 123 (normal 98-107). Urinalysis shows a very dilute urine. Further testing involves a gene named aquaporin-2 that has several transmembrane domains demarcated by β turns. Which of the following β-turn amino acids are most likely to be mutated in patients with nephrogenic diabetes insipidus?

a. Arginine and lysine
b. Aspartic acid and glutamic acid
c. Leucine and valine
d. Glycine and proline
e. Tryptophan and tyrosine

99. A 14-year-old Hispanic adolescent presents with acute abdominal pain and is noted to have mildly yellow whites of the eyes (scleral icterus). Blood counts indicate a low hemoglobin concentration and the blood smear shows sphere-shaped instead of biconcave red blood cells. The girl's mother reports that she, her father, and several other relatives have anemia, and that they have been diagnosed with a form of spherocytosis (MIM*182900) that is caused by mutations in the ankyrin structural protein of erythrocytes. The student on the case is asked to prepare discussion of clinical-molecular correlation on morning rounds, and downloads a diagram of ankyrin structure and amino acid sequence. The structure has domains of antiparallel α-helices, which facilitate stacking of ankyrins into ordered arrays. As the student attempts correlation of ankyrin sequence and structure, α-helical domains could be best identified by the absence of which of the following amino acids?

a. Alanine
b. Cysteine
c. Histidine
d. Proline
e. Glycine

100. A 1-year-old Caucasian girl presents to a pediatrician after being removed from her parents because of severe neglect. The pediatrician notes the child is undersized with sparse hair, boggy subcutaneous tissue, and a hopeless, depressed look. Marasmus is suspected, and supported with laboratory studies that include a low serum protein concentration. The pediatrician institutes a gradual regimen of increased calories and nutrition, gradual because rapid feeding will produce diarrhea and further protein loss. This is because long-term starvation leads to low protein concentrations, reduced osmotic pressure, and acidosis in the tissues, producing the extra tissue fluid (edema) and catabolic state of marasmus. Marasmus and related starvation conditions (like the swollen abdomen and reddish hair of kwashiorkor) demonstrate the importance of proteins in maintaining tissue hydration and pH. The greatest buffering capacity at physiologic pH would be provided by a protein rich in which of the following amino acids?

a. Lysine
b. Histidine
c. Aspartic acid
d. Valine
e. Leucine

101. A 1-year-old Caucasian boy presents with several fractures, and a protective services investigation ensues. Laboratory evaluation shows mild anemia, a serum pH of 7.2, and a urine pH that is anomalously high at 8.5. Review of the radiographs shows some increased bone density of the skull and limbs, and the diagnosis is changed from battered child to a form of osteopetrosis (MIM*259730). This condition is caused by a nonfunctional mutation in the gene for one form of carbonic anhydrase, the enzyme catalyzing reversible hydration of carbon dioxide $CO_2 + H_2O \leftrightarrows H_2CO_2 \leftrightarrows H^+ + HCO_3^-$. The discrepant blood and urine pH values in the patient are best explained by which of the following?

a. Decreased renal carbonic anhydrase with increased conversion and excretion of bicarbonate in urine
b. Increased renal carbonic anhydrase with reduced conversion and excretion of bicarbonate into urine
c. Decreased renal carbonic anhydrase with reduced formation and excretion of hydrogen ion into urine
d. Decreased renal carbonic anhydrase with increased formation and excretion of hydrogen ion into urine
e. Increased renal carbonic anhydrase with reduced formation and excretion of hydrogen ion into urine

102. A 2-year-old African American girl has been healthy until she developed a severe gastroenteritis with progressive sleepiness and fatigue. On presentation to her pediatrician, she has obvious signs of dehydration with no tears on crying, dry mucous membranes, tenting of her skin (retention of a skin fold when pinched), and lack of urination. Her respiratory rate is normal and her lips pink, suggestive of good aeration. Initial laboratory values indicate a low glucose with normal electrolyte values in mEq/L (sodium 140, potassium 4.5, chloride 110) except for bicarbonate (8, normal 20-28) and pH (7.1). She does not have glucose or ketones in her urine by color tests. The clinical scenario and electrolyte values are most consistent with which of the following?

a. A first episode of diabetes mellitus
b. Respiratory acidosis due to lethargy and poor breathing
c. Respiratory acidosis suggestive of a toxic ingestion
d. Metabolic acidosis with increased anion gap suggesting buildup of a negatively charged metabolite
e. Metabolic acidosis without increased anion gap suggesting high ammonium ion

103. A newborn African American girl is resuscitated during delivery and found to have a very small chest with deformed ribs, multiple rib and shoulder girdle fractures occurring during delivery, short limbs, and bluish-gray sclerae (whites of the eyes). A diagnosis of severe osteogenesis imperfecta (MIM*166210) is made and the parents are counseled regarding a lethal disease best managed with palliative care. A skin biopsy is taken before death so that the responsible type I collagen chains can be examined for amino acid changes. Which of the following shows the repeating 3-amino acid motif most compatible with collagen triple helix formation and the mutation most likely to cause severe osteogenesis imperfecta?

a. Pro-X-Y mutated to Gly-X-Y in one repeat
b. Ala-X-Y mutated to Leu-X-Y in one repeat
c. Ala-X-Y mutated to Gly-X-Y in one repeat
d. Gly-X-Y mutated to Ala-X-Y in one repeat
e. Gly-X-Y mutated to Pro-X-Y in one repeat

104. A firstborn Caucasian male infant does well in the nursery but seems to have a reaction to cereal introduced at age 6 weeks. The infant begins vomiting severely, often spewing vomitus across the crib (projectile vomiting). Concern about food allergy persists until an experienced surgeon sits with her hand over the infant's stomach for 20 minutes at the bedside, feeling a small oval shape that has been described as an olive. The surgeon obtains electrolytes and blood gases preparatory to anesthesia. Which of the combinations of laboratory results below and their interpretations are most likely for this infant?

a. ↓ P_{CO_2}, normal bicarbonate, normal chloride, ↑ pH—pure respiratory alkalosis
b. ↓ Low P_{CO_2}, ↓ low bicarbonate, ↓ low pH, ↓ low chloride—compensated metabolic acidosis
c. Normal P_{CO_2}, ↓ low bicarbonate, ↓ low pH, normal chloride—pure metabolic acidosis
d. ↑ High P_{CO_2}, normal bicarbonate, low pH, normal chloride—pure respiratory acidosis
e. Normal P_{CO_2}, high bicarbonate, ↑ high pH, ↓ low chloride—pure metabolic alkalosis

105. A 1-year-old Caucasian girl presents with growth failure and mild elevation of blood urea nitrogen and creatinine (suggesting decreased kidney function). No hormonal or dietary causes of her growth failure are found, and her mother informs her pediatrician that the child seems to avoid light. Referral to an ophthalmologist reveals unusual crystals in her cornea. Measurement of her blood amino acids reveals an unusual peak, which on analysis breaks down into an amino acid with a sulfhydryl group. The derived amino acid furthermore seems to have an ionizable side group with a pK of about 8.3. Which of the following is the most likely amino acid?

a. Lysine
b. Methionine
c. Cysteine
d. Arginine
e. Glutamine

106. A 60-year-old Caucasian male is brought to his physician from an institution for severe mental deficiency. The physician reviews his family history and finds he has an older sister in the same institution. Their parents are deceased but reportedly had normal intelligence and no chronic diseases. The man sits in an odd position as though he was sewing, prompting the physician to obtain a ferric chloride test on the man's urine. This test turns color with aromatic (ring) compounds, including certain amino acids, and a green color confirms the physician's diagnosis. Which of the following amino acids was most likely detected in the man's urine?

a. Glycine
b. Serine
c. Glutamine
d. Phenylalanine
e. Methionine

107. A 2-year-old Caucasian boy is admitted for failure to gain weight. His hair has turned reddish brown and his extremities are swollen with extra subcutaneous fluid water (edema). Initial studies show a serum albumin of 1.5 g/dL (normal for age 3.3-5.8) and total protein 2.7 g/dL (normal for age 5.3-8.1). Which of the following statements best explains the reason for the child's edema?

a. Water forms strong covalent bonds with sodium salts
b. Proteins form hydrogen bonds with water and exert osmotic pressure to retain intravascular volume.
c. Surface valine and isoleucine on proteins bind water and exert osmotic pressure.
d. Surface glutamic and aspartic acid on proteins form hydrogen bonds with water and become impermeable to capillary walls.
e. Surface hydroxyl groups due to protein serines and threonines form aggregates through hydrogen bonding with water and cannot pass capillary membranes.

108. A 25-year-old African American female displays decreased appetite, increased urinary frequency, and thirst. Her physician suspects new-onset diabetes mellitus (MIM*222100) and confirms that she has elevated urine glucose and ketones. Which of the following blood values is most compatible with diabetic ketoacidosis?

	pH	Bicarbonate (mM)	Arterial P_{CO_2}
a.	7.05	16.0	52
b.	7.25	20.0	41
c.	7.40	24.5	39
d.	7.66	37.0	30
e.	7.33	12.0	21

109. A 2-year-old Caucasian girl presents with severe vomiting, dehydration, and fever. Initial blood studies show acidosis with a low bicarbonate and an anion gap (the sum of sodium plus potassium minus chloride plus bicarbonate is 40 and larger than the normal 12 ± 2). Preliminary results from the blood amino acid screen show two elevated amino acids, both with nonpolar side chains. A titration curve performed on one of the elevated species shows two ionizable groups with approximate pKs of 2 and 9.5. Which of the following pairs of elevated amino acids is most likely elevated?

a. Aspartic acid and glutamine
b. Glutamic acid and threonine
c. Histidine and valine
d. Leucine and isoleucine
e. Glutamine and isoleucine

110. A 12-month-old girl presents for evaluation of extreme irritability without fever. She came to Texas shortly after birth as a Somalian refugee, and seemed to feed and grow well with a slight falloff in weight recently. Physical examination reveals a slightly enlarged liver, a palpable spleen, and tenderness over her extremities. A peripheral smear shows sickle-shaped red blood cells and subsequent studies confirm a diagnosis of sickle cell anemia (MIM*603903). When told this is a genetic disorder, the parents are skeptical because she had been so healthy early in life. Which of the following explanations concerning hemoglobin chain structure best explains her lack of symptoms the first few months after birth?

a. The $(\alpha_1-\alpha_2)(\beta_1-\beta_2)$ subunit structure shifts to $(\alpha_1-\beta_1)-(\alpha_2-\beta_2)$ at puberty.
b. The $\alpha_1-\alpha_2-\alpha_3-\alpha_4$ subunit structure switches to $(\alpha_1-\beta_1)-(\alpha_2-\beta_2)$ during pregnancy.
c. $\beta-\beta-\beta-\alpha$ Subunit structure switches to $(\alpha_1-\beta_1)-(\alpha_2-\beta_2)$ during infancy.
d. The $(\beta_1-\beta_2-\beta_3-\alpha_1)$ subunit structure switches to $(\alpha_1-\beta_1)-(\alpha_2-\beta_2)$ during pregnancy.
e. The $(\alpha_1-\gamma_1)-(\alpha_2-\gamma_2)$ subunit structure switches to $(\alpha_1-\beta_1)-(\alpha_2-\beta_2)$ at 2 to 6 months.

111. A 2-year-old Hispanic boy presents with frequent sinus and ear infections, including one, which progressed to staphylococcal bacteria in the blood (bacteremia) and bone infection (osteomyelitis). Family history indicated that his mother had a brother who died young of sepsis and that her mother had two brothers who died young. Suspicion of an X-linked immunoglobulin deficiency led to assay for a phosphokinase that is known to be deficient in Bruton X-linked agammaglobulinemia (MIM*300300). Which of the following amino acids could be used as an acceptor for the phosphate group in the Bruton kinase assay?

a. Cysteine
b. Leucine
c. Methionine
d. Tyrosine
e. Tryptophan

112. Blood is drawn from a 21-year-old African American female with severe anemia and the globin protein is degraded for peptide and amino acid analysis. Of the results below, which change in globin primary structure is most likely to correlate with the clinical phenotype of anemia?

a. Ile-Leu-Val to Ile-Ile-Val
b. Leu-Glu-Ile to Leu-Val-Ile
c. Gly-Ile-Gly to Gly-Val-Gly
d. Gly-Asp-Gly to Gly-Glu-Gly
e. Val-Val-Val to Val-Leu-Val

113. A 35-year-old female with heavy menstrual periods (metrorrhagia) has anemia but does not respond to iron supplementation. Blood is drawn and the red cell hemoglobin is analyzed. Which of the following results is most likely if the patient has an altered hemoglobin molecule (hemoglobinopathy)?

a. Several proteins but only one red protein detected by high-performance liquid chromatography (HPLC)
b. Two proteins detected in normal amounts by Western blotting
c. Several proteins and two red proteins separated by native gel electrophoresis
d. Two labeled bands a slight distance apart after SDS-gel electrophoresis and reaction with labeled antibody to α- and β-globin
e. A reddish mixture of proteins retained within a dialysis membrane

114. A 15-year-old Caucasian adolescent presents with chest pain on exertion. He is noted to be very tall and thin, with lax joints that enable him to do tricks for his friends. His chest is very concave (pectus excavatum), and he has flat feet. His physician suspects Marfan syndrome (MIM*154700) and orders DNA testing for fibrillin, the gene that causes Marfan syndrome. The physician explains that fibrillin gene testing is not very sensitive, because it is a large gene with many variations, and each Marfan family tends to have a different type of mutation. Which of the following amino acid changes (derived from the DNA sequence) would be most likely to represent a pathogenetic mutation rather than benign variation (polymorphism)?

a. gly-ser-ala to gly-ser-ser
b. gly-ser-ala to gly-ser-arg
c. gly-ser-ala to gly-ser-gly
d. gly-ser-ala to gly-ser-tyr
e. gly-ser-ala to gly-ser-val

115. A 3-year-old Asian boy presents with multiple blisters over his extremities, first in response to scrapes or bruises, but then appearing regularly with illnesses or at contact sites for clothes, etc. The group of heritable diseases called epidermolysis bullosa (blistering skin—eg, MIM*131900) is suspected, and the diagnosis is confirmed by DNA testing with a mutation in the gene encoding type 5 keratin. The keratins are notable for their high content of which of the following?

a. Tyrosine
b. Proline
c. Cystine
d. Melanin
e. Serine

116. Parents bring in a 2-week-old Caucasian male infant fearful that he has ingested a poison. They had delayed disposing one of the child's diapers, and noted a black discoloration where the urine had collected. Later, they realized that all of the child's diapers would turn black if stored as waste for a day or so. Knowing that phenol groups can complex to form colors, which of the following amino acid pathways are implicated in this phenomenon?

a. The phenylalanine, tyrosine, and homogentisate pathway
b. The histidine pathway
c. The leucine, isoleucine, and valine pathway
d. The methionine and homocystine pathway
e. The arginine and citrulline pathway (urea cycle)

117. A 2-year-old Caucasian girl is brought for evaluation after being found neglected in a trailer with no kitchen facilities. She has extreme irritability due to thin and bleeding gums with tender forearms and lower legs. A diagnosis of scurvy is made among other deficiencies and her vitamin C levels are low. Which of the following amino acids will be deficient in her bone proteins?

a. Hydroxytryptophan
b. Hydroxytyrosine
c. Hydroxyhistidine
d. Hydroxyalanine
e. Hydroxyproline

118. A newborn African American girl has a large and distorted cranium, short and deformed limbs, and very blue scleras (whites of the eyes). Radiographs demonstrate multiple limb fractures and suggest a diagnosis of osteogenesis imperfecta (brittle bone disease-MIM*155210). Analysis of type I collagen protein, a triple helix formed from two α_1- and one α_2-collagen chains, shows a 50% reduction in the amount of type I collagen in the baby's skin. DNA analysis demonstrates the presence of two normal α_1-alleles and one normal α_2-allele. These results are best explained by which of the following?

a. Deficiency of α_1-collagen peptide synthesis
b. Inability of α_1-chains to incorporate into triple helix
c. Defective α_1-chains that interrupt triple helix formation
d. Incorporation of defective α_2-chains that cause instability and degradation of the triple helix
e. A missense mutation that alters the synthesis of α_1-chains

119. A 12-year-old African American girl, who has tall stature, loose joints, and detached retinas, is found to have a mutation in type II collagen. Recall that collagen consists of a repeating tripeptide motif where the first amino acid of each tripeptide is the same. Which of the following amino acids is the recurring amino acid most likely to be altered in mutations that distort collagen molecules?

a. Glycine
b. Hydroxyproline
c. Hydroxylysine
d. Tyrosine
e. Tryptophan

120. Children with urea cycle disorders present with elevated serum ammonia and consequent neurologic symptoms including altered respiration, lethargy, and coma. Several amino acids are intermediates of the urea cycle, having side ammonia groups that join with free carbon dioxide and ammonia to produce net excretion of ammonia as urea (NH_2CONH_2). Which of the following amino acids has an ammonia group in its side chain and is thus likely to be an intermediate of the urea cycle?

a. Arginine
b. Aspartate
c. Methionine
d. Glutamate
e. Phenylalanine

121. A child who was normal at birth shows developmental delay with coarsened facial features and enlarged liver and spleen by age 1 year. He is suspected of having I-cell disease (inclusion cell disease-MIM*252500), a lysosomal storage disease with progressive accumulation of complex carbohydrates and glycoproteins in organs. Affected individuals lack multiple enzymes in their lysosomes (with excess amounts in serum) because mannose 6-phosphate groups that target enzymes to lysosomes are not correctly synthesized. Which of the following techniques for purification of proteins could be used to isolate the putative lysosomal membrane protein that recognizes mannose 6-phosphate groups and transports enzymes into lysosomes?

a. Dialysis
b. Affinity chromatography
c. Gel filtration chromatography
d. Ion exchange chromatography
e. Electrophoresis

122. An adolescent presents with shortness of breath during exercise and is found to be anemic. A hemoglobin electrophoresis is performed that is depicted in the figure below. The adolescent's sample is run with controls including normal, sickle trait, and sickle cell anemia hemoglobin samples and serum. The adolescent is determined to have an unknown hemoglobinopathy. Which of the following lanes contains the adolescent's sample?

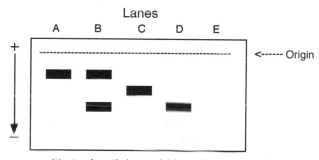

Electrophoretic hemoglobin patterns

a. Lane A
b. Lane B
c. Lane C
d. Lane D
e. Lane E

123. A 2-year-old Arabic boy presents with a large liver and slow growth. His development is normal, and a fasting glucose level is 45 mg/dL (normal 60-100). A mild form of glycogen storage disease is suspected and liver biopsy obtained that shows increased glycogen. Assay of glycogen phosphorylase, deficiency of which can cause one form of glycogen storage disease (MIM*232700), is performed. The specific activity of glycogen phosphorylase is 2.5 units/mg homogenate protein in the patient compared to 24 units/mg homogenate protein in control liver. Which of the following is the correct conclusion based on this information?

a. The yield of enzyme from liver tissue is greater than 80%.
b. The enzyme is deficient in this patient's liver.
c. The enzyme is purified almost 10-fold in the control.
d. The enzyme has undergone structural alteration in the patient.
e. The enzyme has been activated in the control.

124. A 22-year-old Hispanic male college student with a normal medical history collapses during an intramural soccer game. His friends think he is joking, then notice his blue color and call an ambulance. Resuscitation is unsuccessful and the autopsy reveals dilated cardiac chambers with increased thickness of the ventricular walls (hypertrophic, dilated cardiomyopathy). Electron microscopy of the heart muscle shows abnormal thick filaments, and the pathologist suspects a genetic disorder. Genes encoding which of the following proteins would be most likely to reveal the causative mutation?

a. Keratin
b. Lamin
c. Myosin
d. Peripherin
e. Vimentin

125. Which of the following proteolytic enzymes is activated by acid hydrolysis of the proenzyme form?

a. Carboxypeptidase
b. Chymotrypsin
c. Elastase
d. Pepsin
e. Trypsin

126. A 3-day-old African American female infant was normal at birth but becomes lethargic after several feedings; the medical student describes an unusual smell to the urine but is ignored. Infection (sepsis) is suspected, and blood tests show normal white blood cell counts with a serum pH of 7.0. Electrolytes reveal an anion gap, and evaluation for an inborn error of metabolism shows an abnormal amino acid screen. The report states that branch-chain amino acids are strikingly elevated. Which of the following amino acids does the report refer to?

a. Arginine
b. Aspartic acid
c. Isoleucine
d. Lysine
e. Glycine

127. In comparing the secondary structure of proteins, which of the following descriptions applies to both the α-helix and the β-pleated sheet?

a. All peptide bond components participate in hydrogen bonding.
b. N-terminals of chains are together and parallel.
c. The structure is composed of two or more segments of polypeptide chain.
d. N- and C-terminal ends of chains alternate in an antiparallel manner.
e. The chains are almost fully extended.

128. A 6-year-old African American girl with speech delay is found to have a large, abnormal peak when blood amino acids are measured. The abnormal amino acid migrates toward the anode, indicating a positively charged side group in addition to its carboxyl and amino groups. Which of the following amino acids is most probable?

a. Alanine
b. Glycine
c. Histidine
d. Leucine
e. Valine

129. The oxygen carrier of muscle is the globular protein myoglobin. Which of the following amino acids is highly likely to be localized within the interior of the molecule?

a. Arginine
b. Aspartic acid
c. Glutamic acid
d. Valine
e. Lysine

130. A 2-year-old Asian child has stopped progressing in speech and develops coarse facial features with thick mucous drainage. Skeletal deformities including curved spine (kyphosis), thickened and short fingers, and curved limbs appear over the next year, and the child regresses to a vegetative state by age 10 years. The child's urine tests positive for glycosaminoglycans that include which of the following molecules?

a. Collagen
b. γ-Aminobutyric acid
c. Heparan sulfate
d. Glycogen
e. Fibrillin

131. Under normal conditions in blood, which of the following amino acid residues of albumin is neutral?

a. Arginine
b. Aspartate
c. Glutamine
d. Glutamate
e. Histidine

132. Several diseases (osteogenesis imperfecta, Ehlers-Danlos, sensorineural deafness) result from mutations in collagens, a large family of proteins that are important for connective tissue. Different types of collagens occur in bone, ligaments, joints, sclerae (whites of the eyes), and even the inner ear. Collagen peptides have repeating units of gly-X-Y, allowing them to form triple helices that lend structural support to tissues. Which of the following are characteristics of glycine that might account for its use as the initial amino acid in this repeat?

a. Acidic side groups to promote binding
b. Basic side groups to promote binding
c. Hydrophilic to facilitate water incorporation
d. Small molecular diameter compared to other amino acids
e. Optically active with asymmetry to direct the helix

133. Which of the following amino acids is aromatic (ring compound), and in a pathway leading to neurotransmitters and melanin?

a. Arginine
b. Cystine
c. Glutamine
d. Leucine
e. Proline
f. Serine
g. Tyrosine

134. Which of the following substances is primarily found in tendons?

a. Collagen
b. Fibrillin
c. Fibrin
d. Fibronectin
e. Troponin

135. Which of the following is primarily found in the extracellular matrix?

a. Collagen
b. Fibrin
c. Keratin
d. Proteoglycan
e. Troponin

136. The presence of which of the following structural arrangements in a protein strongly suggests that it is a DNA-binding, regulatory protein?

a. α helix
b. β bend
c. β sheet
d. Triple helix
e. Zinc finger

137. During synthesis of mature collagen fibers, which of the following steps occurs within the fibroblast?

a. Hydrolysis of procollagen to form collagen
b. Glycosylation of proline residues
c. Formation of a triple helix
d. Formation of covalent cross-links between molecules
e. Assembly of the collagen fiber

Acid-Base Equilibria, Amino Acids, and Protein Structure

Answers

95. The answer is d. (*Murray, pp 9-13. Scriver, pp 3-45.*) The infant has alkalosis (pH above 7.4) with low P_{CO_2}, eliminating incorrect answers a-c that suggest acidosis and incorrect answer e suggesting metabolic rather than respiratory alkalosis. Brain injury or metabolic diseases that irritate the respiratory center may cause tachypnea in term infants, resulting in respiratory alkalosis. The increased respiratory rate removes ("blows off") carbon dioxide from the lung alveoli and lowers blood CO_2, forcing a shift in the indicated equilibrium toward the left:

$$CO_2 + H_2O \leftrightarrows H_2CO_2 \leftrightarrows H^+ + HCO_3^-$$

Carbonic acid (H_2CO_2) can be ignored because negligible amounts are present at physiologic pH, leaving the equilibrium:

$$CO_2 + H_2O \leftrightarrows H^+ + HCO_3^-$$

The leftward shift to replenish the exhaled CO_2 of rapid breathing decreases the hydrogen ion concentration [H^+] and increases the pH ($-\log_{10}[H^+]$) to produce alkalosis (blood pH above the physiologic norm of 7.4).

The newborn does not have acidosis, defined as a blood pH below 7.4, either from excess blood acids (metabolic acidosis) or from slower or ineffective respiration with increased [CO_2] (respiratory acidosis). The baby also does not have metabolic alkalosis, caused by loss of hydrogen ion from the kidney (eg, with renal tubular disease) or stomach (eg, with severe vomiting). Respiratory alkalosis is best treated by eliminating the underlying disease which will diminish the respiratory rate, elevate blood [CO_2], force the above equilibrium to the right, elevate the [H^+], and decrease the pH.

The infant would prove to have a urea cycle disorder such as citrullinemia (MIM*215700) with neurologic effects (hypotonia, seizures) of high ammonia concentrations. Withdrawal of milk (protein) and other therapies decreased the ammonia, eliminated the seizures, and restored normal respiration.

96. The answer is a. (*Murray, pp 9-13. Scriver, pp 3-45.*) The equilibrium between an acid and its conjugate base is defined by the Henderson-Hasselbalch equation:

$$pH = pK_a + \log \, [base]/[acid] \text{ or } pH = 6.1 + \log \, [HCO_3^-]/[CO_2]$$

in the case of carbonic acid. Note that CO_2 is the effective acid and HCO_3^- the conjugate base for carbonic acid due to its complete dissociation in water. Given a pH of 7.1 in the cyanotic newborn, then $7.1 - 6.1 = 1 = \log \, (10) = \log \, [HCO_3^-]/[CO_2] = \log \, [HCO_3^-]/0.03 \times P_{CO_2}$. Since the $[HCO_3^-]$ is 12 mM, the $P_{CO_2} \times 0.03$ must be 1.2 mM and the P_{CO_2} 40 mm Hg. This normal calculated value for P_{CO_2} means that the baby must have metabolic acidosis, a common accompaniment of hypoxia (low P_{O_2}) that can be treated by providing oxygen or administering alkali to ameliorate the acidosis. A test administration of 100% oxygen is often given to see if an increase in P_{O_2} is obtained, because children with heart defects (like transposition of the great arteries) may have separate pulmonary and systemic circulations connected by a small shunt (patent ductus arteriosus) that allows minimal delivery of pulmonary oxygen to the tissues. Children who do not respond to oxygen will require extracorporeal membrane oxygen (ECMO) and immediate surgery to create a palliative shunt between circulations (eg, widened foramen ovale).

Other answers are eliminated because a baby with respiratory acidosis, would have elevated P_{CO_2}, treated by restoring ventilation to blow off CO_2. Renal treatment of acidosis by increasing acid excretion or alkali retention is not effective for severe hypoxia.

97. The answer is b. (*Murray, pp 9-13. Scriver, pp 1471-1488.*) The man is acidotic as defined by the pH lower than the normal 7.4. His hyperventilation with Kussmaul respirations can be interpreted as compensation by the lungs to blow off CO_2, lower P_{CO_2}, increase $[HCO_3^-]/[CO_2]$ ratio, and raise pH. The correct answer therefore includes a low

P_{CO_2}, eliminating choices c through e. Using the Henderson-Hasselbalch equation indicates that the pH minus the pK for carbonic acid (7.3 − 6.1 = 1.2) equals log [15]/[0.03 × 30 mm Hg] or log [15/0.9]. These values correspond to those in choice b. The man has compensated his metabolic acidosis (caused by the accumulation of ketone bodies such as acetoacetic acid) by increasing his respiratory rate and volume. The treatment of diabetes is administration of insulin to restore glucose entry into cells, fluids to reverse dehydration, and potassium and/or phosphate administration to correct deficits caused by poor renal perfusion.

98. The answer is d. (*Murray, pp 9-13. Scriver, pp 3-45.*) A β-turn structure consists of four amino acids in which the first residue is hydrogen bonded to the fourth residue of the turn. Glycine residues are small and flexible, while proline residues assume a cis or flattened conformation, making these residues amenable to tight turns as opposed to the other amino acids listed (incorrect answers a-c and e). Transport proteins often have several membrane-spanning domains demarcated by β turns that allow them to exit and return back into the membrane. These transmembrane domains form channels that regulate transport of ions and water in organs like lung, gut, and kidney. Nephrogenic diabetes insipidus results when the kidney is less responsive to antidiuretic hormone excreted by the posterior pituitary, causing abnormal water excretion, dehydration, and electrolyte disturbances. Treatment is difficult and in part utilizes the paradoxical effect of some diuretics (eg, chlorothiazide or Diuril) in restoring sodium balance.

99. The answer is d. (*Murray, pp 9-13. Scriver, pp 3-45. Lewis, pp 194-199.*) A stable α helix requires hydrogen bonding between peptide bonds at four amino acid intervals. Proline is uncommon in α helices because it destabilizes the helix by introducing a kink that will not hydrogen bond with other residues; proline is common in β turns while the other amino acids listed are common in α-helical regions (incorrect answers a-c, e). Other residues with negative (glutamates, aspartates) or positive (lysine, arginine) charges will also destabilize the helix if present in large blocks. Ankyrin mutations that cause spherocytosis disrupt the α-helical domains and interfere with ankyrin stacking that contributes to red cell shape. The altered shape reduces red cell survival, increases hemolysis, and increases the amount of heme converted to bilirubin. Increased bilirubin may be seen in the whites of the eyes (sclerae) or skin as a yellow color (jaundice). Increased storage of bilirubin in the gall bladder may cause gall stones and inflammation (cholecystitis), leading to acute abdominal pain and sometimes requiring gall bladder removal (cholecystectomy).

100. The answer is b. (*Murray, pp 9-13. Scriver, pp 3-45.*) Proteins can be effective buffers of body and intracellular fluids. Buffering capacity is dependent on the presence of amino acids having ionizable side chains with pKas near physiologic pH. In the example given, only histidine has an ionizable imidazolium group that has a pK close to neutrality (pK = 6.0). Valine and leucine (incorrect answers d, e) are amino acids with uncharged, branched side chains while lysine (incorrect answer a) has a basic amino group (pK = 10.5) and aspartic acid (incorrect answer c) has a side chain carboxyl (pK = 3.8) that is negative at pH 7.

101. The answer is c. (*Murray, pp 9-13. Scriver, pp 3-45.*) A nonfunctional mutation in the gene for carbonic anhydrase will reduce amounts of the renal enzyme (incorrect answers b, e) and reduce hydrogen ion formation (incorrect answer d) as well as that of bicarbonate (incorrect answer a). Several forms of carbonic anhydrase exist in human tissues, functioning to catalyze the reversible conversion of carbon dioxide and water to carbonic acid (which in turn dissociates into hydrogen ion and bicarbonate). The concentrations of carbon dioxide will be different among tissues, requiring carbonic anhydrases with different K_{ms} and catalytic properties. The enzyme in renal tubular tissue is important for converting serum and tissue carbon dioxide into hydrogen ion and bicarbonate, allowing for excretion of hydrogen ion in diseases with acidosis. When the kidney cannot excrete hydrogen ion appropriately, a primary renal tubular acidosis ensues with paradoxically high urine pH (lower hydrogen ion concentration and higher pH) compared to serum pH. Renal tubular acidosis has secondary effects on calcification and bone resorption, causing the brittle and dense bones (literally, petrified bones) in the rare recessive osteopetrosis and renal tubular acidosis due to carbonic anhydrase deficiency (MIM*259730).

102. The answer is d. (*Murray, pp 9-13. Scriver, pp 3-45.*) The normal aeration eliminates answers b and c positing respiratory acidosis, and the lack of urine glucose eliminates diabetes mellitus (incorrect answer a). The sum of measured cations (Na 140 + K 4.5 = 144.5) is greater than the sum of measured anions (Cl 110 + bicarbonate 8 = 118) by 26.5, creating an anion gap greater than the normal of 12 to 14 mEq/L due to unmeasured phosphates or sulfates in serum. Ammonium ion is positively charged and would not increase a negative ion gap (incorrect answer e). Fatty or organic acids that build up due to missing enzymes in inborn errors of metabolism are hidden anions in serum and cause the kidney to excrete bicarbonate in an effort to balance the serum pH. Anion gaps over 20 and lowering of the pH to cause acidosis (7.1 in this case) indicate the kidney can no longer compensate. Such changes can occur in neonates with inborn errors of organic acid metabolism or older children with disorders of fatty acid oxidation who have a routine illness, stop eating, and accumulate a fatty acid anion when they attempt to switch from glucose to fat metabolism.

Separate enzyme pathways exist for breakdown of long, medium, or short chain fatty acids, so deficiency in one (like medium chain fatty acyl-CoA dehydrogenase or MCAD) may not compromise the child until there are severe demands for fat breakdown and energy once carbohydrates and glycogen are depleted (3-4 hours after feeds on average). Depletion of glycogen and inability to maintain glucose through gluconeogenesis may lead to low serum glucose (hypoglycemia), and ineffective fatty acid/organic acid breakdown will not yield the ketones seen in hypoglycemia from other causes or in diabetes mellitus where glucose cannot enter cells. Fatty acids that build up due to the enzyme block manifest as hidden anions. If the disorder is suspected, feeding or infusion of glucose is curative by preventing the need for fat oxidation to provide energy. A child similar to this was not recognized in time, leading the politically connected parents to advocate for expanded newborn screening that is becoming the standard in most states.

103. The answer is c. (*Lewis, pp 219-232. Murray, pp 31-42. Scriver, pp 5241-5286.*) The presence of glycine-X-Y repeats (not pro-X-Y or ala-X-Y for incorrect answers a-c) allows for very tight packing and association of three chains to form a triple helix. Mutations substituting larger or differently configured amino acids for a glycine within one repeat would disrupt the tight packing, alter triple helix conformation; and cause weakness leading to bone deformation and easy fractures. Alanine substitutions for glycine (incorrect answer d) would be less disruptive than proline.

Collagen is the most abundant fibrous protein and is found in connective tissue, bone, cartilage, skin, ligaments, and tendons as well as other tissues. Collagen consists of three peptide chains arranged in a triple helix, exemplified by the two α_1- and one α_2-chains that make up type I collagen that is predominant in bone and mutated in the various forms of osteogenesis imperfecta (MIM*166210). Substitutions of amino acids for glycine are most disruptive, causing severe, neonatal, and often lethal forms of osteogenesis imperfecta. Those at the X-Y positions of a repeat or those affecting the α_2 rather than the α_1-chain (two copies per helix) are less severe, allowing thicker bones with fewer fractures and thicker sclerae with more normal color of the eye whites (thin sclerae allow the underlying blue choroid to show through).

104. The answer is e. (*Murray, pp 9-13. Scriver, pp 3-45.*) Pure metabolic acidosis (incorrect answer c) or pure metabolic alkalosis (incorrect answer e) exhibits abnormal bicarbonate and normal lung function. Pure respiratory acidosis (incorrect answer d) or alkalosis (incorrect answer a) is associated with normal renal function (and normal blood acids) with a normal bicarbonate and abnormal P_{CO_2}. Incorrect answer b must involve compensation, since both the P_{CO_2} and bicarbonate are abnormal. The infant is affected with pyloric stenosis (MIM*179010), blocking the exit of stomach contents into the duodenum and causing vomiting. The blockage is caused by failure of pyloric tissue to regress by cell death during development, leaving a ball of muscular tissue surrounding the pyloric valve (gastro-duodenal junction). The preferred treatment is surgical, slicing the excess tissue (pyloromyotomy) to relieve the blockage. When diagnosis is delayed, infants can die because of severe metabolic alkalosis caused by expulsion of hydrochloric acid in stomach fluid.

105. The answer is c. (*Murray, pp 9-13. Scriver, pp 3-45. Lewis, pp 188-194.*) The amino acid cystine, essentially a dimer of cysteine, accumulates in the lysosomes of patients with cystinosis (MIM*219800). It has a sulfhydryl side group with a pKa of 8.3 that is different from the amino side groups of lysine, arginine, and glutamine (pKas 9-12). These patients exhibit progressive vision problems and renal failure, but these problems can be forestalled by cysteamine treatment, which complexes with cystine and allows egress from lysosomes.

106. The answer is d. (*Murray, pp 9-13. Scriver, pp 3-45. Lewis, pp 194-199.*) Phenylalanine, with its benzene ring, is an essential amino acid that is converted to tyrosine by phenylhydroxylase, the enzyme (or its cofactor biopterin) that is deficient in phenylketonuria (PKU-MIM*261600). The other amino acid choices (incorrect answers a-c and e) do not have aromatic (benzene ring) side chains—serine has a hydroxyl group, glutamine an amino group, and methionine a sulfydryl group. Deficiency of phenylalanine hydroxylase in PKU causes elevated substrate (phenylalanine) and deficient product (tyrosine), leading to developmental delays and ultimately severe mental retardation if the disease is not recognized. Now children with PKU are detected by newborn screening and placed on low-phenylalanine diets that allow normal brain development. Adults can moderate the greatly restricted and not very tasty diet but may elect to go back on for clear thinking before exams or, in the case of affected females, to prevent birth defects caused by high maternal phenylalanine in pregnancy.

107. The answer is b. (*Murray, pp 9-13. Scriver, pp 3-45. Lewis, pp 215-218.*) Water is an ideal solvent because of its dipole nature ($+H_2O^-$), forming hydrogen bonds and solvating positive (eg, arginine-$NH4^+$) and negative (eg, glutamate-COO^-) groups of proteins. No covalent bonds or protein aggregates are formed (incorrect answers a, e). The solvated proteins exert osmotic pressure of about 25 mm within vessels, causing net return of fluid in veins (outward hydrostatic pressure 17 mm and outward fluid flow in arterioles (outward hydrostatic pressure 37 mm). Hydrophobic amino acids (valine, leucine) resist hydration and cluster internally in proteins while hydrophilic (charged) amino acids (glutamate, aspartate) tend to be on the protein surface (incorrect answers c, d). Nonionic but polar compounds are dissolved in water because of hydrogen bonding between water molecules and groups such as alcohols, aldehydes, and ketones.

108. The answer is e. (*Murray, pp 9-13, 31-42. Scriver, pp 1471-1488. Lewis, pp 188-194.*) In the presence of insulin deficiency, a shift to fatty acid oxidation produces the ketones such as acetoacetate that cause metabolic acidosis. The pH and bicarbonate are low, and there is frequently some respiratory compensation (hyperventilation with deep breaths) to lower the PCO_2, as in correct answer e. A low pH with high PCO_2 would represent respiratory acidosis (incorrect answers a and b—the low-normal bicarbonate values in these choices indicate partial compensation). Incorrect answer d represents respiratory alkalosis as would occur with anxious hyperventilation (high pH and low P_{CO_2}, partial compensation with high bicarbonate). Incorrect answer c illustrates normal values.

109. The answer is d. (*Murray, pp 14-20. Scriver, pp 1971-2006. Lewis, pp 194-199.*) Leucine and isoleucine have nonpolar methyl groups as side chains. As for any amino acid, titration curves obtained by noting the change in pH over the range of 1 to 14 would show a pK of about 2 for the primary carboxyl group and about 9.5 for the primary amino group; there would be no additional pK for an ionizable side chain. Recall that the pK is the point of maximal buffering capacity when the amounts of charged and uncharged species are equal (see answer to Question 104). Aspartic and glutamic acids (second carboxyl group), histidine (imino group), and glutamine (second amino group) all have ionizable side chains that would give an additional pK on the titration curve. The likely diagnosis here is maple syrup urine disease, which involves elevated isoleucine, leucine, and valine together with their ketoacid derivatives. The ketoacid derivatives cause the acidosis, and the fever suggests that the metabolic imbalance was worsened by an infection.

110. The answer is e. (*Murray, pp 14-20. Scriver, pp 3-45. Lewis, pp 194-199.*) Adult hemoglobin (hemoglobin A), is composed of two α-chains and two β-chains held together by noncovalent interactions. The designation (α_1-β_1)-(α_2-β_2), referring to (α_1-β_1) and (α_2-β_2) dimers is the correct way to refer to the quaternary structure of adult hemoglobin (incorrect answers a-d). Fetal hemoglobin (hemoglobin F) has the structure (α_1-γ_1)-(α_2-γ_2) and predominates during later pregnancy and early infancy, so mutations affecting β-chain structure or expression will not present until the switch to hemoglobin F at age 3 to 6 months. Considerable research effort has examined ways to prevent the hemoglobin F to A switch and therefore eliminate β-chain diseases like sickle cell anemia (MIM*603903) or β-thalassemia (MIM*141900).

111. The answer is d. (*Murray, pp 14-20. Scriver, pp 3-45. Lewis, pp 194-199.*) Serine, threonine, and tyrosine can all be phosphorylated on their side-chain hydroxyl group. In addition, histidine, lysine, arginine, and aspartates are common targets for phosphorylation by protein kinases. Phosphorylation by protein kinases and dephosphorylation by protein phosphatases is a common method for regulating protein activity. In Bruton agammaglobulinemia (MIM*300300), deficiency of a tyrosine kinase prevents normal B-cell development. B cells are the arm of the immune system responsible for making immunoglobulins, so children with B-cell deficiencies have frequent and overwhelming bacterial infections with normal T-cell function (resistance to viral infections).

112. The answer is b. (*Murray, pp 14-20. Scriver, pp 3-45. Lewis, pp 194-199.*) Primary protein structures denote the sequence of amino acids held together by peptide bonds (carboxyl groups joined to amino groups to form amide bonds). The types of amino acids then determine the secondary structure of peptide regions within the protein, sometimes forming spiral α_1-helices or flat pleated sheets. These regional peptide secondary structures then determine the overall three-dimensional tertiary structure of a protein, which is vital for its function. Amino acid substitutions that alter the charge of an amino acid side chain, like the change from glutamic acid (charged carboxyl group) to valine (nonpolar methyl groups) in choice b, are most likely to change the secondary and tertiary protein structure. A change in globin structure can cause instability, decreased mean cellular hemoglobin concentration (MCHC), and anemia. A change from glutamic acid to valine at position six in the β-globin chain is the mutation responsible for sickle cell anemia (MIM*602903).

113. The answer is c. (*Murray, pp 43-50. Scriver, pp 3-45. Lewis, pp 194-199.*) In the technique of polyacrylamide gel electrophoresis (PAGE), the distance that a protein is moved by an electrical current is proportional to its charge and inversely proportional to its size. Patients with normal hemoglobin A have two α-globin and two β_1-globin chains, each encoded by a pair of normal globin alleles. Mutation in one α- or β-globin allele alters the primary amino acid sequence of the encoded globin peptide. If the amino acid change alters the charge of the peptide, then the hemoglobin tetramer assembled with the mutant globin peptide has a different charge and electrophoretic migration than the normal hemoglobin tetramer. The electrophoresis of native (undenatured) hemoglobin therefore produces two species (two bands) rather than one, each retaining its heme molecule and red color. If the hemoglobins were first denatured into their α- and β-globin chains as with SDS-polyacrylamide gel electrophoresis, then the similar size of the α- or β-globin peptides would cause them to move closely together as two colorless bands. Identification of these peptides as globin would require use of labeled antibody specific for globin (Western blotting). Because the sodium dodecyl sulfate (SDS) detergent covers the protein surface and causes all proteins to be negatively charged, the distance migrated is solely dependent (inversely proportional) on protein size. High-performance liquid chromatography (HPLC) uses ionic resins to separate proteins by charge. The columns are run under high pressure, rapidly producing a series of proteins that are separated from most negative to most positive (or vice versa, depending on the charge of the ionic resin). A mutant hemoglobin with altered charge should produce a second red protein in the pattern. In dialysis, semipermeable membranes allow smaller proteins to diffuse into the outer fluid, but not larger proteins such as hemoglobin.

114. The answer is b. (*Murray, pp 14-20. Scriver, pp 5241-5286. Lewis, pp 194-199.*) The amino acids gly (glycine), ser (serine), and alanine (ala) have uncharged and small side groups (the serine hydroxyl group will not be ionized at near neutral biological pHs of 7-7.4). Replacement of the alanine group with another small and uncharged amino acid would be less likely to alter fibrillin conformation and function than replacement with a charged amino acid like arginine (ammonium group with positive charge on side chain). Although Marfan syndrome (MIM*154700) is relatively common at 1 in 3000 births, fibrillin DNA testing remains difficult because the gene is large and susceptible to mutations throughout its length. DNA diagnosis thus requires complete sequencing of the gene in suspect patients, which is cost-prohibitive for commercial laboratories. Once a sequence variation is found, its pathogenicity can be assessed by testing for its presence in the normal parents.

115. The answer is c. (*Murray, pp 43-50. Scriver, pp 3-45. Lewis, pp 194-199.*) Keratins are a type of intermediate filament that comprises a large portion of many epithelial cells. The characteristics of skin, nails, and hair are all due to keratins. Keratins contain a large amount of the disulfide amino acid cystine. Approximately 14% of the protein composing human hair is cystine. This is the chemical basis of depilatory creams, which are reducing agents that render keratins soluble by breaking the disulfide bridges of these insoluble proteins. Mutations in keratins also alter the adherent properties of keratins and keratin-rich tissues, causing fragility (epidermolysis with blisters) or aggregation (hyperkeratosis) of skin cells.

116. The answer is a. (*Murray, pp 248-261. Scriver, pp 1971-2006. Lewis, pp 399-402.*) Lack of the enzyme homogentisate oxidase causes the accumulation of homogentisic acid, a metabolite in the pathway of degradation of phenylalanine and tyrosine. Homogentisate, like tyrosine, contains a phenol group. It is excreted in the urine, where it oxidizes and is polymerized to a dark substance upon standing. Under normal conditions, phenylalanine is degraded to tyrosine, which is broken down through a series of steps to fumarate and acetoacetate. The dark pigment melanin is another end product of this pathway. Deficiency of homogentisate oxidase is called alkaptonuria (black urine—MIM*203500), a mild disease discovered by Sir Archibald Garrod, the pioneer of biochemical genetics. Garrod's geneticist colleague, William Bateson, recognized that alkaptonuria, like nearly all enzyme deficiencies, exhibits autosomal recessive inheritance.

117. The answer is e. (*Murray, pp 527-544. Scriver, pp 5241-5286. Lewis, pp 215-218.*) Proline and lysine residues in collagen are modified by hydroxylation in a reaction requiring the reducing agent ascorbic acid (vitamin C—eliminating answers a-d). The enzymes catalyzing the reactions are prolyl hydroxylase and lysyl hydroxylase. In scurvy, which results from a deficiency of vitamin C, insufficient hydroxylation of collagen causes abnormal collagen fibrils. The weakened collagen in teeth, bone, and blood vessels causes tooth loss, brittle bones with fractures, and bleeding tendencies with bruising and bleeding gums.

118. The answer is d. (*Murray, pp 31-42. Scriver, pp 5241-5286. Lewis, pp 215-218.*) Collagen peptides assemble into helical tertiary structures that form quaternary triple helices. The triple helices in turn assemble end to end to form collagen fibrils that are essential for connective tissue strength. Over 15 types of collagen contribute to the connective tissue of various organs, including the contribution of type I collagen to eyes, bones, and skin. The fact that only one of two α_2-alleles is normal in this case implies that a mutant α_2-allele could be responsible for the disease (even if the α_2-locus is on the X chromosome, since the baby is girl with two X chromosomes). The mutant α_2-collagen peptide would be incorporated into half of the type I collagen triple helices, causing a 50% reduction in normal type I collagen. (A mutant α_1-collagen peptide would distort 75% of the molecules because two α_1-peptides go into each triple helix.) The ability of one abnormal collagen peptide allele to alter triple helix structure with subsequent degradation is well documented and colorfully named protein suicide or, more properly, a dominant-negative mutation.

119. The answer is a. (*Murray, pp 31-42. Scriver, pp 3-45. Lewis, pp 215-218.*) The primary structure of collagen peptides consists of repeating tripeptides with a gly-X-Y motif, where gly is glycine and X and Y are any amino acid. The small CH_2 group connecting the amino and carboxyl groups of glycine contrasts with the larger connecting groups and side chains of other amino acids. The small volume of glycine molecules is crucial for the α-helix secondary structure of collagen peptides. This in turn is necessary for their tertiary helical structure and their assembly into quaternary tripeptide, triple-helix structures. The most severe clinical phenotypes caused by amino acid substitutions in collagen peptides are those affecting glycine that prevent a helix formation. The child has a disorder called Stickler syndrome (MIM*108300) that exhibits autosomal dominant inheritance.

120. The answer is a. (*Murray, pp 31-42. Scriver, pp 3-45. Lewis, pp 194-199.*) Arginine is an amino acid used in proteins that is also part of the urea cycle. Citrulline and ornithine are amino acids not used in proteins but important as urea cycle intermediates. Aspartate is condensed with citrulline to form argininosuccinate in the urea cycle, and acetylglutamate is a cofactor in the joining of carbon dioxide with ammonia to form carbamoyl phosphate at the beginning of the urea cycle.

121. The answer is b. (*Murray, pp 31-42. Scriver, pp 3-45. Lewis, pp 194-199.*) Each of the techniques listed separates proteins from each other and from other biologic molecules based on characteristics such as size, solubility, and charge. However, only affinity chromatography can use the high affinity of proteins for specific chemical groups or the specificity of immobilized antibodies for unique proteins. In affinity chromatography, a specific compound that binds to the desired protein—such as an antibody, a polypeptide receptor, or a substrate—is covalently bound to the column material. A mixture of proteins is added to the column under conditions ideal for binding the protein desired, and the column is then washed with buffer to remove unbound proteins. The protein is eluted either by adding a high concentration of the original binding material or by making the conditions unfavorable for binding (eg, changing the pH). The other techniques are less specific than affinity binding for isolating proteins. Dialysis separates large proteins from small molecules. Ion exchange chromatography separates proteins with an overall charge of one sort from proteins with an opposite charge (eg, negative from positive). Gel filtration chromatography separates on the basis of size. Electrophoresis separates proteins on the principle that net charge influences the rate of migration in an electric field.

Inclusion-cell disease (mucolipidosis II—MIM*252500) can result from deficiency in either of two phosphotransferase enzymes that put mannose-6-phosphate groups on degradative enzymes, targeting them to lysosomes. Mucolipidosis II with multiple mistargeted enzymes is thus similar to but more severe than disorders like Hunter syndrome (iduronate sulfatase deficiency—MIM*309900) that result from deficiency of a single lysosomal enzyme.

122. The answer is c. (*Murray, pp 31-42. Scriver, pp 3-45. Lewis, pp 194-199.*) Protein electrophoresis is an important laboratory technique for investigating red cell proteins such as hemoglobin or plasma proteins such as the immunoglobulins. The proteins are dissolved in a buffer of low pH where the amino groups of amino acid side chains are positively charged, causing most proteins to migrate toward the negative electrode (anode). Red cell hemolysates are used for hemoglobin electrophoresis, plasma (blood supernatant with unhemolyzed red cells removed) for plasma proteins. Serum (blood supernatant after clotting) would not contain red cells but would contain many blood enzymes and proteins. In sickle cell anemia, the hemoglobin S contains a valine substitution for the glutamic acid at position six in hemoglobin A. Hemoglobin S thus loses two negative charges (loss of a glutamic acid carboxyl group on each of two β-globin chains) compared to hemoglobin A. Hemoglobin S is thus more positively charged and migrates more rapidly toward the anode than hemoglobin A (figure below Question 122). Lane B must represent the heterozygote with sickle cell trait (hemoglobins S and A), establishing lane A as the normal and lane D as the sickle cell anemia sample. The hemoglobin in lane C migrates differently from normal and hemoglobin S, as would befit an abnormal hemoglobin that is different from S. Lane E must be serum, which does not contain red blood cells.

123. The answer is b. (*Murray, pp 31-42. Scriver, pp 3-45. Lewis, pp 194-199.*) The activity of tissue enzymes must be compared based on equivalent amounts of tissue protein, expressed as units (micromoles substrate converted or product produced per minute of reaction) over milligram of tissue protein added (enzyme specific activity). This avoids error arising from different yields of protein in patient and control (incorrect answer a) and compares enzyme activity, not degree of purity (incorrect answer c). The specific activity does not give information about enzyme structure (incorrect answer d) or activation (incorrect answer e) unless it is correlated with other measures (eg, migration by electrophoresis, increased/decreased by the presence of phosphorylation, etc).

124. The answer is c. (*Murray, pp 31-42, 545-565. Scriver, pp 5433-5432.*) Incorrect answers a-b and d-e are intermediate filament proteins that anchor the cytoskeleton. Cardiac and skeletal muscles are similar in that both are striated and contain two kinds of interacting protein filaments. The thick filaments (15 nm in diameter) contain primarily myosin, while the thin filaments (7 nm in diameter) contain actin, troponin, and tropomyosin. The thick and thin filaments slide past one another during muscle contraction. Myosins are a family of proteins with heavy and light chains, and muscle myosins function as ATPases that bind to thin filaments during contraction. A particular cardiomyopathy (MIM*160760) is caused by mutations in the myosin 7 heavy chain gene, one of many causes of acute life-threatening events (ALTE) that can affect previously asymptomatic adults. ALTE are adult equivalents of sudden infant death syndrome (SIDS) or, more inclusively, sudden unexplained death syndrome (SUDS) that affect children. Congenital defects in muscle filaments, potassium channels, and the like, that affect cardiac contractility are substantial contributors to these tragic and unexpected disease categories—important reasons for annual and transitional (sports, precollege) physical examinations.

125. The answer is d. (*Murray, pp 31-42, 459-468. Scriver, pp 3-45. Lewis, pp 182-201.*) Pepsin is secreted in a proenzyme form in the stomach. Unlike the majority of proenzymes, it is not activated by protease hydrolysis. Instead, spontaneous acid hydrolysis at pH 2 or lower converts pepsinogen to pepsin. Hydrochloric acid secreted by the stomach lining creates the acid environment. All the enzymes secreted by the pancreas are activated at the same time upon entrance into the duodenum. This is accomplished by trypsin hydrolysis of the inactive proenzymes trypsinogen, chymotrypsinogen, procarboxypeptidase, and proelastase. Primer amounts of trypsin is derived from trypsinogen by the action of enteropeptidase secreted by the cells of the duodenum.

126. The answer is c. (*Murray, pp 31-42. Scriver, pp 3-45. Lewis, pp 194-199.*) The carbon next to a carboxyl (C=O) group may be designated as the α-carbon, with subsequent carbons as β, γ, δ, etc. α-Amino acids contain an amino group on their α-carbon, as distinguished from compounds like γ-aminobutyric acid, in which the amino group is two carbons down (γ-carbon). In α-amino acids the amino acid, carboxylic acid, and the side chain or R group are all bound to the central α-carbon, which is thus asymmetric (except when R is hydrogen, as for glycine). Amino acids are classified as acidic, neutral hydrophobic, neutral hydrophilic, or basic, depending on the charge or partial charge on the R group at pH 7. Hydrophobic (water-hating) groups are carbon-hydrogen chains like those of leucine, isoleucine, glycine, or valine. Basic R groups, such as those of lysine and arginine, carry a positive charge at physiologic pH owing to protonated amide groups, whereas acidic R groups, such as glutamic acid, carry a negative charge owing to ionized carboxyl groups. Glycine has no side chain and is neutral at physiologic pH.

Leucine, isoleucine, and valine are amino acids with branched side groups, and they share a pathway for degradation that is deficient in children with maple syrup urine disease (MIM*248600). Their amino groups can be removed, but the resulting carboxy-acids accumulate with resulting acidosis, coma, and death unless a diet free of branch-chained amino acids is instituted.

127. The answer is a. (*Murray, pp 31-42. Scriver, pp 3-45. Lewis, pp 194-199.*) Regular arrangements of groups of amino acids located near each other in the linear sequence of a polypeptide are the secondary structure of a protein. The α helix, β sheet, and β bend are the secondary structures usually observed in proteins. In both the α helix and the β sheet, all the peptide bond components participate in hydrogen bonding. That is, the oxygen components of the peptide bond form hydrogen bonds with the amide hydrogens. In the case of the α helix, all hydrogen bonding is intrachain and stabilizes the helix. In the case of β sheets, the bonds are interchain when formed between the polypeptide backbones of separate polypeptide chains and intrachain when the β sheet is formed by a single polypeptide chain folding back on itself. While the spiral of the α helix prevents the chain from being fully extended, the chains of β sheets are almost fully extended and relatively flat. The chains of β sheets can be either parallel or antiparallel. When the N-terminals of chains run together, the chain or segment is considered parallel. In contrast, when N- and C-terminal ends of the chains alternate, the β strand is considered antiparallel.

128. The answer is c. (*Murray, pp 14-30. Scriver, pp 3-45. Lewis, pp 194-199.*) Except for terminal amino acids, all α-amino groups and all α-carboxyl groups are utilized in peptide bonds. Thus only the side chains of amino acids may be ionizable in proteins. Seven of the twenty common amino acids have easily ionizable side chains. Lysine, arginine, and histidine have basic side chains (yielding a positive charge at neutral pH); aspartate and glutamate have acidic side chains (yielding a negative charge at neutral pH); and tyrosine and cysteine have hydroxyl/sulfydryl groups (ionizing only at basic pHs or within special environments of protein/ enzyme active sites/channels).

Histidinemia (MIM*235800) is one of several abnormalities discovered when advances in ion exchange chromatography and paper electrophoresis made screening of blood and urine amino acids distributions feasible for patients. These diagnostic tests allowed confirmation of clinically defined disorders like phenylketonuria (MIM*261600), and revealed a host of new disorders like histidinemia or hyperprolinemia (MIM*239500). Although the latter disorders have been traced to specific enzyme deficiencies, their clinical significance is uncertain because many individuals with elevated screens do not have disease.

129. The answer is d. (*Murray, pp 31-42. Scriver, pp 3-45. Lewis, pp 194-199.*) The structure of myoglobin is illustrative of most water-soluble proteins. Globular proteins tend to fold into compact configurations with nonpolar cores. The interior of myoglobin is composed almost exclusively of nonpolar, hydrophobic amino acids like valine, leucine, phenylalanine, and methionine. In contrast, polar hydrophilic residues such as arginine, aspartic acid, glutamic acid, and lysine are found mostly on the surface of the water-soluble protein.

130. The answer is c. (*Murray, pp 31-42. Scriver, pp 3421-3452. Lewis, pp 194-199.*) Glycosaminoglycans (mucopolysaccharides) are polysaccharide chains that may be bound to proteins as proteoglycans. Each proteoglycan is a complex molecule with a core protein that is covalently bound to glycosaminoglycans—repeating units of disaccharides. The amino sugars forming the disaccharides contain negatively charged sulfate or carboxylate groups. The primary glycosaminoglycans found in mammals are hyaluronic acid, heparin, heparan sulfate, chondroitin sulfate, and keratan sulfate. Inborn errors of glycosaminoglycan degradation cause neurodegeneration and physical stigmata described by the outmoded term "gargoylism"—exemplified by Hurler syndrome (MIM*252800). Glycogen is a polysaccharide of glucose used for energy storage and has no sulfate groups. Collagen and fibrillin are important proteins in connective tissue. γ-Aminobutyric acid is a γ-amino acid involved in neurotransmission.

131. The answer is c. (*Murray, pp 14-20. Scriver, pp 3-45. Lewis, pp 194-199.*) In blood and other solutions at physiologic pH (approximately 7), only terminal carboxyl groups, terminal amino groups, and ionizable side chains of amino acid residues in proteins have charges. The basic amino acids lysine, arginine, and histidine have positive charges (protonated amines). The acidic amino acids aspartate and glutamate have negative charges (ionized carboxyls). Glutamine possesses an uncharged but hydrophilic side chain.

132. The answer is d. (*Murray, pp 31-42. Scriver, pp 3-45. Lewis, pp 194-199.*) All α-amino acids have an asymmetric α-carbon atom to which an α-carboxyl group, an α-amino group, and an α-side chain are attached. Levorotary (L) isomers of amino acids compose proteins in nature. Glycine has no side chain, and its two hydrogens (plus the amino carboxyl groups) on the α-carbon makes it uniquely symmetrical (optically inactive) among the amino acids. Side chains contribute the distinctive properties at physiological pH to each amino acid (and hence proteins), which include: basic (positive); acidic (negative); neutral polar; neutral nonpolar; sulfur-containing (thiol); hydroxyl-containing; aromatic; hydrophobic; hydrophilic; branched; or straight-chained. Glycine is not a positively or negatively charged amino acid nor is it hydrophobic. Instead, glycine offers great flexibility to a peptide chain because of its small hydrogen side chain; thus, glycine is found in β turns in proteins like the collagens.

133. The answer is g. (*Murray, pp 14-30. Scriver, pp 3-45. Lewis, pp 194-199.*) Amino acids are composed of an α-carbon atom bonded to carboxyl, amino, and side chain R groups. The α-carbon is so named because it is adjacent to the carboxyl group. The distinctive R side chains, with their variation in charge, shape, size, and reactivity, account for the diversity of protein conformations and functions. Aliphatic amino acids contain carbon chains as side groups (eg, leucine, isoleucine, and valine). Aromatic amino acids have rings in their side groups, like phenylalanine and tyrosine. Those with carbon chains or rings are hydrophobic in nature, causing them to sequester together away from water in the interior of proteins. Polar amino acids have ionizable groups on their side chains, including basic amino acids (positively charged at neutral pH—lysine, arginine, histidine) and acidic amino acids (negatively charged at neutral pH—glutamate, aspartate). Polar amino acids are located on the outsides of proteins and moderate interactions of proteins with themselves and smaller molecules. Aromatic rings interact to produce colors, and the benzene ring of tyrosine is incorporated into melanin. Other branches of this pathway produce important neurotransmitters such as catecholamines and dopamine. External amino acids also provide substrates for enzymic modification of protein conformation and function, illustrated by the phosphorylation of tyrosine by kinases.

134. The answer is a. (*Murray, pp 31-42. Scriver, pp 3-45. Lewis, pp 194-199.*) Collagens are insoluble proteins that have great tensile strength. They are the main fibers composing the connective tissue elements of skin, bone, teeth, tendons, and cartilage. Collagen is composed of tropocollagen, a triple-stranded helical rod rich in glycine, proline, and hydroxyproline residues. Troponin is found in muscle, fibrillin in heart valves, blood vessels, and ligaments (it is defective in Marfan syndrome [MIM*154700]). Fibrin is a component of blood clots and fibronectin is a component of extracellular matrix.

135. The answer is d. (*Murray, pp 31-42. Scriver, pp 3-45. Lewis, pp 194-199.*) The major macromolecular components of ground substance are proteoglycans, which are made up of polysaccharide chains attached to core proteins. The polysaccharide chains are made up of repeats of negatively charged disaccharide units. This polyanionic quality of proteoglycans allows them to bind water and cations and thus determines the viscoelastic properties of connective tissues. Collagen is the other major component of connective tissue besides ground substance. The cornified layer of epidermis derives its toughness and waterproof nature from keratin. Keratins are disulfide-rich proteins that compose the cytoskeletal elements known as intermediate filaments. Hair and animal horns are also composed of keratin. Troponin is a component of muscle, fibrin of blood clots.

136. The answer is e. (*Murray, pp 31-42. Scriver, pp 3-45. Lewis, pp 194-199.*) Regulatory proteins must bind with great specificity and high affinity to the correct portion of DNA. Several structural motifs have been discovered in DNA-regulatory proteins: the zinc finger, the leucine zipper, and the helix-turn-helix (found in homeotic proteins). Because of the uniqueness of these structural arrangements, their presence in a protein indicates that the protein might bind to DNA. The β sheet, β bend, and α helix are secondary structures found in polypeptide chains, and the triple helix is a tertiary structure composed of three polypeptides as in collagen.

137. The answer is c. (*Murray, pp 31-42. Scriver, pp 3-45. Lewis, pp 194-199.*) The connective tissue fiber collagen is synthesized by fibroblasts. However, because the length of the finished collagen fibers is many times greater than that of the cell of origin, a portion of assembly occurs extracellularly. The intracellular formation of the biosynthetic precursor of collagen, procollagen peptides pro-α_1(I) and pro-α_2, occurs in the following steps: (1) synthesis of polypeptides, (2) hydroxylation of proline and lysine residues, (3) glycosylation of lysine residues (proline residues are not glycosylated), (4) formation of the triple helix, and (5) secretion. Once outside the fibroblasts, procollagen molecules are activated by fibroblast-specific procollagen peptidases. Before specific proteolytic cleavage of procollagen, tropocollagen bundles do not assemble into collagen fibers. Once the collagen fibers are formed, cross-links between lysine and histidine covalently bind the collagen chains to one another. The extent and type of cross-linking determines the flexibility and strength of the collagen mass formed.

Protein Structure/Function

Questions

138. A 72-year-old African American female with emphysema presents to the emergency room with fatigue and respiratory distress. Which of the following sets of arterial blood gas values would represent her condition and reflect a shift of the hemoglobin oxygen-dissociation curve to the right?

a. pH 7.05, bicarbonate 35 mEq/L, P_{CO_2} 60, P_{O_2} 88
b. pH 7.35, bicarbonate 10 mEq/L, P_{CO_2} 30, P_{O_2} 98
c. pH 7.35, bicarbonate 15 mEq/L, P_{CO_2} 30, P_{O_2} 98
d. pH 7.4, bicarbonate 24 mEq/L, P_{CO_2} 60, P_{O_2} 88
e. pH 7.45, bicarbonate 15 mEq/L, P_{CO_2} 60, P_{O_2} 88

139. The small town doctor in the movie *Doc Hollywood* impresses the aspiring plastic surgeon by treating a cyanotic child with a soft drink, knowing the child has reduced hemoglobin from drinking well water. The ability of hemoglobin to serve as an effective transporter of oxygen and carbon dioxide between lungs and tissues is explained by which of the following properties?

a. The isolated heme group with ferrous iron binds oxygen much more avidly than carbon dioxide.
b. The α- and β-globin chains of hemoglobin have very different primary structures than myoglobin.
c. Hemoglobin utilizes oxidized ferric iron to bind oxygen, in contrast to the ferrous ion of myoglobin.
d. In contrast to myoglobin, hemoglobin exhibits greater changes in secondary and tertiary structure after oxygen binding.
e. Hemoglobin binds proportionately more oxygen at low oxygen tension than does myoglobin.

140. A 65-year-old obese Caucasian male presents with pain radiating down the left arm and shortness of breath. A serum lactate dehydrogenase (LDH) level is obtained to evaluate possible myocardial infarction, and its activity is only slightly elevated. Shortly thereafter the laboratory calls, saying that a more detailed analysis of LDH does suggest myocardial damage. The managing physician knows that lactate dehydrogenase is composed of two different polypeptide chains arranged in the form of a tetramer. Which of the following is the likely correlation between LDH measures and the likelihood of myocardial infarction?

a. LDH is an enzyme specific to the endocardium.
b. LDH is mainly localized in liver, and its elevation in cardiac disease occurs because of heart failure.
c. LDH isozymes are composed of different subunit combinations, some released during inflammation following heart attacks.
d. LDH isozymes are composed of different subunit combinations, some specific for heart and released with myocardial damage.
e. LDH isozymes are composed of different subunit combinations, some specific for vascular endothelium and released with infarction.

141. A 28-year-old Caucasian female presents to her obstetrician at week 23 of pregnancy, complaining of extreme fatigue. Evaluations of serum iron level and fetal well-being are normal, but the nurse notices a weak and irregular pulse. Chest x-ray reveals an enlarged heart and the electrocardiogram reveals a short PR interval and prolonged QRS interval, including a slurred-up stroke of the R wave called a delta wave. The ECG is read as showing Wolff-Parkinson-White syndrome, a condition with risks for paroxysmal supraventricular tachycardia. The physician considers treatment with calcium channel regulators, balancing their risks to mother and fetus. Contraction of cardiac and skeletal muscle is initiated by the binding of calcium to which of the following substances?

a. Actin
b. Actomyosin
c. Myosin
d. Tropomyosin
e. Troponin

142. A previously healthy 2-year-old Caucasian boy becomes gray and dusky looking and is brought to his physician with suspicion of heart disease. Rather than doing a cardiac evaluation, the physician asks about the family's water supply and notes they are farmers using well water. The physician then provides some oxygen and vitamin C with rapid improvement of the child's color. The child's problem was most likely due to which of the following?

a. Nitrates in well water cause reduced hemoglobin (methemoglobin) and cyanosis in all families exposed.
b. Cyanide in well water poisoning the respiratory chain.
c. Nitrates in well water interacting with heterozygous methemoglobin reductase deficiency to produce methemoglobin.
d. Nitrates in well water competing for hemoglobin oxygen binding, producing a sigmoidal binding curve.
e. Carbon dioxide released by methane fuels causing decreased hemoglobin O_2 affinity.

143. A 17-year-old African American adolescent is evaluated for anemia and is found to have increased indirect bilirubin in serum and plasma-free hemoglobin suggestive of hemolysis (lysis of red blood cells). Enzyme assays reveal deficiency of bisphosphoglycerate mutase (MIM*222800) with low concentrations of 2,3-bisphosphoglycerate (BPG) in her red blood cells. The teenager shows greater respiratory distress than expected for the degree of anemia. Which of the following statements best explains the consequences of this enzyme deficiency?

a. BPG shifts the curve to the right, so less BPG will cause greater release of oxygen to tissues.
b. BPG shifts the curve to the right, so less BPG will cause lesser release of oxygen to tissues.
c. BPG shifts the curve to the left, so less BPG will cause greater release of oxygen to tissues
d. BPG shifts the curve to the left, so less BPG will cause lesser release of oxygen to tissues.
e. BPG binds oxygen directly and has no effect on the curve.

144. A 43-year-old Caucasian male is rushed to the hospital with crushing chest pain radiating to his left arm and a probable heart attack. His cholesterol is 420 mg/dL despite prior use of statin medicines and he has familial hypercholesterolemia (MIM*143890). Which of the following treatments should be considered?

a. A platelet transfusion
b. Heparin infusion
c. Thrombin infusion
d. Fibrinogen infusion
e. Tissue plasminogen activator infusion

145. A 21-year-old Caucasian male college student presents to the health clinic with symptoms of increased urination (polyuria), avid thirst and water drinking (polydipsia), and weight loss without dieting. Significant in the family history is his father's death at age 42 of what was said to be "acute diabetes." His father's sister and a paternal aunt also have diabetes, described as adult onset or type II. Laboratory evaluation reveals increased glucose in blood (hyperglycemia), urine (glucosuria), and urinary ketones. However, Western blotting of insulin species shows normal amounts of protein with a higher molecular size than usual. Which of the following is the most likely explanation?

a. Defective processing of proinsulin to insulin, causing decreased insulin action and diabetes mellitus
b. Defective insulin-like growth factors that must act in concert with insulin
c. Defective insulin receptors with reduced insulin action
d. Progressive fibrosis of pancreatic β-cells, leading to insulin deficiency
e. Defect in processing of a pituitary hormone that contains the insulin peptide

146. Sickle cell anemia (MIM*604903) was one of the first disorders selected for newborn screening despite concerns about stigmatization from the African American community. The disease results from homozygous mutation causing substitution of valine for glutamate at position 6 on the β chain of hemoglobin, producing hemoglobin S. Which of the following techniques might be considered for hemoglobin S screening?

a. Decreased polymerization of deoxyhemoglobin
b. Altered electrophoretic mobility
c. Increased solubility of deoxyhemoglobin
d. More flexible red blood cells
e. Unchanged primary structure

147. An increased affinity of hemoglobin for O_2 may result from which of the following?

a. Acidosis
b. Lower 2,3-bisphosphoglycerate (BPG) levels within erythrocytes
c. High CO_2 levels
d. More ferric ion
e. Initial binding of O_2 to one of the four sites available in each deoxyhemoglobin molecule

148. A middle-aged man is brought to the emergency room in coma, well known to the medical staff because of alcoholism and progressive liver disease. His current measure of serum glutamine-oxalate aminotransferase (AST), an enzyme used as a marker of liver cell damage, is reported as 1500 μmol/min per mg protein, elevated but not as high as previous values in the 20,000 range. The lower AST activity contrasts with other measures of liver disease, including a serum ammonia in the 750 range (normal less than 30) and decreased amounts of coagulation factor proteins (these changes respectively account for the coma and bleeding tendencies of advanced liver disease). A call to the laboratory reveals an inexperienced technologist is on duty, who emphasizes he has performed the assay in the standard way. Which of the following is the most likely reason for the lower AST activity?

a. Measure of activity rather than specific activity
b. Inappropriate units for measure of specific activity
c. Substrate concentration similar to value of K_m
d. Lack of dilution with too much enzyme for substrate
e. Lack of dilution with too much substrate for enzyme

149. The functions of many enzymes, membrane transporters, and other proteins can be quickly activated or deactivated by phosphorylation of specific amino acid residues catalyzed by enzymes called what?

a. Cyclases
b. Kinases
c. Phosphatases
d. Proteases
e. Zymogens

150. A 65-year-old Hispanic female delays evaluation of a breast lump and presents to her physician with a fungating surface cancer. She also has severe diabetes and heart disease that prevent radical surgery, so her physician decides upon local surgery with surface chemotherapy that includes the drug fluorouracil. This agent blocks the activity of thymidylate synthase by which of the following mechanisms?

a. Allosteric inhibition
b. Competitive inhibition
c. Irreversible inhibition
d. Noncovalent inhibition
e. Noncatalytic inhibition

151. A 28-year-old female presents for evaluation after failing to become pregnant after 3 years of marriage. Her husband's sperm counts and her uterine sonogram plus clotting and hormone studies are all normal, and tubal insufflation has failed to influence fertility. Her physician then notes a positive urine reducing substance that turns out to be galactose, and orders testing of the GALT enzyme that converts UDP-galactose (substrate) to UDP-glucose (product) and is responsible for classical galactosemia (MIM*230400). The result shows a slightly low value for GALT activity with none of the common mutant alleles detected by DNA sequencing. The physician recalls the occurrence of ovarian dysfunction in galactosemia and invites collaboration with the pathologist to measure the K_m of the female's GALT enzyme to see if an alteration might justify detailed DNA sequencing studies. The amount of UDP-galactose to UDP-glucose conversion in 1 minute is measured using the same amount of enzyme (E) at 6 increasing UDP-galactose concentrations. Which of the following analyses would be most useful for determining the K_m?

a. Plot of E against S
b. Plot of $1/Vi$ versus $1/S$
c. Plot of Vi versus S
d. Plot of $1/E$ versus $1/S$
e. Plot of V_{max} versus $1/S$

152. A 28-year-old African American female develops extreme fatigue with vomiting and anorexia after eating oysters and her husband notes a yellow hue to the whites of her eyes. Her physician recognizes her jaundiced sclerae and does laboratory testing that shows a serum aspartate aminotransaminase (AST or SGOT) level of 3000 U/L (normal 15-45) along with other abnormalities that suggest liver disease. Antigen studies confirm a diagnosis of hepatitis A and the physician follows his patient with AST levels of 3050 U/L at day 2, 3075 at day 4, and 2950 at day 6. The physician is puzzled because the similar AST levels seem to show no progression of hepatitis, yet his patient has developed severe liver disease with coma due to high ammonia levels and copious bleeding from coagulopathy. Which of the following is the most likely explanation?

a. Constant liver cell death with selective effects on coagulation proteins
b. Assay of ALT enzyme with inadequate substrate levels
c. Assay of ALT enzyme with inadequate product levels
d. Inappropriate assay of ALT enzyme from dilute serum
e. Inappropriate assay of ALT enzyme from undialyzed serum

153. In the study of enzymes, a sigmoidal plot of substrate concentration ([S]) versus initial reaction velocity (V_i) may indicate which of the following?

a. Michaelis-Menten kinetics
b. Competitive inhibition
c. Noncompetitive inhibition
d. Cooperative binding
e. Suicidal inhibition where the enzyme catalyzes formation of inhibitor

154. A noncompetitive inhibitor of an enzyme does which of the following?

a. Decreases V_{max}
b. Increases V_{max}
c. Decreases K_m and decreases V_{max}
d. Increases K_m and increases V_{max}
e. Increases K_m with no or little change in V_{max}

155. In the 1980s, biochemically oriented researchers focused on the enzyme superoxide dismutase (SOD) as a potential cause of Down syndrome. The trisomy (three doses) of chromosome 21 in that disorder would produce three copies of the *SOD* gene that is located on chromosome 21. SOD acts to remove superoxide anion free radical, catalyzing the reaction of two superoxide radicals with two hydrogen ions to form hydrogen peroxide and oxygen. Reasoning that the increased SOD activity and its excess peroxide products might cause embryonic birth defects, researchers constructed a mouse with three doses of the gene encoding SOD. Instead of simulating the multiple developmental changes of Down syndrome, mice with triplicated SOD loci had no abnormalities at all. Which of the following is the most likely fallacy in this research approach?

a. SOD enzyme assays with inadequate substrate concentration.
b. Lack of attention to the concept of enzyme reserve, where most enzymes are present in excess of in vivo substrate concentrations.
c. Lack of attention to colinked peroxidase loci that will also be increased in Down syndrome.
d. Effects of human genetic mutations cannot be replicated in mice.
e. Lack of attention to potential repressive mechanisms that negate extra doses of enzyme-encoding loci.

156. A 2-year-old Caucasian girl presents with mildly enlarged liver, history of low blood sugar (hypoglycemia) on several occasions, and growth just below the third percentile for age. Evaluation for glycogen storage disease includes glycogen phosphorylase enzyme assay, which is low-normal and does not increase with addition of cyclic AMP. Which of the following is most likely?

a. Glycogen phosphorylase is activated by a cyclic AMP-regulated enzyme that is deficient in the patient.
b. Glycogen phosphorylase is an allosteric enzyme regulated by a cyclic AMP binding site that is mutated in the patient.
c. Glycogen phosphorylase gave a false normal value in the patient because it was not properly diluted to give excess substrate.
d. Glycogen phosphorylase is subject to feedback inhibition by its product cyclic AMP.
e. Glycogen is a complex substrate, so a linear relation of enzyme amount and activity cannot be expected.

157. Which of the following enzymes is regulated primarily through allosteric interaction?

a. Aspartate transcarbamoylase
b. Chymotrypsin
c. Glycogen phosphorylase
d. Glycogen synthase
e. Pyruvate dehydrogenase

158. A 28-year-old African American female and her husband have serial ultrasound studies during their last month of pregnancy because their fetus has short limbs. Their maternal-fetal medicine specialist suspects the diagnosis of achondroplasia (MIM*100800), a moderate form of dwarfism caused by mutation within the receptor domain of the fibroblast growth factor-3 receptor (*FGFR3*) gene. Unfortunately, the findings after birth suggest a more severe dwarfism with very short limbs and a small chest that does not allow adequate oxygenation. After death, a lys650-to-glu change in the FGFR3 tyrosine kinase domain is found that is consistent with the severe phenotype called thanatophoric (death-loving) dwarfism (MIM*187600). Both of these phenotypes exhibit autosomal dominant inheritance, requiring one abnormal allele at the FGFR3 locus on chromosome 4. Which of the following is a likely molecular explanation for their difference in severity?

a. Mutation at the tyrosine kinase domain rather than the saturable ligand-binding domain will have more severe effects.
b. Signal transduction through tyrosine phosphorylation is an enzyme-mediated process requiring two abnormal alleles for phenotypic effects (recessive inheritance).
c. Fibroblast growth factor-3 is a large molecule and cannot achieve saturating concentrations that would overcome receptor mutations.
d. Binding of ligands to receptors is a linear process that is independent of ligand or receptor concentration.
e. Binding of tyrosine phosphate to FGFR3 is an allosteric effect.

159. Digestive enzymes such as pepsin, trypsin, and chymotrypsin are synthesized as inactive precursors. What are the preproteins of the active enzymes termed?

a. Kinases
b. Inducers
c. Isozymes
d. Phosphatases
e. Zymogens

160. Which of the following enzymes exhibits a hyperbolic curve when initial reaction velocity is plotted against substrate concentration?

a. Aspartate transcarbamoylase
b. Phosphofructokinase
c. Hexokinase
d. Pyruvate kinase
e. Lactate dehydrogenase

161. A 7-month-old Caucasian girl has stopped growing and evaluation reveals a blood urea nitrogen (BUN) level of 36 mg/dL (normal 5-18) and a creatinine of 2.1 mg/dL (normal 0.3-0.7). She also seems sensitive to sunlight, and ophthalmologic slit lamp examination shows crystals in the eye lenses. A diagnosis of cystinosis (MIM*219800) is considered reflecting growth delay, photosensitivity with crystals in the lens of the eye, and progressive renal failure due to accumulation of cystine in cellular lysosomes. The defect involves a specific lysosomal membrane receptor that facilitates cystine egress, and an effective therapy has been found using oral cysteamine, a compound similar in structure to cystine. This therapy reflects the general principle that competitive inhibitors typically resemble the structure of which of the following?

a. Structure of enzyme or receptor protein
b. Structure of substrates or ligands that bind the enzyme/receptor
c. Structure of enzyme reaction products
d. Structure of the transition state in enzyme-catalyzed reactions
e. Structure of an allosteric regulator of enzyme/receptor activity

162. Which of the following is an accurate description for the process of rigor mortis?

a. Intracellular levels of ATP drop so ATP is not available to bind the S1 head of myosin; thus, actin does not dissociate from myosin.
b. Intracellular levels of ATP drop so ATP is not available to bind the S1 head of myosin; thus, actin dissociates from myosin.
c. Intracellular levels of ATP rise so ATP is available to bind the S1 head of myosin; thus, actin dissociates from myosin.
d. Intracellular levels of ATP rise so ATP is available to bind the S1 head of myosin; thus, actin does not dissociate from myosin.
e. Intracellular levels of ATP rise, producing more ADP that counteracts relaxation.

163. A group of congenital disorders exhibit multiple joint contractures at birth, described by the term 'arthrogryposis' (arthro = joint, gryposis = contracture). A subgroup involves decreased fetal muscle function with resulting deformation (contracture) of the limbs by surrounding uterine forces to produce deviated hands, club feet, etc. Mutations, in which of the following proteins or protein fragments would be most likely in an otherwise normal neonate with arthrogryposis due to skeletal muscle dysfunction?

a. Light meromyosin component of myosin II
b. S-2 fragment of myosin-II
c. Troponin complex proteins
d. Tropomyosin
e. Myosin-I.

164. Inherited deficiency of the enzyme methylmalonyl-CoA mutase (MMACoA mutase, MIM*251000) causes serum and urine accumulation of methylmalonic acid with acidosis, neurologic degeneration, and death. Recognition that pernicious anemia (due to deficiency of vitamin B_{12}) can involve accumulation of methylmalonic acid led to successful treatment of some patients with MMACoA mutase deficiency using excess B_{12}. Studies of purified MMACoA mutase enzyme from normal patients then showed enhanced mutase activity when B_{12} was added to the reaction mixture. These facts are best reconciled by which of the following explanations?

a. Vitamin B_{12} is a precursor for methylmalonic acid synthesis.
b. Vitamin B_{12} is a prosthetic group for the enzyme MMACoA mutase.
c. Vitamin B_{12} is a cofactor for the MMACoA mutase enzyme.
d. Vitamin B_{12} is a competitive inhibitor of MMACoA mutase enzyme.
e. Vitamin B_{12} is a feedback inhibitor of MMACoA mutase enzyme.

Protein Structure/Function

Answers

138. The answer is a. (*Murray, pp 43-50, 545-565. Scriver, pp 4571-4636.*) The female would exhibit respiratory acidosis due to shortness of breath and decreased efficiency of gas exchange in the lungs. This would yield low oxygen saturation with retention of carbon dioxide (incorrect answers b and c) and lower pH (incorrect answers d and e). Emphysema involves dilated and dysfunctional alveoli from alveolar tissue damage, usually secondary to cigarette smoking. The hypoxia leads to tissue deoxygenation and acidosis, exacerbated by the hypercarbia (CO_2 accumulation) that distinguishes respiratory acidosis (higher bicarbonate than expected) from metabolic acidosis (very low bicarbonate, usually with low P_{CO_2} due to compensatory hyperventilation). The increased temperature and BPG in exercising muscle have similar effects.

The tetrameric structure of hemoglobin allows cooperative binding of oxygen in that binding of oxygen to the heme molecule of the first subunit facilitates binding to the other three. This enhanced binding is due to allosteric changes of the hemoglobin molecule, accounting for its S-shaped oxygen-saturation curve as compared with that of myoglobin (see Fig. 8 of the High-Yield Facts). At the lower oxygen saturations in peripheral tissues (P_{O_2} 30-40), hemoglobin releases much more oxygen (up to 50% desaturated) than myoglobin with its single polypeptide structure. The amount of oxygen released (and CO_2 absorbed as carboxyhemoglobin) is further increased by the Bohr effect—increasing hydrogen ion (H^+) concentration (lowering pH) and increasing CO_2 partial pressure (P_{CO_2}) shift the sigmoidal-shaped oxygen-binding curve for hemoglobin further to the right.

139. The answer is d. (*Murray, pp 43-50. Scriver, pp 4571-4636.*) Successive binding of oxygen atoms to hemoglobin progressively changes the tertiary and quaternary structure to produce cooperative kinetics and a sigmoidal oxygen-binding curve. This cooperativity does not occur with the subunits of myoglobin despite similar primary and secondary protein structure (incorrect answer b). Hemoglobin thus binds proportionately less oxygen within the capillaries of low-oxygen peripheral tissues and allows more oxygen delivery to these tissues (incorrect answer e). Isolated heme binds carbon dioxide 25,000 times more strongly than oxygen, but in myoglobin and each hemoglobin chain, a histidine group interferes with the preferred mode of carbon dioxide binding such that oxygen is favored (incorrect answer a). Oxidation of the ferrous iron in myoglobin or hemoglobin to ferric ion abolishes oxygen binding, in contrast to the case with other proteins like cytochromes or catalase, where oxidation/reduction of iron modulates their function (incorrect answer c). Nitrates in well water inhibit methemoglobin reductase and increase the percentage of hemoglobin with ferric ion (methemoglobin). Some mutant hemoglobins like hemoglobin M stabilize the ferric ion and produce more peripheral cyanosis.

140. The answer is d. (*Murray, pp 31-42. Scriver, pp 4571-4636.*) Isozymes are multiple forms of a given enzyme that occur within a given species. Since isozymes are composed of different proteins, analysis by electrophoretic separation can be done. Lactate dehydrogenase is a tetramer composed of any combination of two different polypeptides, H and M. Thus the possible combinations are H4, H3M1, H2M2, H1M3, and M4. Although each combination is found in most tissues, M4 predominates in the liver and skeletal muscle, whereas H4 is the predominant form in the heart. White and red blood cells as well as brain cells contain primarily intermediate forms. The M4 forms of the isozyme seem to have a higher affinity for pyruvate compared with the H4 form. Following a myocardial infarction, the H4 (LDH1) type of lactate dehydrogenase rises and reaches a peak approximately 36 hours later. Elevated LDH1 levels (increased H4 relative to other isoforms) may signal myocardial disease even when the total lactate dehydrogenase level is normal.

141. The answer is e. (*Murray, pp 545-565. Scriver, pp 4571-4636.*) Calcium ions are the regulators of contraction of skeletal muscle. Calcium is actively sequestered in sarcoplasmic reticulum by an ATP pump during relaxation of muscle. Nervous stimulation leads to the release of calcium into the cytosol and raises the concentration from less than 1 mM to about 10 mM. The calcium binds to troponin C. The calcium-troponin complex undergoes a conformational change, which is transmitted to tropomyosin and causes tropomyosin to shift position. The shift of tropomyosin allows actin to interact with myosin and contraction to proceed.

Mutations affecting proteins involved in muscle contraction can present with low muscle tone and developmental delay in childhood, as chronic muscle cramps or fatigue, or with cardiomyopathies due to weakened heart muscle. Since cardiac muscle contraction is coordinated by electrical conduction from the sinus and atrioventricular nodes, muscle protein abnormalities can also interfere with cardiac rhythm. A specific mutation in troponin I can cause cardiomyopathy and the irregular cardiac rhythm known as Wolff-Parkinson-White syndrome (MIM*600858).

142. The answer is c. *(Murray, pp 43-50. Scriver, pp 4571-4636.)* Oxidizing agents can convert hemoglobin from its ferrous iron (Fe^{2+}) form to the ferric ion (Fe^{3+}) form (methemoglobinemia) that has poor oxygen-carrying capacity. Methemoglobin reductases in the red cell (with NADP or NADPH and cytochrome cofactors) keep the hemoglobin reduced. Autosomal dominant-acting mutations in the globin peptides, autosomal recessive deficiencies of methemoglobin reductase (eg, MIM*250800), or exogenous oxidizing agents (nitrates in well water) can produce significant amounts of methemoglobinemia with reduced blood oxygen and cyanosis. Vitamins C, E, and other antioxidants can oppose the action of oxidizing agents. Children who get severe methemoglobinemia from well-water nitrates are heterozygotes (carriers) for methemoglobin reductase deficiency.

143. The answer is b. *(Murray, pp 43-50. Scriver, pp 4571-4636.)* BPG (2,3 bisphosphoglycerate) binds to and stabilizes deoxyhemoglobin (incorrect answer e), shifting the oxygen-dissociation curve of hemoglobin to the right (incorrect answers c, d) and allowing more oxygen delivery to tissues where oxygen tensions are low (incorrect answer a). Individuals with lower levels of BPG mutase cannot increase erythrocyte BPG in low-oxygen tissues and thus have less oxygen delivery.

The oxygen-binding curve of myoglobin and hemoglobin, percent oxygen saturation on the y-axis is plotted against the partial pressure of oxygen (PO_2), see Fig. 8 of High-Yield Facts. At a low oxygen pressure, that is, 20 mm Hg, hemoglobin has much less oxygen (less oxygen saturated) than myoglobin, allowing that oxygen to be displaced from red blood cells to the surrounding tissues. Low oxygen conditions as in the peripheral tissues stimulates BPG mutase and increases 2,3-bisphosphoglycerate (BPG), cross-linking deoxyhemoglobin and aiding the shift of oxygen to peripheral tissue (shift of the oxygen-dissociation curve to the right. Other factors include increased H^+ ions (lower pH in tissues) and increased CO_2 that enhance the release of O_2 from hemoglobin with shift of the curve to the right and better oxygen delivery. Conversely, the lower H^+ levels with increasing pH and decreasing CO_2 shift the curve leftward. Fetal hemoglobin has a greater affinity for O_2 that facilitates materno-fetal transfer.

144. The answer is e. *(Murray, pp 583-592. Scriver, pp 2863-2914.)* Many enzymes interact to regulate blood clotting. Plasmin is activated by proteolytic cleavage of its zymogen, plasminogen. The activating protease is called tissue plasminogen activator (tPA). Plasmin hydrolyzes fibrin clots to form soluble products and is used to dissolve clots in coronary arteries that cause myocardial infarction. Platelets, thrombin, and fibrinogen promote clotting through the intrinsic pathway and would be contraindicated in myocardial infarction. Platelets form a plug at the site of bleeding and bind prothrombin to facilitate its conversion to thrombin. Fibrinogen is the substrate acted on by thrombin to yield the fibrin mesh of blood clots. Heparin is a mucopolysaccharide that terminates clot formation by interfering with a number of steps in the coagulation cascade. Heparin inhibits the formation of clots, but cannot dissolve clots that have already formed.

145. The answer is a. *(Murray, pp 43-50. Scriver, pp 4571-4636.)* The higher molecular size suggests an abnormally processed insulin rather than reduced synthesis or signaling implied by answers b to d; insulin is produced in the pancreas rather than the pituitary (incorrect answer e). Insulin is secreted from the pancreatic β-cells as a propeptide called proinsulin with contiguous N-terminal A peptide, internal C peptide, and C-terminal B peptide. During processing, the C peptide is removed with joining of the A and B peptides (at sulfhydryl bonds) to form mature insulin. C peptide is thus a marker for endogenous insulin production rather than synthetic, exogenous insulins that will have the A and B peptides. Rare families will exhibit autosomal dominant inheritance of mild, adult-onset diabetes due to decreased proinsulin processing and reduced amounts of insulin. They will have increased amounts of proinsulin in their blood, so the disease is called hyperproinsulinemia (MIM*176730). These individuals will be like juvenile diabetics who do not make insulin, but milder because they have one allele defective in the putative peptidase that processes proinsulin and another allele that is normal. They will respond normally to insulin, unlike many type II adult-onset diabetics who exhibit insulin resistance in their tissues.

146. The answer is b. (*Murray, pp 43-50. Scriver, pp 4571-4636.*) Substitution of uncharged valine for glutamate (change of primary structure eliminating answer e) by mutation produces sickle cell hemoglobin, which is less negatively charged and has an increased electrophoretic mobility. Increased polymerization of the deoxygenated form of sickle hemoglobin (incorrect answer a) occurs owing to the alteration of primary structure caused by the valine substitution. The polymerized hemoglobin is more insoluble (incorrect answer c) and produces less flexible erythrocytes (incorrect answer d) that become rigid and sickle shaped. Newborn screening must rely on blood spots placed on filter paper through heel sticks, so detection of small amounts of hemoglobin S in the presence of excess fetal hemoglobin requires sensitive high pressure liquid chromatography.

147. The answer is e. (*Murray, pp 43-50. Scriver, pp 4571-4636.*) The addition of each O_2 molecule to deoxyhemoglobin requires the breakage of salt links, such as those formed by 2,3-BPG. Each subsequent O_2 molecule requires the breakage of fewer salt links. Thus, initial O_2 binding actually results in an increased affinity for subsequent O_2 binding, which in turn produces "cooperativity" and a sigmoidal shape to the oxygen-binding curve. The lower pH of acidosis (incorrect answer b), higher carbon dioxide levels (incorrect answer c), lower BPG levels (incorrect answer b), and more ferric ion (incorrect answer d) all cause less affinity for oxygen—all but the latter option occur in peripheral tissues to facilitate oxygen delivery.

BPG binds specifically to deoxyhemoglobin; that is, BPG cross-links positively charged residues on the β chain, thereby decreasing oxygen affinity and stabilizing the deoxygenated form of hemoglobin. CO_2 reacts reversibly with the amino acid terminals of hemoglobin to create carbaminohemoglobin, which is negatively charged and which forms salt bridges, stabilizing deoxyhemoglobin. Hence, CO_2 binding lowers the affinity of hemoglobin for O_2.

148. The answer is d. (*Murray, pp 62-74. Scriver, pp 4571-4636.*) Enzyme assays require excess substrate such that the initial conversion of substrate to product will be maximal (V_{max}) and linear with time (substrate concentration [S] much above that concentration giving half-maximal reaction velocity = K_m). Substrate concentrations are usually expressed in terms of molarity, for example, M = moles per liter, mM = millimoles per liter, μM = micromoles per liter. K_m, the Michaelis constant, is expressed in terms of substrate concentration. Under these reaction conditions, each unit of enzyme activity represents the amount of enzyme that converts a specific amount of substrate to a product within a given time. The standard units of activity are micromoles of substrate per minute. Specific activity relates the units of enzyme activity to the amount of protein present in the reaction, expressed as units of enzyme activity per milligram of protein. If the enzyme is pure (no proteins except the assayed enzyme are present), then the specific activity is maximal and constant for that particular enzyme (units of activity per milligram of enzyme). Serum contains a complex mixture of enzymes and proteins, so the specific activity of enzymes like AST is related to milligrams of total serum protein. In severe liver disease with hepatocellular damage, large amounts of AST enzyme is released, causing excess enzyme in the amount of serum protein aliquoted into the standard assay. The hyperbolic relation of enzyme amount with reaction rate results in a plateau with excess enzyme, requiring that the serum be serially diluted until SGOT activity is linear with time. Without dilution, all enzyme amounts above the saturating value will measure as the same limiting activity, giving an underestimate of true AST activity. Other factors affecting AST activity will include small overestimates as the total serum protein decreases with liver disease (most proteins are synthesized in the liver) and eventual destruction of all liver cells (cirrhosis) so that there is no new enzyme to be released.

149. The answer is b. (*Murray, pp 75-83. Scriver, pp 4571-4636.*) A variety of highly regulated protein kinases can cause activation or deactivation of certain key regulatory proteins by covalent modification of specific serine, threonine, or tyrosine hydroxyl residues by phosphorylation. For example, skeletal muscle glycogen phosphorylase b is activated by phosphorylation of a single serine residue (serine 14) in each subunit of the dimers composing the enzyme. The phosphorylation reaction itself is catalyzed by phosphorylase kinase. Protein phosphatases can quickly reverse such effects. Activated muscle glycogen phosphorylase a is deactivated by a specific phosphatase that hydrolyzes the phosphoryl group of serine 14. Whether the phosphorylated or dephosphorylated form of a protein predominates depends on the relative activities of the kinase versus the phosphatase.

150. The answer is c. (*Murray, pp 75-83. Scriver, pp 4571-4636.*) Rapidly multiplying cancer cells spend increased time in S phase with DNA replication and are thus dependent on the synthesis of deoxythymidylate (dTMP) from deoxyuridylate (dUMP), the enzyme catalyzing this step (thymidylate kinase) is a prime target in cancer therapy. The anticancer drug fluorouracil is converted in vivo to fluorodeoxyuridylate (FdUMP), which is an analogue of dUMP. FdUMP irreversibly forms a covalent complex with the enzyme thymidylate synthase and its cofactor N5,N10-methylene-tetrahydrofolate (eliminating answers a-b, d-e). This is a case of suicide inhibition, where an enzyme actually participates in the change of a substrate into a covalently linked inhibitor that irreversibly inhibits its catalytic activity.

151. The answer is b. (*Murray, pp 62-74. Scriver, pp 4571-4636.*) Clinical measures of enzyme activity must ensure excess substrate and brief assay periods to ensure maximal reaction velocity. This ensures the measured activity is proportionate to the amount of enzyme in a given tissue or fluid and reflects the catalytic efficiency of the enzyme. Measure of reaction velocity during brief periods provides an initial reaction velocity (V_i) before substrate concentration (S) is depleted, and measuring V_i with increasing substrate concentrations gives a hyperbolic saturation curve that asymptotically approaches maximal reaction velocity (V_{max}) for that amount of enzyme (see Fig. 9A of the High-Yield Facts). Measure of the substrate concentration S that gives half-maximal reaction velocity (K_m) requires estimation of V_{max} from the asymptote (incorrect answer c) and is thus more accurate using the reciprocal Lineweaver-Burk plot of $1/V_i$ versus $1/S$ (Fig. 9B) where $1/V_{max}$ is the intercept on the y-axis and $-1/K_m$ the intercept on the x-axis (eliminating answers a, d, e). Mutations affecting enzyme conformation and/or its binding site with substrate alter the K_m and reduce the reaction velocity at usual tissue substrate levels. Removal of lactose from the diet of patients with galactosemia prevents mental retardation and liver disease but not female infertility.

152. The answer is b. (*Murray, pp 62-74. Scriver, pp 4571-4636.*) In order to use enzyme activity as a measure of enzyme amount, substrate must be in sufficient excess to saturate the enzyme (incorrect answer c). Fluids with high enzyme concentrations must be diluted to ensure adequate substrate excess (incorrect answer d), and dialysis of serum would remove small molecular weight inhibitors but would not dilute serum AST to ensure saturating substrate levels (incorrect answer e). If substrate concentrations are not saturating and limit the initial reaction velocity, then increasing enzyme amounts will not produce increased activity. Liver cell death and release of

AST enzyme in hepatitis may peak to accurately reflect enzyme. Adequate dilution of serum until the AST activity was proportionate to serum protein added would reveal increasing AST activity proportionate to increased AST released by progressive liver cell death in hepatitis (incorrect answer a). Severe liver damage will reduce liver protein synthesis that is essential to produce several coagulation factors. Clinical measures of enzyme activity often look for deficient/ineffective enzyme as with inborn errors of metabolism or abnormal levels of serum enzymes as a marker of tissue death; each requires saturating substrate (at the asymptotic part of the curve in Fig. 9A of the High-Yield Facts) so that activity reflects enzyme amounts.

153. The answer is d. *(Murray, pp 62-74. Scriver, pp 4571-4636.)* Allosteric enzymes often have several binding sites for substrate and/or cofactors, such that one active site positively affects another active site in the same molecule. This leads to cooperativity and sigmoidal enzyme kinetics in a plot of substrate [S] versus initial reaction velocity [Vi]. The terms competitive inhibition and noncompetitive inhibition apply to Michaelis-Menten kinetics and not to allosteric enzymes (incorrect answers a-c). Suicidal inhibition where a substrate is converted to inhibitor would simulate competitive inhibition with Michaelis-Menten kinetics (incorrect answer d).

154. The answer is a. *(Murray, pp 62-74. Scriver, pp 4571-4636.)* In contrast to competitive inhibitors, noncompetitive inhibitors are not structural analogues of the substrate. Consequently, noncompetitive inhibitors bind to enzymes in locations remote from the active site. For this reason, the degree of inhibition is based solely upon the concentration of inhibitor and increasing the substrate concentrations do not compete with or change the inhibition. Therefore, unlike the increase in K_m seen with competitive inhibition, in noncompetitive inhibition V_{max} decreases while K_m usually remains the same. While competitive inhibitors can be overcome at sufficiently high concentration of substrate, noncompetitive inhibition is irreversible.

155. The answer is b. *(Murray, pp 62-74. Scriver, pp 4571-4636.)* Nearly all enzymes in mammalian cells are present in excess of that needed for maximal reaction rates with in vivo substrate concentrations, a state called enzyme reserve. This is why nearly all metabolic disorders caused by enzyme deficiencies are inherited as autosomal recessive; mutation of one allele leaves another normal allele with 50% of enzyme amounts, still enough for maximal reaction. Although many human genes are conserved in mice, differences in gene regulation/interaction can cause even simple disease mutations (eg, those causing cystic fibrosis, sickle cell anemia) to have minimal effects in mice.

156. The answer is a. *(Murray, pp 62-74. Scriver, pp 4571-4636.)* Phosphorylase kinase is a cyclic AMP-regulated enzyme that converts inactive phosphorylase b to active phosphorylase a. (incorrect answers c-e). Phosphorylase kinase is an allosteric enzyme regulated by cAMP but phosphorylase is activated or deactivated by kinases that add (phosphorylase kinase) or remove (phosphoprotein phosphatase) a phosphate from the enzyme. Glycogen phosphorylase is thus directly regulated by phosphorylation through allosteric modulation of phosphorylase kinase activity (incorrect answer b). In liver, glucagon triggered by low glucose levels increases cAMP and phosphorylase kinase activity; in muscle, norepinephrine released by stress (flight or fright) stimulates phosphorylase kinase to activate phosphorylase and release glucose for muscle activity. Several types of mutations alter activity of glycogen phosphorylase or its kinase including those of glycogen storage disease type IV (MIM*232700).

157. The answer is a. *(Murray, pp 75-83. Scriver, pp 4571-4636.)* Aspartate transcarbamoylase, which controls the rate of pyrimidine synthesis in mammals, is negatively inhibited by the allosteric effector cytidine triphosphate, an end product of pyrimidine synthesis. The allosteric modulation occurs via the binding of effectors at the regulatory site of the enzyme. Noncovalent bonds are formed during the binding between effector and enzyme. In contrast, all the other enzymes are activated or deactivated by covalent modification. Chymotrypsinogen is secreted as an inactive proenzyme (zymogen) in pancreatic juice and is irreversibly activated by trypsin cleavage of a specific peptide bond. Glycogen phosphorylase is reversibly activated by phosphorylation of a specific serine residue. At the same time, glycogen synthase is reversibly deactivated by phosphorylation of a specific serine residue, thereby preventing a futile cycle of breakdown and resynthesis of glycogen. Pyruvate dehydrogenase also is reversibly inactivated by phosphorylation of a specific serine residue. In all four enzymes, a single, discrete, covalent modification leads to conformational changes that allow the switching on or off of enzyme activity.

158. The answer is a. (*Murray, pp 75-83. Scriver, pp 4571-4636.*) Binding of ligands like FGFR3 to their receptors is a saturable process like enzyme-substrate binding; mutations affecting the receptor are thus better compensated by increased ligand concentration as opposed to those in the tyrosine kinase site that interrupt signal transduction (incorrect answers b-e). The single abnormal allele implied by autosomal dominant inheritance is likely to be more severe when it affects the kinase site (as in thanatophoric dwarfism, MIM*187600) than when it affects the receptor site (as in achondroplasia, MIM*100800). Ligand-receptor reciprocal plots analogous to those for enzyme reactions can reveal saturating ligand concentrations and the number of ligand molecules bound per receptor molecule. Reduction in the number of FGF3 receptors by 50% may be compensated by higher extracellular ligand concentrations as opposed to a 50% reduction in functional kinase sites that may not be sufficient for the all-or-none process of signal transduction.

Many events of cell growth/metabolism, including those of differentiation and embryonic development, are controlled by signal transduction. A smaller signal molecule (ligand) interacts with membrane, intracellular, or nuclear receptors to initiate a cascade of protein changes. Ligand binding can initiate conformational changes in the receptor, activating processes like DNA binding (transcriptional activation/repression), membrane permeability (transport, conductivity), or cascades of protein phosphorylation (ATP, GTP, cAMP-mediated kinase reactions). Protein conformational changes are rapid, with cascades "channeled" within protein complexes so as to be obligate and unresponsive to surrounding metabolites.

159. The answer is e. (*Murray, pp 75-83*) These digestive enzymes are proteases and are secreted as inactive zymogens; the active site of the enzyme is masked by a small region of its peptide chain, which is removed by hydrolysis of a specific peptide bond. Synthesis of proteases as zymogens is a mechanism that ensures that proteases will only be active when and where they are needed as inappropriate protease activity would be expected to have a very deleterious effect on the cell.

160. The answer is e. (*Murray, pp 75-83. Scriver, pp 4571-4636.*) Nonregulatory enzymes, such as lactate dehydrogenase, typically exhibit a hyperbolic saturation curve when initial velocity is plotted against substrate concentration (see Fig. 9A of the High-Yield Facts). Enzymes at key points in metabolic pathways are typically allosteric—their velocities at a given substrate concentration may be altered due to effects of metabolites in the pathway. Allosteric enzymes typically exhibit sigmoidal kinetics. Examples of allosteric enzymes include aspartate transcarbamoylase, which is inhibited by cytidine triphosphate (CTP); phosphofructokinase, which is inhibited by adenosine triphosphate (ATP) and activated by fructose 2,6-bisphosphate; hexokinase, which is inhibited by glucose-6-phosphate; and pyruvate kinase, which is inhibited by ATP. Allosteric enzymes produce sigmoidal kinetics when substrate concentration is plotted against reaction velocity. In contrast, hyperbolic plots are observed with Michaelis-Menten enzymes. The binding of effector molecules, such as end products or second messengers, to regulatory subunits of allosteric enzymes can either positively or negatively regulate catalytic subunits.

161. The answer is b. (*Murray, pp 75-83.*) Ligand-receptor and substrate-enzyme reactions are both saturable processes with similar dependence of reaction rate on ligand/substrate and receptor/substrate concentrations. Competitive inhibitors function by resembling to the substrate, binding to the active site without undergoing catalysis or transport, and thereby blocking access to the substrate (incorrect answers a, c-e). Thus, the structures of competitive inhibitors tend to resemble the structures of the substrate and are often called substrate or ligand analogues. The effects of competitive inhibitors can be overcome by raising the concentration of the substrate, and Lineweaver-Burk plots like those in Fig. 10 of the High-Yield Facts can distinguish competitive inhibitors that can be overcome to yield the same V_{max} (different K_m for substrate when inhibitor is present) from noncompetitive inhibitors that act outside the substrate-binding site (same substrate K_m but lower V_{max} in the presence of inhibitor).

The amount the substrate must be increased to overcome inhibition is dependent on the concentration of the inhibitor, the affinity of the inhibitor for the enzyme, and the affinity of the substrate for the enzyme. For membrane receptors like that in the lysosome that is defective in cystinosis (MIM*219800), the reaction may be one of membrane transport such that internal substrate/ligand is in equilibrium with external substrate/ligand. Thus lysosome-internal cystine is substrate and lysosomal-external cystine a product, in a sense, such that lysosomal-external cysteamine will effectively decrease external cystine concentration and lead to egress of lysosomal cystine through its defective transporter.

162. The answer is a. (*Murray, pp 545-565. Scriver, pp 5493-5496.*) Rigor mortis is the stiffening of the body that occurs after death. Intracellular levels of ATP drop after death so that ATP is not available to bind the S1 head of myosin (incorrect answers c-e). Actin then cannot dissociate and remains bound to myosin (incorrect answer b); skeletal muscle remains contracted because relaxation (where ATP bound to myosin complex is hydrolyzed to ADP and P_i) cannot occur.

163. The answer is c. (*Murray, pp 545-565. Scriver, pp 5493-5496.*) Among 12 classes of myosin found in the human genome, myosin-II is in skeletal muscle while myosin-I binds to cell membranes and connects with cell adhesion components (incorrect answer e). Trypsin cleavage of myosin-II from skeletal muscle yields light meromyosin and the S-2 fragment that have no ATPase activity (incorrect answers a, b), plus the S-1 fragment and heavy meromyosin that do have ATPase activity and participate more directly in the contraction/relaxation cycle. Tropomyosin is present in all muscle-like structures, so mutations would disrupt function outside of skeletal muscle (incorrect answer d). The troponin complex is unique to skeletal muscle, including troponin C that is a calcium-binding protein.

In the relaxation phase of skeletal muscle contraction, the S1 head of myosin hydrolyzes ATP to ADP and P_i, but the products remain bound. When contraction is stimulated (via the regulatory role of calcium (mediated by troponin C), actin becomes accessible and the actin-myosin ADP-P_i complex is formed. Conformational change in the head of myosin results in the power stroke with sliding of thick and thin filaments across one another through cross-bridges.

164. The answer is c. (*Murray, pp 75-83.*) Small molecules may be integral parts of enzymes (prosthetic groups) or cofactors that participate in enzyme-substrate interaction or conversion. Prosthetic groups cannot be dissociated from the enzyme by dilution and thus will not be obvious components of the enzyme reaction when reconstituted in the test tube. Cofactors, like vitamin B_{12} for methylmalonyl-CoA mutase, associate reversibly with enzymes or substrates and can be added in vitro to obtain enhancement of the catalyzed reaction(s). Competitive or feedback inhibitors interact at substrate or allosteric binding sites of the enzyme, reducing effective substrate concentration and reaction rate or converting the enzyme to a less active conformation. Vitamin B_{12} (cyanocobalamin) is a cofactor for MMACoA mutase, accelerating the conversion of methylmalonic acid to succinyl-CoA through activity of its cobalt group. Certain defects in MMA-CoA mutase can be ameliorated by intramuscular B_{12} injections so that effective B_{12} concentration and mutase activity are increased.

Carbohydrate Metabolism

Questions

165. A previously normal 2-month-old Caucasian girl is evaluated because of jittery spells (trembling, irritability) several hours after meals. A low blood glucose value is noted, and physical examination demonstrates a liver edge some two finger breadths below the right costal margin. Percussion of the right chest and abdomen confirms that the liver width is slightly enlarged. Hospital testing reveals that the infant can increase her blood glucose after breast-feeding but that it is not maintained at normal levels 3 to 4 hours after feeding. Which of the following is the most likely diagnosis?

a. Intestinal malabsorption of lactose
b. Galactosemia with inability to convert lactose to glucose
c. Fructosemia with inability to liberate sucrose from glucose
d. Glycogen storage disease
e. Diabetes mellitus with inability to maintain glucose

166. Diarrhea from infection or malnutrition is the world's most prevalent killer of children. A 2-month-old Caucasian girl develops chronic diarrhea and liver inflammation in early infancy when the mother begins using formula that includes corn syrup. Evaluation of the child demonstrates sensitivity to fructose in the diet. Which of the following glycosides contains fructose and therefore should be avoided when feeding or treating this infant?

a. Sucrose
b. Ouabain
c. Lactose
d. Maltose
e. Streptomycin

167. Which of the following carbohydrates would be most abundant in the diet of strict vegetarians?

a. Amylose
b. Lactose
c. Cellulose
d. Maltose
e. Glycogen

168. A 13-year-old African American adolescent is brought in by his parents after his physical education teacher gives him a failing grade. The teacher has scolded him for malingering because he drops out of activities after a few minutes of exercise, complaining of leg cramps and fatigue. A stress test is arranged with sampling of blood metabolites and monitoring of exercise performance. Which of the following results after exercise would support a diagnosis of glycogen storage disease in this teenager?

a. Increased oxaloacetate, decreased glucose
b. Increased glycerol and glucose
c. Increased lactate and glucose
d. Increased pyruvate and stable glucose
e. Stable lactate and glucose

169. Alcohol abuse affects over 13% of adults in the United States, costing more health care dollars ($184 billion annually) than cancer ($107 billion) or obesity ($100 billion) in some studies. In 2001, 47% of those between ages 12 and 20 years reported drinking, 30% of these to binge drinking in the past month. Chronic alcoholics require more ethanol than do non-drinkers to become intoxicated because of a higher level of a specific enzyme. However, independent of specific enzyme levels, the availability of what other substance is rate-limiting in the clearance of ethanol?

a. NADH
b. NAD$^+$
c. FADH
d. FAD$^+$
e. NADPH

170. In lung diseases such as emphysema or chronic bronchitis, there is chronic hypoxia that is particularly obvious in vascular tissues such as the lips or nail beds (cyanosis). Certain genetic diseases like α_1-antitrypsin deficiency (MIM*107400) predispose to emphysema, as do environmental exposures like cigarette smoking or asbestos. Poorly perfused areas exposed to chronic hypoxia have decreased metabolic energy for tissue maintenance and repair. Which of the following is an important reason for this?

a. Increased hexokinase activity owing to increased oxidative phosphorylation
b. Increased ethanol formation from pyruvate on changing from anaerobic to aerobic metabolism
c. Increased glucose utilization via the pentose phosphate pathway on changing from anaerobic to aerobic metabolism
d. Decreased ATP generation and increased glucose utilization on changing from aerobic to anaerobic metabolism
e. Decreased respiratory quotient on changing from carbohydrate to fat as the major metabolic fuel

171. Following a fad diet meal of skim milk and yogurt, a 15-year-old African American adolescent experiences abdominal distention, nausea, cramping, and pain followed by a watery diarrhea. This set of symptoms is observed each time the meal is consumed. Which of the following is the most likely diagnosis?

a. Steatorrhea
b. Lactase deficiency
c. Maltose deficiency
d. Sialidase deficiency
e. Lipoprotein lipase deficiency

172. An 18-year-old Korean college student attends a fraternity party and is embarrassed because he becomes flushed and sick to his stomach after his first drink of alcohol. He learns that this reaction is due to genetic variation in some Asians and Native Americans that affects metabolism of a metabolite of alcohol. Which of the following is the variably degraded metabolite?

a. Methanol
b. Acetone
c. Acetaldehyde
d. Hydrogen peroxide
e. Glycerol

173. A 6-month-old Caucasian girl is hospitalized for evaluation of short stature, enlarged liver, and intermittent lethargy/irritability that on a recent emergency room visit was accompanied by low blood glucose (hypoglycemia). In the same ward is a 6-year-old African American boy who is being evaluated for severe muscle cramping that raised suspicions for sickle cell disease. The family history is unremarkable for these children; each has a normal sibling and normal parents. Both children are given diagnoses of glycogen storage disease with the infant girl having type I (MIM*232200) affecting liver and the older boy type V (McArdle disease, MIM*232600) affecting mainly muscle. Which of the following conversions explains the difference in these presentations?

a. Glycogen to lactate in liver
b. Glycogen and lactate to glucose in liver
c. Glycogen to glucose in muscle
d. Glycogen to alanine in muscle
e. Glycogen to glucose 6-phosphate in liver

174. An 18-year-old African American female is evaluated for her first prenatal visit and is found to have chronic anemia, a slightly enlarged spleen, increased reticulocyte count, and mild elevation of indirect-reacting (unconjugated) bilirubin in serum. Incubation of the female's red cells with glucose yields decreased amounts of ATP as compared to controls, even in the presence of oxygen. The female's anemia is explained by the fact that ATP is produced by which of the following pathways?

a. Glycogen breakdown
b. Glycolysis
c. Oxidative phosphorylation
d. Pentose phosphate cycle
e. Lactate conversion to glucose (Cori cycle)

175. A 3-day-old boy from an Iraqi refugee family exhibits severe tissue swelling (edema), rapid heart rate (tachycardia), enlargement of liver and spleen (hepatosplenomegaly), and jaundice of the eyes and skin. The couple had two prior female infants who are alive and well, and the wife relates that she lost a brother in infancy with severe hemolysis induced after a viral infection. Blood tests show hemoglobin of 5 g/dL (normal neonate mean 18.5) with reticulocyte count of 15% (normal 1.8-4.6). Exchange transfusion is attempted but the child suffers cardiac arrest. Postmortem assay of red cell enzymes confirms the suspected diagnosis of glucose-6-phosphate dehydrogenase deficiency (MIM*305900), implying defective synthesis of which of the following compounds?

a. Deoxyribose and NADP
b. Glucose and lactate
c. Lactose and NADPH
d. Ribose and NADPH
e. Sucrose and NAD

176. A 2-day-old Caucasian girl begins vomiting after feeding, becomes severely jaundiced, has liver disease, and cloudy lenses of the eyes suggestive of cataracts. Treatment for possible sepsis is initiated, and the urine is found to have reducing substances. A blood screen for galactosemia (MIM*230400) is positive, and lactose-containing substances are removed from the diet. Lactose is toxic in this case because of which of the following?

a. Excess glucose accumulates in the blood.
b. Galactose is converted to the toxic substance galactitol (dulcitol).
c. Galactose competes for glucose during hepatic glycogen synthesis.
d. Galactose is itself toxic in even small amounts.
e. Glucose metabolism is shut down by excess galactose.

177. Which of the following best explains why fructose was formerly recommended for patients with diabetes mellitus?

a. Fructose is a better substrate for hexokinase.
b. Fructose stimulates residual insulin release.
c. Fructose has a specific kinase in liver that allows bypass of phosphofructokinase.
d. Fructose is phosphorylated and cleaved to triose phosphates, which cannot be used for gluconeogenesis.
e. Hexokinase phosphorylates fructose in extrahepatic tissues, and its activity will not be affected by high glucose concentrations in diabetes.

178. A 6-month-old Hispanic female infant begins having trembling with irritability (jittery spells) and vomiting after certain meals including baby food containing fruits. She showed a falloff in growth when pureed fruits and vegetables were introduced at age 4 months. She is hospitalized for evaluation, and blood obtained for testing when she exhibits tremors and irritability after a typical feeding. Serum glucose is 40 g/dL (normal 60-100) and plasma lactate 35 g/dL (normal 5-20), causing her physician to suspect hereditary fructose intolerance (MIM*229600—a deficiency of the enzyme aldolase B). The symptoms and serum abnormalities of this disease are due to which of the following?

a. Accumulation of hexose phosphates, phosphate and ATP depletion, defective electron transport, and glycogen phosphorylase inhibition
b. Accumulation of triose phosphates, phosphate and ATP excess, defective glycolysis, and glycogen synthase inhibition
c. Accumulation of triose phosphates, phosphate and ATP depletion, defective electron transport, and glycogen synthase inhibition
d. Accumulation of hexose phosphates, phosphate and ATP depletion, defective electron transport, and glycogen phosphorylase stimulation
e. Accumulation of hexose phosphates, phosphate and ATP excess, defective electron transport, and glycogen phosphorylase stimulation

179. A 2-month-old Caucasian girl is evaluated for hypoglycemia and lactic acidosis and noted to have an enlarged liver. Biopsy reveals stored glycogen, and a glycogen storage disease is suspected. Assay of usual glycogen enzyme deficiencies in the liver specimen is normal, so the metabolic consultant recommends assay of rarer enzyme deficiencies that influence glycogen metabolism. These enzymes would most likely include which of the following?

a. Hexokinase
b. cAMP-dependent protein kinase
c. Glucose-6-phosphate dehydrogenase
d. Phosphofructokinase
e. Fructose-1,6-diphosphatase

180. An 11-month-old infant with hypoglycemia and a palpable liver is evaluated for possible glycogen storage disease. The parents have immigrated from Russia, and report that the child's older brother was diagnosed with a "debrancher" enzyme deficiency with similar glycogen storage. This diagnosis would imply accumulation of glycogen with which type of glucose linkages?

a.   Linear $\alpha 1 \rightarrow 4$ linkages with branching $\alpha 1 \rightarrow 6$ linkages
b.   Linear $\alpha 1 \rightarrow 6$ linkages with branching $\beta 1 \rightarrow 4$ linkages
c.   Linear $\beta 1 \rightarrow 4$ linkages only
d.   Linear $\beta 1 \rightarrow 6$ linkages only
e.   Branching $\beta 1 \rightarrow 6$ linkages only

181. A 7-year-old obese Hispanic girl presents with dehydration after 3 days of vomiting and diarrhea. Her parents mention that a sibling was diagnosed with a type of diabetes that spilled sugar into the urine but did not need treatment. Urine reagent strip test for reducing sugars is strongly positive. The physician obtains a blood glucose level that is normal and a urine glucose oxidase test on the urine is also negative for glucose. Further analysis of the urine reveals a small amount of fructose and a large amount of an unidentified pentose that is most likely which of the following?

a.   Galactose
b.   Glucose
c.   Lactose
d.   Mannose
e.   Xylulose

182. A 2-week-old Caucasian boy returns to his pediatrician for evaluation of increased jaundice during his nursery stay and to follow-up on a positive newborn screen for galactosemia (MIM*230400). Clinical assessment suggests the child's jaundice has resolved and he has a good weight gain with no feeding concerns. The pediatrician obtains a repeat newborn screen, but recalls that certain carbohydrates can be recognized as reducing substances in urine by the Clinitest reaction that produces a green color. The urine reagent strip test is positive and physician suggests a switch to nonlactose formula until the nurse mentions that she spilled the urine and performed the test on a tabletop where sugar for coffee had been spilled. Among the following C6 isomers of glucose, which is a ketose and reducing substance?

a. Fructose
b. Galactose
c. Glucofuranose
d. Glucopyranose
e. Mannose

183. After a term uncomplicated gestation, normal delivery, and unremarkable nursery stay, a 10-day-old African American girl is readmitted to the hospital because of poor feeding, weight loss, and rapid heart rate. Antibiotics are started as a precaution against sepsis, and initial testing indicates an unusual echocardiogram with a very short PR interval and a large heart on x-ray. Initial concern about a cardiac arrhythmia changes when a large tongue is noted, causing concern about glycogen storage disease type II (Pompe disease—MIM*232300). Which of the following best explains why Pompe disease is more severe and lethal compared to other glycogen storage diseases?

a. The deficiency is a degradative rather than synthetic enzyme
b. The deficiency involves a liver enzyme
c. The deficiency involves a lysosomal enzyme
d. The deficiency causes associated neutropenia
e. The deficiency involves a serum enzyme

184. Which of the following explains why individuals with hyperlipidemia and/or gout should minimize their intake of sucrose and high-fructose syrups?

a. Fructose can bypass phosphofructokinase using a fructokinase in liver.
b. Fructose can be phosphorylated by hexokinase in liver cells.
c. Fructose is converted to UDP-fructose in liver.
d. Fructose is ultimately converted to galactose in liver.
e. Fructose can be phosphorylated by hexokinase in adipose cells.

185. A 14-year-old Caucasian adolescent with past history of drug/alcohol abuse is brought to the emergency room after she cannot be aroused for school; her parents think that a bottle of acetaminophen (Tylenol) in their medicine cabinet has fewer tablets than they remember. The ER physician notes that cellulose is listed as the solid binder in the particular brand of acetaminophen. Since liver-protective N-acetylcysteamine therapy must be started within 16 hours of potential toxicity, the physician suggests that a rapid test for cellulose ingestion would be helpful in ascertaining if the child took the acetaminophen. Which of the following tests would be most informative regarding cellulose ingestion?

a.   Serum glucose to reflect intestinal digestion and absorption of cellulose
b.   Serum glucose after hydrolysis to break up cellulose $\beta1 \rightarrow 4$ bonds
c.   Stool glucose after hydrolysis to break up cellulose $\beta1 \rightarrow 4$ bonds
d.   Stool glucose to reflect intestinal digestion of ingested cellulose
e.   Stool glucose to reflect intestinal digestion of $\beta1 \rightarrow 4$ bonds distal to $\beta1 \rightarrow 6$ branching points in cellulose

186. The Warburg effect refers to the seemingly paradoxical preference for glycolysis over oxidative phosphorylation in many cancer tissues. Which of the following statements best reflects this paradox?

a.   Glycolysis consumes 4 ATP early in the pathway, produces 2 ATP later, and the net of -2 ATP per glucose is less than the 2 ATP produced per oxidation of citrate.
b.   Glycolysis consumes 2 ATP early in the pathway, produces 4 ATP later, and the net of 2 ATP per glucose is less than 1/6 of that produced by oxidative phosphorylation.
c.   Glycolysis consumes 4 ATP early in the pathway, produces 6 ATP later, and the net of 2 ATP per glucose is less than 1/6 of that produced by oxidative phosphorylation.
d.   Glycolysis consumes 2 ATP early in the pathway, produces 4 ATP later, and the net of 2 ATP per glucose is less than the 3 produced by oxidative phosphorylation.
e.   Glycolysis consumes 6 ATP early in the pathway, produces 12 ATP later, and the net of 6 ATP per glucose is less than the 8 produced by oxidative phosphorylation.

187. A frequent presentation in the newborn period is transient hypo-glycemia as the child adapts to separation from maternal glucose controls. Blood glucose is generally maintained at concentrations of 4.5 to 5.5 mmol/L but may rise to 6.5 to 7.2 mmol/L after feeding or decrease to 3.3 to 3.9 mmol/L in the fasting state. Which of the following enzymes plays an important role in regulating blood glucose levels after feeding?

a. Glucokinase
b. Glucose-6-phosphatase
c. Phosphofructokinase
d. Pyruvate kinase
e. Glucose-6-phosphate dehydrogenase

188. A 25-year-old Nigerian medical student studying in the United States develops hemolytic anemia after taking the oxidizing antimalarial drug pri-maquine. Which of the following is the most likely cause of this severe reaction?

a. Glucose-6-phosphate dehydrogenase deficiency
b. Concomitant scurvy
c. Vitamin C deficiency
d. Diabetes
e. Glycogen phosphorylase deficiency

189. A 5-year-old African American girl is brought to the emergency room with tonic-clonic seizures. Laboratory studies are drawn as anticonvulsants given do not completely stop the seizures. A blood glucose of 30 mg/dL (normal 60-100) is found, prompting administration of 25% dextrose intravenously and 1 mg of glucagon intramuscularly. Which of the following events will occur in response to glucagon?

a. CO_2 is consumed
b. Inorganic phosphate is consumed
c. Acetyl-CoA is utilized
d. ATP is generated
e. GTP is generated

190. A 6-month-old Caucasian boy has exhibited somewhat slow growth but becomes very ill after contracting influenza from an older sibling. A plasma lactate level of 55 mg/dL is found that suggests underlying mitochondrial disease, and mitochondrial DNA studies confirm a large deletion that affects several oxidative-phosphorylation complexes. Exacerbation of routine illness by the child's reduced energy reserves would most affect which of the following reactions of the citric acid cycle?

a. Citrate → α-ketoglutarate
b. α-Ketoglutarate → succinate
c. Succinate → fumarate
d. Fumarate → malate
e. Malate → oxaloacetate

191. A 45-year-old African American female is found unconscious at her desk and rushed to the emergency room via ambulance. She is a known diabetic and an injectable insulin pen was found on her desk. Serum glucose was less than 20 g/dL as read by glucometer on the way to the hospital. Which of the following statements reflects the pathogenesis of her hypoglycemia?

a. Her liver was suddenly permeable to glucose after added insulin.
b. Her insulin increased glucose import into extrahepatic tissues using various glucose transporters.
c. Her insulin stimulated liver glucokinase which phosphorylates glucose only at low glucose concentrations.
d. Her extrahepatic tissues became permeable to glucose through the opposing action of glucagon.
e. Insulin stimulated glucose uptake into her liver even when the serum glucose became low.

192. Which of the following two compounds are the primary products of the pentose phosphate pathway?

a. NAD⁺ and ribose
b. NADH and ribose
c. NADP⁺ and ribose
d. NADPH and ribose
e. NAD⁺ and glucose
f. NADH and glucose
g. NADP⁺ and glucose
h. NADPH and glucose

193. Which of the following is an energy-requiring step of glycolysis?

a. Glucokinase
b. Lactate dehydrogenase
c. Phosphoglycerate kinase
d. Pyruvate kinase
e. Phosphohexose isomerase

194. Which of the following are primary substrates for gluconeogenesis?

a. Galactose and fructose
b. Glycerol and alanine
c. Acetyl-CoA and succinyl-CoA
d. Sucrose and lactose
e. GTP and biotin

195. A 2-year-old Caucasian girl has ingested cyanide from her parents' garage and is rushed to the emergency room. Which of the following components of the citric acid cycle will be depleted first in this child?

a. NAD$^+$ cofactor
b. Citrate synthase
c. Aconitase
d. Citrate production
e. Acetyl-CoA production

196. A 6-month-old Caucasian boy becomes ill after fruits and vegetables are added to his diet of breast milk. Mother feels that he used to become colicky when she ate fruit, although her pediatrician did not think this was significant. After 1 month of these new foods, the child has stopped gaining weight and the pediatrician feels an enlarged liver. Initial blood tests show a mild acidosis (pH 7.2) with increased lactic acid and low blood glucose. The urine reagent strip test reaction is positive for reducing substances in the urine, but the glucose oxidase test is negative for glucosuria. A glycogen storage disease is suspected, and a liver biopsy dose shows mildly increased glycogen with marked cellular damage suggestive of early cirrhosis. Assays for type IV glycogen storage disease are negative, and the initial frozen urine sample is reanalyzed and found to contain fructose. The most likely diagnosis and the reasons for hypoglycemia and glycogen accumulation is which of the following?

a. Hereditary fructose intolerance with inhibition of liver phosphorylase
b. Hereditary fructose intolerance with inhibition of glycogen synthase
c. Essential fructosuria with inhibition of glycogen synthase
d. Essential pentosuria with inhibition of liver phosphorylase
e. Essential fructosuria with allosteric stimulation of glycogen synthase

197. Disorders with abnormalities of the respiratory chain present with central nervous system and muscle symptoms (seizures, low tone) due to energy deficiency. A preliminary test to decide if a patient may have a mitochondrial electron transport disorders examines the ratio of pyruvate to that of its product under resting conditions. What is the ratio and how would it be affected by abnormal electron transport?

a. Pyruvate/Acetyl-CoA —increased
b. Pyruvate/Acetyl-CoA—decreased
c. Pyruvate/Glucose—decreased
d. Pyruvate/Lactate—increased
e. Pyruvate/Lactate—decreased

198. A 24-year-old Caucasian female of Swedish origin requests evaluation for frequent early fatigue, heart palpitations, and muscle cramping during exercise. Her symptoms have been present since childhood but have become more aggravating since she has taken up jogging for exercise. Blood testing during exercise demonstrates a rapid increase in succinate, alanine, lactate, and pyruvate. Her physician suspects an inherited enzyme deficiency that interferes with oxidative-phosphorylation in muscle. Which of the following pathways, enzyme reaction, and associated product levels are most likely deficient?

a. Glycolysis, pyruvate kinase, coenzyme A
b. Glycolysis, hexokinase, glucose 1-phosphate
c. Gluconeogenesis, pyruvate carboxylase, carbon dioxide
d. Gluconeogenesis, pyruvate carboxylase, ATP
e. Citric acid cycle, fumarase, succinyl-CoA
f. Citric acid cycle, succinate dehydrogenase, $FADH_2$

199. A 55-year-old Caucasian male exhibits progressive neurologic symptoms of deteriorating handwriting, declining sports performance, and increased clumsiness that has caused accidents in his construction work. Hospital studies reveal he has increased muscle fatigue accompanied by rising lactic acid and decreased glucose. Which of the following compounds would be the best candidate for therapy if successfully delivered to muscle?

a. Fumarate
b. Citrate
c. Oxaloacetate
d. Succinate
e. Alanine

200. A 3-month-old Caucasian girl presents with low blood glucose (hypoglycemia), enlarged liver (hepatomegaly), and excess fat deposition in the cheeks (cherubic facies). A liver biopsy reveals excess glycogen in hepatocytes. Deficiency of which of the following enzymes best explains this phenotype?

a. α-1,1-glucosidase
b. α-1,1-galactosidase
c. α-1,4-glucosidase
d. α-1,4-galactosidase
e. α-1,6-galactosidase

201. An 18-year-old Hispanic female is evaluated for fainting spells that tend to occur when she has not eaten due to illness or work. Her body mass index (weight in kg/height in meters^2 is over 29 (<26 desirable) and the initial history makes anxiety or blood pressure changes unlikely. Several random blood samples demonstrate lower glucose than normal and a glucose tolerance test is abnormal, showing a slow decrease in administered glucose that is suggestive of diabetes mellitus. Glucagon proves effective in helping her fainting spells, and a dietician places her on a moderate, low-carbohydrate diet with monitoring of glucose by glucometer and use of glucagon when symptomatic. What is the role of glucagon in this situation?

a. To stimulate the citric acid cycle when tissue resistance leads to excess insulin
b. To stimulate gluconeogenesis when tissue resistance leads to excess insulin
c. To stimulate glycolysis in the presence of decreased insulin secretion
d. To stimulate the pentose phosphate pathway in the presence of decreased insulin secretion
e. To stimulate glycogenolysis in the presence of decreased insulin secretion

202. Fasting is observed in many religions and occurs with food shortages or fad diets. A man goes on a hunger strike and confines himself to a liquid diet with minimal calories. Which of the following would occur after 4 to 5 hours?

a. Decreased cyclic AMP and increased liver glycogen synthesis
b. Increased cyclic AMP and increased liver glycogenolysis
c. Decreased epinephrine levels and increased liver glycogenolysis
d. Increased Ca^{2+} in muscle and decreased glycogenolysis
e. Decreased Ca^{2+} in muscle and decreased glycogenolysis

203. A 2-year-old African American boy is evaluated for short stature (height below the 3rd percentile with weight and head circumference at the 20th percentile for age), irritability between meals accompanied by low glucose levels, enlarged liver, and easy bruisability. Liver biopsy reveals excess glycogen and deficiency of the α1 → 6 branching enzyme is documented for a diagnosis of type IV glycogen storage disease (MIM*232500). This disorder causes variable liver and neuromuscular symptoms but can be lethal due to progressive liver scarring (cirrhosis) because of the presence of abnormal glycogen. Conventional therapy with continuous glucose supply (eg, nocturnal cornstarch by tube) to minimize the need for glycogen breakdown is often not effective, and additional agents to minimize synthesis of abnormal glycogen have been considered. Inhibition of glycogen synthesis might target which of the following molecules?

a. UDP-glucose 1-phosphate
b. UDP-glucose
c. UDP-glucose 6-phosphate
d. Glucose 6-phosphate
e. Glucose 1-phosphate

204. Which of the following statements best describes the structure of glycogen?

a. Glycogen is a copolymer of glucose and galactose.
b. There are more branch residues than residues in straight chains.
c. Branch points contain α1-4 glycosidic linkages.
d. New glucose molecules are added to the C1 aldehyde group of chain termini, forming a hemiacetal.
e. The monosaccharide residues alternate between D- and L-glucose.

205. An 8-year-old Caucasian boy presents with ataxia (poor muscle coordination with abnormal gait) and anemia that are suggestive of a mitochondrial disorder called Pearson syndrome (MIM*557000). This disorder is caused by a large mitochondrial DNA deletion, rendering multiple mitochondrial pathways ineffective. Which of the following conversions would be most affected in this child?

a. Glucose to glucose 6-phosphate
b. UDP-glucose to glycogen
c. D-glucuronate to L-gulonate to ascorbate
d. Oxaloacetate to citrate
e. D-glyceraldehyde to glyceraldehyde 3-phosphate

206. A 25-year-old African American male notices increased fatigue and decreased performance when playing outfield for his office softball team. After a game in hot weather with many fielding chances, he has severe muscle pains and cramps that keep him awake and notices his urine is dark that night. His physician suspects McArdle disease (type V glycogen storage disease—MIM*232600) and has him run on a treadmill breathing air with reduced oxygen. The man develops severe cramps after this ischemic exercise, further supporting the presumptive diagnosis. A diagnostic muscle biopsy is likely to show which of the following?

a. Increased normal glycogen with deficient hexokinase
b. Increased normal glycogen with deficient glycogen synthase
c. Increased normal glycogen with deficient phosphorylase
d. Decreased muscle glycogen with decreased glycogen synthase
e. Decreased muscle glycogen with decreased debranching enzyme

207. The 10-year experience of a biochemical genetics laboratory includes 5 patients who had a positive urine reagent dipstick reaction for reducing sugars. Two of these were young females evaluated for vomiting and failure to thrive while three were from a boy and two girls who were studied as part of a control population. Mass spectrometry profiles had shown that a urine chemical with six carbons and a ketone group. Which of the following metabolites satisfy these chemical criteria and accumulate in specific inborn errors?

a. Fructose, fructose 1-phosphate
b. Galactose, galactose 1-phosphate
c. Glucose, glucose 1-phosphate
d. Ribulose, ribose 1-phosphate
e. Xylulose, xylose 1-phosphate

Carbohydrate Metabolism

Answers

165. The answer is d. (*Murray, pp 113-120, 459-468. Scriver, pp 1521-1551.*) The infant had been previously normal, excluding severe diseases like galactosemia (answer b) or early diabetes (answer e) that should have elevated glucose in addition to times of hypoglycemia. The ability to digest breast milk lactose with absorption and conversion to glucose makes malabsorption unlikely (answer a) and sucrose is a disaccharide of glucose-fructose (answer c). Low glucose during fasting and liver enlargement implies altered regulation of glycogen synthesis/release due to one of the enzyme deficiencies within the category of glycogen storage disease.

Important carbohydrates include the disaccharides maltose (glucose-glucose), sucrose (glucose-fructose), and lactose (galactose-glucose), and the glucose polymers starch (cereals, potatoes, vegetables) and glycogen (animal tissues). Humans must convert dietary carbohydrates to simple sugars (mainly glucose) for fuel, employing intestinal enzymes and transport systems for enzymatic digestion and absorption. Simple sugars (galactose, fructose) are converted to glucose by liver enzymes, and the glucose is reversibly stored as glycogen. Enzymatic deficiencies in intestinal digestion (eg, lactase deficiency in those with lactose intolerance), in sugar to glucose conversion (eg, galactose to glucose conversion in galactosemia) or in glycogenesis/glycogenolysis (eg, in those glycogen storage diseases) result in glucose deficiencies (low blood glucose or hypoglycemia) with potential accumulation and toxicity to hepatic tissues.

166. The answer is a. (*Murray, pp 113-120. Scriver, pp 1489-1520.*) Glycosides are formed by condensation of the aldehyde or ketone group of a carbohydrate with a hydroxyl group of another compound. Other linked groups (aglycones) include steroids with hydroxyl groups (eg, cardiac glycosides such as digitalis or ouabain) or other chemicals (eg, antibiotics such as streptomycin). Sucrose (α-D-glucose-β-1 $\rightarrow$ 2-D-fructose), maltose (α-D-glucose-α-1 $\rightarrow$ 4-D-glucose), and lactose (α-D-galactose-β-1 $\rightarrow$ 4-D-glucose) are important disaccharides. Fructose is among several carbohydrate groups known as ketoses because it possesses a ketone group. The ketone group is at carbon 2 in fructose, and its alcohol group at carbon 1 (also at carbon 6) allows ketal formation to produce pyranose and furanose rings as with glucose. Most of the fructose found in the diet of North Americans is derived from the disaccharide sucrose (common table sugar). Sucrose is cleaved into equimolar amounts of glucose and fructose in the small intestine by the action of the pancreatic enzyme sucrase. Deficiency of sucrase can also cause chronic diarrhea. Hereditary fructose intolerance (MIM*229600) is caused by deficiency of the liver enzyme aldolase B, which hydrolyzes fructose 1-phosphate.

167. The answer is c. *(Murray, pp 113-120. Scriver, pp 1521-1552.)* Cellulose, the most abundant compound known, is the structural fiber of plants and bacterial walls. It is a polysaccharide consisting of chains of glucose residues linked by β1 → 4 bonds. Since humans do not have intestinal hydrolases that attack β1 → 4 linkages, cellulose cannot be digested but forms an important source of "bulk" in the diet. Lactose is a disaccharide of glucose and galactose found in milk. Amylose is an unbranched polymer of glucose residues in β1 → 4 linkages. Glycogen is a branched polymer of glucose with both β1 → 4 and β1 → 6 linkages. Maltose is a disaccharide of glucose, which is usually the breakdown product of amylose.

168. The answer is e. *(Scriver, pp 1521-1551. Murray, pp 157-164.)* In muscle, glycogenolysis is synchronized with contraction by epinephrine (through cyclic AMP) and calcium activation of muscle glycogen phosphorylase. In those with a muscle-specific phosphorylase defects (McArdle disease or glycogen storage disease type V MIM*232600), glucose is not mobilized as efficiently from glycogen, causing decreased contractile efficiency (cramping, fatigue), decreased yield of lactate from glycolysis, and maintenance of serum glucose by compensating liver metabolism. All of the other substances listed—oxaloacetate, glycerol, and pyruvate—can be made into glucose by the liver.

Under circumstances of intense muscular contraction, the rate of formation of NADH by glycolysis exceeds the capacity of mitochondria to reoxidize it. Consequently, pyruvate produced by glycolysis is reduced to lactate, thereby regenerating NAD^+. Since erythrocytes have no mitochondria, accumulation of lactate occurs normally. Lactate goes to the liver via the blood, is formed into glucose by gluconeogenesis, and then reenters the bloodstream to be reutilized by erythrocytes or muscle. This recycling of lactate to glucose is called the Cori cycle. A somewhat similar phenomenon using alanine generated by muscles during starvation is called the glucose-alanine cycle.

169. The answer is b. *(Murray, pp 212-223. Scriver, pp 1521-1552.)* In humans, ethanol is cleared from the body by oxidation catalyzed by two NAD$^+$-linked enzymes: alcohol dehydrogenase and acetaldehyde dehydrogenase (eliminating answers a, c-e). These enzymes act mainly in the liver to convert alcohol to acetaldehyde and acetate, respectively. In chronic alcoholics, alcohol dehydrogenase may be elevated somewhat. The NADH level is significantly increased in the liver during oxidation of alcohol, owing to the consumption of NAD$^+$. This leads to a swamping of the normal means of regenerating NAD$^+$. Thus, NAD$^+$ becomes the rate-limiting factor in oxidation of excess alcohol.

170. The answer is d. *(Murray, pp 593-615. Scriver, pp 5559-5586.)* The exposure of tissues to chronic hypoxia makes them rely more on anaerobic metabolism for the generation of energy as ATP and other high-energy phosphates. Most tissues except for red blood cells can metabolize glucose under anaerobic or aerobic conditions (red blood cells do not have mitochondria for electron transport and must rely on other tissues to generate glucose back from lactate). In most tissues, a switch from aerobic to anaerobic metabolism greatly increases glucose utilization and decreases energy production. (Increased glucose utilization under anaerobic conditions in bacteria is known as the Pasteur effect after its discoverer.) Under aerobic conditions, the cell can produce a net gain in moles of ATP formed per mole of glucose utilized that can be as high as 18 times that produced under anaerobic conditions. Thus the cell generates more energy and requires less glucose under aerobic conditions. Such increased ATP concentrations, together with the release of citrate from the citric acid cycle under aerobic conditions, allosterically inhibit the key regulatory enzyme of the glycolytic pathway, phosphofructokinase. Decreased phosphofructokinase activity decreases metabolism of glucose by glycolysis.

171. The answer is b. *(Murray, pp 459-468. Scriver, pp 1521-1552.)* In many populations, a majority of adults are deficient in lactase and hence intolerant to the lactose in milk. In all populations, at least some adults have lactase deficiency (MIM*223000). Since virtually all children are able to digest lactose, this deficiency obviously develops in adulthood. In lactase-deficient adults, lactose accumulates in the small intestine because no transports exist for the disaccharide. An outflow of water into the gut owing to the osmotic effect of the milk sugar causes the clinical symptoms. Steatorrhea, or fatty stools, is caused by unabsorbed fat, which can occur following a fatty meal in persons with a deficiency of lipoprotein lipase (MIM*238600). Sialidase deficiency (MIM*256550) causes accumulation of sialic acid–containing proteoglycans and neurodegeneration.

172. The answer is c. (*Murray, pp 212-223. Scriver, pp 1521-1552.*) The principal pathway for hepatic metabolism of ethanol is thought to be oxidation to acetaldehyde in the cytoplasm by alcohol dehydrogenase. Acetaldehyde is then oxidized, chiefly by acetaldehyde dehydrogenase within the mitochondrion, to yield acetate. Acetone, methanol, hydrogen peroxide, and glycerol do not appear in this biodegradation pathway, eliminating answers a-b, d-e). The genetic variations of acetaldehyde dehydrogenase have few phenotypic effects aside from sensitivity to alcoholic beverages and are extremely common in the affected populations. These characteristics qualify acetaldehyde dehydrogenase variation as an example of enzyme polymorphism.

173. The answer is b. (*Murray, pp 157-164. Scriver, pp 1521-1551.*) Glycolysis in muscle produces lactate, which must be converted to glucose by liver or kidney via the Cori cycle (incorrect answers a, c, e). Defects in liver glycogen metabolism therefore impair glucose 6-phosphate production or gluconeogenesis (alanine is also a substrate for gluconeogenesis—incorrect answer d) with resulting hypoglycemia and liver glycogen storage with or without toxicity (cirrhosis). Defects in muscle glycogen metabolism impair contraction (cramps, fatigue) with decreased serum lactate production during exercise and muscle glycogen accumulation (progressive weakness and atrophy).

Glucose 1-phosphate is the first intermediate in the conversion of glycogen to glucose. The enzyme glycogen phosphorylase catalyzes this first step. The second intermediate, glucose-6-phosphate is subsequently converted to glucose by the enzyme glucose-6-phosphatase. This enzyme is found only in the liver and kidney; thus, these are the only tissues able to break down glycogen for use by other tissues. In tissues such as muscle, glycogen can be broken down to glucose 6-phosphate but can only be used in the cell in which it was produced.

174. The answer is b. (*Murray, pp 149-156. Scriver, pp 4637-4664.*) Anaerobic tissues (like muscle during exercise) or those without mitochondria (like erythrocytes) are dependent on glucose metabolism by glycolysis to lactate (through pyruvate) for production of ATP and energy. Glycolysis is the major source of ATP in cells lacking mitochondria, but is a minor source of ATP in tissues undergoing active oxidative phosphorylation (incorrect answers c, e). Lactate produced by red cells and exercising muscle is not reused by those tissues but routed to the liver for conversion to glucose (incorrect answer d); glycogen breakdown is prominent in liver and muscle rather than red blood cells (incorrect answer a), and the pentose phosphate cycle reduces glucose 6-phosphate using NADP (as opposed to NAD in glycolysis) while generating no ATP (incorrect answer d).

Defects in glycolytic enzymes (like hexokinase deficiency—MIM*235700) reduce ATP production in erythrocytes, shortening red cell life span with increased cell death (hemolysis). The increased hemolysis decreases red cell counts (anemia) with increased heme conversion to bilirubin, increased jaundice, and splenomegaly due to red cell storage. The increased heme load prior to liver metabolism increases indirect-reacting (unconjugated) bilirubin rather than increased conjugated or direct-reacting bilirubin from defective liver/gall bladder metabolism.

175. The answer is d. (*Scriver, pp 4517-4554. Murray, pp 174-183.*) Glucose-6-phosphate dehydrogenase (G6PD) is the first enzyme of the pentose phosphate pathway, a pathway that metabolizes glucose to produce ribose and NADPH (eliminating answers a-c, e). Its deficiency (MIM*305900) is the most common enzymopathy, affecting 400 million people worldwide. It contrasts with glycolysis in its use of NADP rather than NAD for oxidation, its production of carbon dioxide, its production of pentoses (ribose, ribulose, xylulose), and its production of the high-energy compound PRPP (5-phosphoribosyl-1-pyrophosphate) rather than ATP. Production of NADPH by the pentose phosphate pathway is crucial for reduction of glutathione, which in turn removes hydrogen peroxide via glutathione peroxidase. Erythrocytes are particularly susceptible to hydrogen peroxide accumulation, which oxidizes red cell membranes and produces hemolysis. Stresses like newborn adjustment, infection, or certain drugs can increase red cell hemolysis in G6PD-deficient individuals, leading to severe anemia, jaundice, plugging of renal tubules with released hemoglobin, renal failure, heart failure, and death. Since the locus encoding

G6PD is on the X chromosome, the deficiency exhibits X-linked recessive inheritance with severe affliction in males and transmission through asymptomatic female carriers. Ribose 5-phosphate produced by the pentose phosphate pathway is an important precursor for ribonucleotide synthesis, but alternative routes from fructose 6-phosphate allow ribose synthesis in tissues without the complete cohort of pentose phosphate enzymes or with G6PD deficiency. The complete pentose phosphate pathway is active in liver, adipose tissue, adrenal cortex, thyroid, erythrocytes, testis, and lactating mammary gland. Skeletal muscle has only low levels of some of the enzymes of the pathway but is still able to synthesize ribose through fructose 6-phosphate.

176. The answer is b. (*Murray, pp 174-183. Scriver, pp 1553-1588.*) The severe symptoms of galactosemia (MIM*230400) are caused by the reduction of galactose to galactitol (dulcitol) in the presence of the enzyme aldose reductase (eliminating answers a, c-e). Galactose derives from lactose (glucose-galactose disaccharide) in breast milk and infant formula that is cleaved by intestinal lactase to the efficiently absorbed glucose and galactose. In galactosemia (MIM*230400), deficiency of galactose-1-phosphate uridyl transferase prevents the conversion of galactose into glucose 6-phosphate by the liver or erythrocytes. Most other organs do not metabolize galactose. The accumulation of galactose yields higher levels of galactitol that cause cataracts, accumulation of galactose 1-phosphate that contributes to liver disease, and accumulation of galactose metabolites in urine that measure positive for reducing substances by the Clinitest method. Carbohydrates including glucose with a C1 aldehyde group or fructose with a C2 ketone group register as reducing substances by Clinitest; the Dextrostix test that uses glucose oxidase on the reagent strip to specifically measure glucose can be used as a control to differentiate common glucosuria (prematurity, diabetes, renal diseases) from uncommon carbohydrates in urine.

In normal children, galactose is first phosphorylated by ATP to produce galactose 1-phosphate in the presence of galactokinase. Next, galactose-1-phosphate uridyl transferase transfers UDP from UDP-glucose to form UDP-galactose and glucose 1-phosphate. Under the action of UDP-galactose-4-epimerase, UDP-galactose is epimerized to UDP-glucose. Finally, glucose 1-phosphate is isomerized to glucose 6-phosphate by phosphoglucomutase. Infants with suspected galactosemia must be withdrawn from breast-feeding or lactose formulas and placed on nonlactose formulas such as Isomil.

177. The answer is c. (*Murray, pp 174-183. Scriver, pp 1489-1520.*) A special pathway for fructose metabolism (a specific fructokinase plus aldolase B and triokinase) is present in liver, kidney, and small intestine (incorrect answers a, b, d, e). Foods high in sucrose (glucose-fructose) such as syrups, beverages, or diabetic substitutes yield high concentrations of fructose in the portal vein. Fructose is catabolized more rapidly than glucose by its specific fructokinase, bypassing hexokinase that is regulated by fasting and insulin. While providing a fuel for glycolysis, fructose also increases fatty acid, VLDL, and cholesterol-LDL production that are also side effects of diabetes mellitus due to the necessary shift to fat oxidation when intracellular glucose is less available. Recent data also suggests that fructose in soft drinks and other foods promote insulin resistance and type II diabetes. For these reasons, the American Diabetic Association (www.diabetes.org) now suggests avoidance of fructose with the exception of naturally occurring fructose in fruits.

Fructose metabolism begins when fructokinase catalyzes the phosphorylation of fructose to fructose 1-phosphate, which is then split to D-glyceraldehyde and dihydroxyacetone by aldolase B. Triokinase converts D-glyceraldehyde to glyceraldehyde 3-phosphate, which can be metabolized further by glycolysis or be condensed with dihydroxyacetone phosphate by adolase to form fructose 1,6-diphosphate, glucose 6-phosphate, and glucose through gluconeogenesis.

178. The answer is a. (*Murray, pp 157-164. Scriver, pp 1489-1520.*) Hereditary fructose intolerance (MIM*229600) with deficiency of aldolase B causes accumulation of fructose 1-phosphate and other hexose phosphates (incorrect answers b-c). The accumulated hexose phosphates deplete cellular phosphate pools (incorrect answer e), inhibiting generation of ATP through glycolysis or oxidative-phosphorylation (with increased lactate). Altered AMP/ATP ratios cause increased uric acid formation, and inhibition of glycogen phosphorylase (incorrect answer d) by fructose phosphates produces hypoglycemia. Once recognized, hereditary fructose intolerance can be treated by elimination of fructose and sucrose from the diet.

179. The answer is b. (*Murray, pp 157-164. Scriver, pp 1521-1552.*) Glycogen synthesis and breakdown (glycogenolysis) are accomplished by separate pathways rather than reversible reactions. Glycogen synthase is active when dephosphorylated; glycogen phosphorylase is active when phosphorylated by a cyclic AMP-dependent protein kinase (incorrect answers a, c-e). These enzyme phosphorylations and dephosphorylations integrate glycogen synthesis/breakdown with food and glucose availability (refer to Fig. 14 in the High-Yield Facts).

Glycogen storage diseases are a group of inherited enzyme deficiencies that cause accumulation of glycogen in liver, heart, or muscle. Glucose is the primary source of energy for most cells and excess glucose is stored as glycogen. Glycogen provides for short-term high-energy consumption in muscle and is an emergency energy supply for the brain. Glycogen stored in the liver can be converted back to glucose for release into the blood stream for use by other tissues. Deficiency of adenylyl kinase or cAMP-dependent protein kinase can alter glycogenesis/glycogenolysis regulation and produce glycogen storage (refer to Table 6, High-Yield Facts).

180. The answer is a. (*Murray, pp 157-164. Scriver, pp 1521-1552.*) Normal glycogen is composed of glucose residues joined in straight chains by $\beta1 \rightarrow 4$ linkages. At 4- to 10-residue intervals, a branch of $\beta1 \rightarrow 4$ linkages is initiated at an $\beta1 \rightarrow 6$ linkage (incorrect answers b-e). Glycogen particles can contain up to 60,000 glucose residues. In the absence of the debrancher enzyme, glycogen can be degraded only to the branch points, inhibiting release of glucose into the serum and causing glycogen storage. As noted in High-Yield Facts, Table 6, Forbes/Cori or type 3 glycogen storage disease (MIM*232400) involves deficiency of debranching enzyme.

181. The answer is e. (*Murray, pp 157-164. Scriver, pp 1489-1520.*) It is important to differentiate glucosuria due to diabetes mellitus or renal tubular problems from other sugars in the urine, like galactose in galactosemia or fructose/xylulose in essential fructosuria (all these are reducing sugars that are positive with Clinitest but only glucose is positive with the glucose oxidase reagent strip Dextrostix). The uronic acid pathway, like the pentose phosphate pathway, provides an alternate fate for glucose without generating ATP. Glucose 6-phosphate is converted to glucose 1-phosphate and reacted with UTP to form the higher energy compound UDP-glucose. UDP-glucose is converted to UDP-glucuronic acid that is a precursor for glucuronide units in proteoglycan polymers. Unused glucuronic acid is converted to xylulose (incorrect answers a-d) and then to xylitol by a xylulose reductase, the enzyme deficiency in essential pentosuria (MIM*260800). In this "disease," which is better called a trait, excess xylulose is excreted into urine but causes no pathology. Pentoses (5-carbon sugars) are important in the pentose phosphate and uronic acid pathways, providing ribose for nucleic acid metabolism. The other sugars listed as options except for lactose are 6-carbon hexoses.

182. The answer is a. (*Murray, pp 113-120.*) 6-Carbon hexoses with a C1 aldehyde group and four asymmetric carbons can generate 16 isomeric forms including ketoses with a C2 ketone group (eg, fructose—incorrect answers b-e) and aldoses with a C1 aldehyde group (glucose, galactose, and mannose). All are reducing sugars that will give a positive reducing substance reaction by urine dipstick, including fructose from the sucrose in table sugar. Glucofuranose and glucopyranose are ring structures of glucose, with the majority of glucose in solution in the glucopyranose form.

183. The answer is c. (*Murray, pp 113-120. Scriver, pp 1521-1552.*) Pompe disease has an early and severe onset compared to the other glycogen storage diseases listed in High-Yield Facts, Table 6 because the defective α-glucosidase is a lysosomal enzyme. Accumulation of substances in the lysosome often leads to a more severe and progressive course, illustrated by the mucopolysaccharidoses like Hurler syndrome (MIM*607014) or the neurolipi doses like Tay-Sachs disease (MIM*272800). Patients with Pompe disease exhibit lysosomal glycogen accumulation in muscle (muscle weakness or hypotonia), brain (with developmental retardation), and heart (with a short PR interval and heart failure). The other glycogen storage diseases lead to glycogen accumulation in liver or muscle with correspondingly milder symptoms.

184. The answer is a. (*Murray, pp 113-120. Scriver, pp 1521-1552.*) Fructose is taken in by humans as sucrose, sucrose-containing syrups, and the free sugar. In liver, fructose is phosphorylated to fructose 1-phosphate by liver fructokinase, allowing it to bypass the ATP-regulated phosphofructokinase, yield glyceraldehyde and dihydroxyacetone phosphate by aldolase cleavage, and increase triglyceride/lipid biosynthesis (incorrect answers b-d). Fructose phosphorylation can also deplete liver cell ATP, lessening its inhibition of adenine nucleotide degradation and increasing uric acid that is the problem in gout. In adipocytes, fructose can be alternatively phosphorylated by hexokinase to fructose 6-phosphate. However, this reaction is competitively inhibited by appreciable amounts of glucose, as it is in other tissues.

185. The answer is c. *(Murray, pp 113-120.)* Glucose (glucopyranose) residues in cellulose are linked by $\beta 1 \rightarrow 4$ bonds in straight chains that humans cannot hydrolyze because they do not possess an enzyme to carry out this function. Cellulose is a structural constituent of plants that is insoluble and provides a source of fiber in the diet. Humans do have intestinal lactase to cleave galactose $\beta 1 \rightarrow 4$ glucose (lactose) bonds, maltase to cleave glucose $\beta 1 \rightarrow 4$ glucose (maltose) bonds, and sucrose to cleave glucose $\beta 1 \rightarrow 4$ fructose (sucrose) bonds. N-acetylcysteamine therapy must be started within 8 hours of acetaminophen ingestion to prevent and within 16 hours to ameliorate liver toxicity, a severe potentially lethal result if over 10 times the therapeutic dose of 5 mg/kg acetaminophen is ingested.

186. The answer is b. *(Murray, pp 149-156. Scriver, pp 1471-1488.)* Two ATPs are expended in the first steps of glycolysis and four ATPs generated by later steps, yielding a net of two ATP molecules generated by glycolysis of one glucose molecule (incorrect answers a, c, e). The citric acid cycle produces 3 ATP from each of 3 molecules of NADH produced, 2 from a molecule of $FADH_2$, and 1 ATP at substrate level from conversion of succinyl-CoA to succinate (12 ATP total—incorrect answer d). The rapid proliferation and high density of cancer cells, along with need for rapid cytoplasmic energy conversion (as in muscle), may explain their preference for glycolysis. ATP hydrolysis occurs during phosphorylation of glucose to glucose 6-phosphate by glucokinase (hexokinase) and phosphorylation of fructose 6-phosphate to fructose 1,6-bisphosphate by phosphofructokinase. ATP is generated during conversion of 1,3-bisphosphoglycerate to 3-phosphoglycerate by phosphoglycerate kinase and in the conversion of phosphoenolpyruvate to pyruvate by pyruvate kinase. Since two molecules of 1,3-bisphosphoglycerate are generated from one glucose molecule (and subsequently two molecules of phosphoenolpyruvate are generated), each of these steps results in generation of 2 ATPs.

187. The answer is a. *(Murray, pp 149-156. Scriver, pp 1471-1488.)* Glucokinase promotes uptake of large amounts of glucose by the liver while the other enzymes are present in pathways active after glucose uptake (incorrect answers b-e). At normal glucose levels, the liver produces glucose from glycogen, but as glucose levels rise after feeding, the liver stops converting glycogen and instead takes up glucose. Insulin also plays a role in regulating blood glucose levels. Pancreatic β-cells produce insulin in response to hyperglycemia. Glucose uptake by the β-cells and phosphorylation by glucokinase stimulates secretion of insulin, which enhances glucose transport into adipose tissues and muscle and thus lowers blood glucose levels.

188. The answer is a. (*Murray, pp 174-183, 593-615. Scriver, pp 4517-4554.*) One of the world's most common enzyme deficiencies is glucose-6-phosphate-dehydrogenase deficiency (MIM*305900); deficiencies of vitamin C, diabetes, or glycogen phosphorylase do not cause severe anemia (incorrect answers b-e). G6PD deficiency in erythrocytes is particularly prevalent among African and Mediterranean males. A deficiency in glucose-6-phosphate dehydrogenase blocks the pentose phosphate pathway and NADPH production. Without NADPH to maintain glutathione in its reduced form, erythrocytes have no protection from oxidizing agents. This X-linked recessive deficiency is often diagnosed when patients develop hemolytic anemia after receiving oxidizing drugs such as primaquine or after eating oxidizing substances such as fava beans.

189. The answer is a. (*Murray, pp 165-173. Scriver, pp 1521-1552.*) Glucagon will stimulate gluconeogenesis and glycogenolysis in liver by increasing cAMP concentrations, thus raising blood glucose levels. The first step of gluconeogenesis is catalyzed by pyruvate carboxylase with consumption of carbon dioxide and utilization of one high-energy ATP phosphate bond (incorrect answers b-d):

$$\text{pyruvate} + \text{ATP} + CO_2 \rightarrow \text{oxaloacetate} + \text{ADP} + P_i$$

Acetyl-CoA activates pyruvate carboxylase and inhibits pyruvate kinase activity of glycolysis but is not utilized in the reactions (incorrect answer c). The second step of gluconeogenesis is catalyzed by phosphoenolpyruvate carboxykinase using energy from GTP which is produced by succinate thiokinase of the citric acid cycle in liver and kidney (rather than ATP in most other tissues):

$$\text{oxaloacetate} + \text{GTP} \rightarrow \text{phosphoenolpyruvate} + \text{GDP} + CO_2$$

Two high-energy phosphates are thus employed for pyruvate to glucose conversion by gluconeogenesis that circumvents irreversible glucose to phosphoenolpyruvate to pyruvate reactions of glycolysis.

190. The answer is b. (*Murray, pp 143-148. Scriver, pp 1521-1552.*) During conversion of α-ketoglutarate to succinate, a molecule of GTP is synthesized from GDP and phosphate using energy from the hydrolysis of succinyl-CoA to produce succinate and CoA (incorrect answers a, c-e). This constitutes substrate-level phosphorylation, and, in contrast to oxidative phosphorylation, this is the only reaction in the citric acid cycle that directly yields a high-energy phosphate bond. The sequence of reactions from α-ketoglutarate to succinate is catalyzed by the α-ketoglutarate dehydrogenase complex and succinate thiokinase, respectively.

$$\alpha\text{-ketoglutarate} + NAD^+ + \text{acetyl-CoA} \rightarrow \text{succinyl-CoA} + CO_2 + NADH$$

$$\text{succinyl-CoA} + P_i + GDP \rightarrow \text{succinate} + GTP + \text{acetyl-CoA}$$

191. The answer is b. (*Murray, pp 143-148. Scriver, pp 1521-1552.*) Liver cells are permeable to glucose while extrahepatic tissues require insulin for glucose entry, reflecting different glucose transporters (GLUT) in different tissues (incorrect answers a, d, e). Liver hexokinase has a low K_m for glucose and acts at a constant rate, while glucokinase has a higher K_m for glucose and promotes glucose uptake at high concentrations as found in the portal vein after meals (incorrect answer c). The liver releases glucose at normal serum glucose concentrations but takes up glucose at high serum glucose concentrations. Insulin and glucagon act in opposing fashion to regulate serum glucose concentration. Insulin, secreted by the pancreatic β-cell in response to internal increases in glucose, ATP, and calcium influx, increases glucose uptake by muscle and adipose cells by recruiting glucose transporters to their plasma membranes. Glucagon, secreted by the pancreatic α-cells, stimulates cyclic AMP synthesis with increased gluconeogenesis and glycogenolysis to increase serum glucose concentrations.

192. The answer is d. (*Murray, pp 174-183. Scriver, pp 1434-1436.*) The pentose phosphate cycle does not produce ATP, but instead produces ribose and NADPH. $NADP^+$ is the hydrogen acceptor instead of NAD^+, as in glycolysis. In the oxidative phase of the pentose phosphate pathway, NADPH is generated by glucose-6-phosphate dehydrogenase. NADPH is also generated by 6-phosphogluconate dehydrogenase. Ribose is generated in the nonoxidative phase.

193. The answer is a. (*Murray, pp 165-173. Scriver, pp 1433-1436.*) Glucokinase catalyzes the conversion of glucose to glucose 6-phosphate in the energy requiring first step of glycolysis. ATP is also required in the conversion of fructose 6-phosphate to fructose 1,6-bisphosphate by phosphofructokinase. ATP is generated in the conversion of 1,3-bisphosphoglycerate to 3-phosphoglycerate by phosphoglycerate kinase and in the conversion of phosphoenolpyruvate to pyruvate by pyruvate kinase (incorrect answers c-d). No energy is required when lactate dehydrogenase converts pyruvate to lactate (a molecule of NADH is converted to NAD^+–incorrect answer b) or when phosphohexose isomerase converts glucose 6-phosphate to fructose 6-phosphate (incorrect answer e).

194. The answer is b. (*Murray, pp 165-173. Scriver, pp 1471-1478.*) Gluconeogenesis refers to the pathway for converting noncarbohydrate precursors to glucose (incorrect answers a, d), Glycerol, lactate, propionate, and certain amino acids such as alanine are all substrates for gluconeogenesis (substrates will undergo chemical conversion to form carbohydrates rather than serving as regulatory factors, incorrect answers a, d). Biotin is a cofactor for the first step (pyruvate carboxylase) of gluconeogenesis while conversion of succinyl-CoA to acetyl-CoA provides GTP for the second step (phosphoenolpyruvate carboxykinase—incorrect answers c, e). Glycogen is a glucose storage molecule that can readily be converted in the liver back to glucose for maintenance of blood glucose levels between meals.

195. The answer is a. (*Murray, pp 103-112, 143-148. Scriver, pp 2261-2274.*) Cyanide blocks respiration by displacing oxygen from hemoglobin, inhibiting oxidative phosphorylation in the mitochondria because cyanide cannot oxidize (accept electrons) from reduced cofactors like NADH. The citric acid cycle is the major pathway for generating ATP and reducing equivalents (NADH, H^+) from catabolism of carbohydrates, amino acids, and lipids. Inability to regenerate NAD^+ from NADH through mitochondrial oxidative phosphorylation depletes the cell of NAD^+ and inhibits the citric acid cycle. Failure to generate ATP by oxidative phosphorylation using NADH from the citric acid cycle depletes the cell of energy and leads to cell and tissue death (organ failure). Enzymes (citrate synthase, aconitase) and intermediates of the citric acid cycle (citrate, acetyl coenzyme A) need only be present in trace amounts because they are not consumed (incorrect answers b-e)

196. The answer is a. (*Murray, pp 149-156. Scriver, pp 1489-1520.*) Hereditary fructose intolerance (MIM*229600) is caused by deficiency of aldolase B that converts fructose 1-phosphate to dihydroxyacetone phosphate and glyceraldehydes. Fructose can be converted to fructose 1-phosphate (by fructokinase, the block in essential fructosuria, MIM*229800) but accumulates with its phosphate and is diverted to fructose 1,6-bisphosphate. These compounds allosterically inhibit glycogen phosphorylase and cause hypoglycemia in the presence of abundant glycogen stores. The abnormal sequestration of phosphate interferes with ATP generation from AMP, depleting cellular energy sources with severe effects on liver or kidney. Affected individuals become nauseated when eating fructose and exhibit a natural aversion to fruits. If diagnosis is postponed and fructose is not minimized in the diet, they can undergo progressive liver and kidney failure with malnutrition and death. Countries like Belgium that use fructose in hyperalimentation solutions may observe patients with milder fructose intolerance who decompensate in the face of high serum concentrations.

197. The answer is e. (*Murray, pp 143-148. Scriver, pp 2261-2274.*) Under aerobic conditions, pyruvate is oxidized by pyruvate dehydrogenase to acetyl-CoA, which enters the citric acid cycle. The citric acid cycle generates reducing equivalents in the form of FADH and NADH that are converted to oxygen by the electron transport chain to yield abundant ATP. Under anaerobic conditions such as heavy exercise, pyruvate must be converted to lactate to recycle NADH to NAD$^+$ to allow glycolysis to continue. In mitochondrial disorders resulting from mutations in cytochromes or pyruvate dehydrogenase, there is deficient NADH oxidation and ATP production. Lactate will accumulate as it does normally in tissues without mitochondria (erythrocytes) or in tissues with exercise stress (like muscle). The lactate can accumulate in serum, causing a decreased pyruvate to lactate ratio and lactic acidosis that are typical signs of mitochondrial disease. These abnormalities also occur with circulatory failure (shock) or hypoxemia, so they are suspect for inborn errors only when cardiorespiratory function is normal. Glycolysis produces only 2 ATP compared to the coupling of citric acid intermediates with electron transport that produces 12 ATP per cycle; tissues highly dependent on the respiratory chain (nerves, muscle, retina) are predominantly affected in mitochondrial disorders—for example, Leigh disease. Suggestive signs like the decreased pyruvate/lactate ratio must be followed by more specific tests like muscle biopsy (ragged red fibers), eye examination (retinal pigmentation), or mitochondrial DNA analysis (deletions, point mutations) to diagnose highly variable mitochondrial diseases.

198. The answer is f. (*Murray, pp 143-148. Scriver, pp 2327-2356.*) The citric acid cycle is closely associated with oxidative-phosphorylation (ox-phos), producing NADH and $FADH_2$ reducing molecules that are reoxidized to NAD^+ while generating ATP. The dehydrogenases, isocitrate dehydrogenase, α-ketoglutarate dehydrogenase, and malate dehydrogenase each produce one NADH while succinate dehydrogenase produces one molecule of $FADH_2$ per turn of the cycle (incorrect answer e). Glycolysis generates ATP energy under anaerobic conditions when oxygen is not available for coupling with phosphorylation (incorrect answers a, b). Gluconeogenesis consumes ATP/GTP energy to generate glucose necessary for brain and other tissues (incorrect answers c, d). Reoxidation of each NADH results in formation of 3 ATP, and reoxidation of $FADH_2$ results in production of 2 ATP for each molecule of coenzyme A entering the citric acid cycle. Succinate dehydrogenase deficiency (MIM*255125) is a rare muscle disorder (myopathy) that impairs flow through the citric acid cycle, coupling of $FADH_2$ with ATP production, oxidative-phosphorylation, and energy production. Although these processes are sufficient under low-energy conditions, stress in muscle (exercise) with ineffective ox-phos due to succinate dehydrogenase deficiency simulates anaerobic conditions with high lactate, less ATP and energy, less creatinine-phosphate shuttled to muscle cytoplasm, and higher amino acids like alanine that usually are converted by transamination to citric acid cycle intermediates, then to oxaloacetate, then to glucose through gluconeogenesis.

199. The answer is c. (*Murray, pp 143-148. Scriver, pp 2327-2356.*) Oxaloacetate could theoretically stimulate two pathways that may be deficient in the patients (answers a-b, d-e incorrect). Oxaloacetate participates in the first step of the citric acid cycle by accepting an acetyl group from acetyl-CoA to form citrate. Citrate is subsequently metabolized to succinate and back to oxaloacetate, making oxaloacetate a catalyst for the citric acid cycle. Oxaloacetate can also be converted to phosphoenolpyruvate by phosphoenolpyruvate carboxykinase and thus becomes a substrate for production of glucose through gluconeogenesis.

200. The answer is c. (*Murray, pp 157-164. Scriver, pp 1521-1552.*) The child has symptoms of glycogen storage disease. Glycogen is a glucose polymer with linear regions linked through the C1 aldehyde of one glucose to the C4 alcohol of the next (α-1,4-glucoside linkage). There are also branches from the linear glycogen polymer that have α-1,6-glucoside linkages. Glycogen is synthesized during times of carbohydrate and energy surplus, but must be degraded during fasting to provide energy. Separate enzymes for breakdown include phosphorylases (α-1,4-glucosidases) that cleave linear regions of glycogen and debranching enzymes (α-1,6-glucosidases) that cleave branch points. Glucose 6-phosphatase is needed in the liver to liberate free glucose from glucose 6-phosphate, providing fuel for other organs. There is no glucose 6-phosphatase in muscle, and muscle glycogenolysis provides energy just for muscle with production of lactate. Deficiencies of more than eight enzymes involved in glycogenolysis, including those mentioned, can produce glycogen storage disease.

201. The answer is b. (*Murray, pp 165-173. Scriver, pp 1471-1488.*) Glucagon responds to decreases in blood glucose by increasing liver cAMP, gluconeogenesis, and glycogenolysis. High cAMP levels activate cAMP-dependent protein kinases that inactivate glycolytic enzymes pyruvate kinase and phosphofructokinase and activate glycogen phosphorylase by phosphorylation (incorrect answers a, c, d). Obesity most commonly causes type II diabetes mellitus due to tissue resistance rather than decreased insulin secretion by the pancreas (incorrect answer e). Early stages of diabetes mellitus may be accompanied by periodic hypoglycemia due to high insulin levels trying to overcome tissue resistance or to periodic bursts of insulin secretion from failing pancreatic β-cells. Glucagon antagonizes insulin by increasing gluconeogenesis and glycogenolysis, both by increased action of cAMP kinases and through allosteric regulation of enzymes—for example, reciprocal activation of pyruvate carboxylase (gluconeogenesis) and inactivation of pyruvate dehydrogenase (glycolysis) by acetyl-CoA. Glucagon also inhibits lipolysis.

202. The answer is b. (*Murray, pp 94-97. Scriver, pp 1521-1552.*) In the presence of low blood glucose, epinephrine or norepinephrine interacts with specific receptors to stimulate adenylate cyclase production of cyclic AMP. Cyclic AMP activates protein kinase, which catalyzes phosphorylation and activation of phosphorylase kinase. Activated phosphorylase kinase activates glycogen phosphorylase, which catalyzes the breakdown of glycogen. Phosphorylase kinase can be activated in two ways. Phosphorylation leads to complete activation of phosphorylase kinase. Alternatively, in muscle, the transient increases in levels of Ca^{2+} associated with contraction lead to a partial activation of phosphorylase kinase. Ca^{2+} binds to calmodulin, which is a subunit of phosphorylase kinase. Calmodulin regulates many enzymes in mammalian cells through Ca^{2+} binding.

203. The answer is b. (*Murray, pp 157-164. Scriver, pp 1521-1552.*) UDP-glucose is the high energy compound from which glycogen is synthesized, made by condensing glucose-1-P and UTP using UDP-glucose pyrophosphorylase (incorrect answers a, c-e). Glucose is rapidly converted to glucose 6-phosphate by glucokinase in liver, its high K_m favoring the high concentrations of glucose in the portal vein (route from glucose-absorbing intestinal veins to the liver). Glucose 6-phosphate is converted to glucose 1-phosphate and activated to form UDP-glucose; a molecule that can arise from UDP-galactose through lactose absorption or follow the glucuronic acid pathway to produce ascorbic acid (vitamin C) and building blocks for proteoglycans. UDP-glucose is added to terminal glucose units of glycogen by glycogen synthase in the form of $\alpha1 \rightarrow 4$ linkages. To increase the solubility of glycogen and to increase the number of terminal residues, glycogen-branching enzyme transfers blocks of ~7 glucose residues to branch points via $\alpha1 \rightarrow 6$ linkages. Absence of the branching enzyme, deficient in type IV glycogen storage disease (MIM*232500) produces a less soluble glycogen with fewer termini, thus decreasing glucose release (short stature from less energy, large liver with stored glycogen) and provoking reaction to the abnormal glycogen to cause liver cell death (scarring and cirrhosis).

204. The answer is d. (*Murray, pp 113-120. Scriver, pp 1521-1552.*) Glycogen is a highly branched polymer of α-D-glucose residues joined by $\alpha1 \rightarrow 4$-glycosidic linkage. Under the influence of glycogen synthase, the C4 alcohol of a new glucose is added to the C1 aldehyde group of the chain terminus. The branched chains occur about every 10 residues and are joined in $\alpha1 \rightarrow 6$-glycosidic linkages. Large amounts of glycogen are stored as 100- to 400-Å granules in the cytoplasm of liver and muscle cells. The enzymes responsible for making or breaking the $\alpha1 \rightarrow 4$-glycosidic bonds are contained within the granules. Thus glycogen is a readily mobilized form of glucose.

205. The answer is d. (*Murray, pp 131-142, 2327-2356.*) In addition to the citric acid cycle that includes conversion of oxaloacetate to citrate, mitochondria also house the enzymes for β-oxidation of fatty acids and oxidative phosphorylation. The cytosol is the site for glycolysis (incorrect answers a, e), glycogenesis (incorrect answer b), the uronic acid and pentose phosphate pathways (incorrect answer c), and fatty acid biosynthesis.

206. The answer is c. (*Murray, pp 157-164. Scriver, pp 1521-1552.*) Glycogen storage diseases are caused by abnormal glycogen breakdown with hepatic (hypoglycemia, hepatomegaly, short stature) or muscle (exercise fatigue, cramping) symptoms. The excess glycogen (incorrect answers d, e) usually reflects defective glycogenolytic enzymes or their phosphorylating kinases but some defects of glycogen synthesis (like the type IV with deficient branching enzyme) or alterations of regulatory enzymes like phosphofructokinase can lead to decreased glycogen mobilization (answers d, e incorrect). Types V (phosphorylase deficiency) and VII (phosphofructokinase deficiency of Tarui disease) are due to enzymes with major effects on muscle while others (I, III-VIII) affect enzymes with major effects on liver (some like Type IV can affect both). The compromised phosphorylation of muscle glycogen characteristic of McArdle disease compels the muscles to rely on auxiliary energy sources such as free fatty acids and ambient glucose.

207. The answer is a. (*Murray, pp 113-120.*) Fructose is a 6-carbon hexose with a ketone group (ketose), while ribulose and xylulose have 5 carbons (incorrect answers d, e) while glucose and galactose have aldehyde rather than ketone groups (incorrect answers b, c). Fructose is the substrate for fructokinase that is deficient in asymptomatic fructosuria (MIM*229800) while fructose 1-phosphate is the substrate for aldolase B that is deficient in hereditary fructose intolerance (MIM*229600) with vomiting, lactic acidosis, and, with continued fructose ingestion, failure to thrive and hepatic disease. Glucose isomers can have different orientations of the H and OH groups on the carbon atom adjacent to the CH_2OH group (D- versus L-isomers) and most of the monosaccharides in mammals are in the D form but differ in their configuration of the H and OH groups at the 2, 3, and 4 carbons (epimers). Mannose and galactose are the most biologically important epimers of glucose.

Bioenergetics and Energy Metabolism

Questions

208. A 13-year-old Hispanic adolescent presents to clinic complaining of muscle cramps on exercise. Past history indicates he had some coordination problems in childhood and received occupational therapy. Blood tests show an increased amount of lactic acid at rest, with dramatic increases on exercise testing. Simultaneous measures by a surface pulse-oxygenation probe showed capillary oxygen saturation of 97% at rest and 96% with exercise (normal >95%). The abnormality most likely involves which of the following?

a. Glycolysis in the lysosomes
b. Glycolysis in the cytosol
c. Respiratory chain in the mitochondria
d. Glycogen breakdown in the mitochondria
e. Glycogen synthesis in the cytosol

209. A 2-week-old Caucasian boy returns to his pediatrician for neonatal follow-up after a newborn screen revealed elevation of citric acid cycle intermediates including succinate and fumarate. He has been feeding poorly, and his weight gain is less than the $\frac{1}{2}$ oz per day expected after accounting for the expected 5 to 10% loss from birth weight. Repeat screen again shows elevations of citrate, α-ketoglutarate, and succinate plus a venous lactate of 6.5 mmol/L (normal 0.5-2.2). The infant is referred to a metabolic clinic where skin biopsy and fibroblast studies reveal deficient yield of carbon dioxide, GTP, and NAD$^+$. Which of the steps shown in the following diagram of the citric acid cycle could account for all three deficiencies?

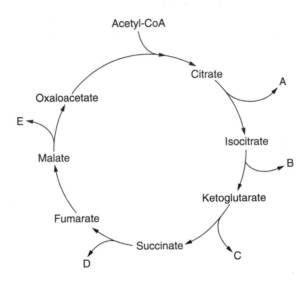

a. Step A
b. Step B
c. Step C
d. Step D
e. Step E

210. A comatose 25-year-old Asian female is brought by ambulance to the emergency room from a campus chemistry laboratory where she works as a teaching assistant. Vital signs reveal a temperature of 40.5°C (105°F) with rapid heart and respiratory rates. Along one arm is a yellow stain and her blood pressure is unobtainable. Two students accompany her and report that she was giving a demonstration on metabolic inhibitors and had an accidental spill on her face, first joking and complaining of blurred vision, then having headaches and shaking movements before passing out. Which of the following is the most likely toxin?

a. Phenobarbital
b. Carboxin
c. Dimercaprol
d. Dinitrophenol
e. Cyanide

211. A 6-year-old boy of Lebanese origin with a past history of mild ane- mia becomes very ill after a wedding celebration, showing pallor, rapid heart rate, shortness of breath, and dark urine. Emergency room evalua- tion shows a hemoglobin of 5 g/dL (mean for age 13.5) with 11% retic- ulocytes (normal 0.5-1). Glucose-6-phosphate dehydrogenase deficiency (MIM*305900) is suspected, known to produce high levels of oxidized glutathione and hydrogen peroxide in red blood cells with consequent membrane damage, hemolysis, and anemia. Which of the following redox pairs, due to its high redox potential, is crucial for glutathione reduction?

a. Fumarate/succinate
b. NADP+/NADPH or NAD/NADH
c. Oxaloacetate/malate
d. Pyruvate/lactate
e. 6-Phosphogluconate/ribulose-5-phosphate

212. A 45-year-old insurance executive is found comatose in his garage with the car engine running and transported by ambulance to the emergency room. He has the typical coal gas breath and red flush to the face and lips with blue (cyanotic) nail beds. Which of the following options indicates the steps of the respiratory chain (as diagramed below) that will be in a reduced state in this patient?

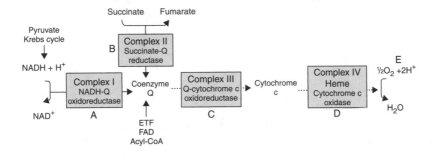

a. Steps A and B
b. Steps A, B, and C
c. Step D alone
d. Step E alone
e. All steps (A-E)

213. Dehydrogenases such as glucose-6-phosphate dehydrogenase serve to transfer H^+ from one substrate to another in coupled oxidation-reduction reactions, ultimately (in the respiratory chain) generating energy by oxygen/water reduction. Dehydrogenases can use which of the following compounds as an electron acceptor?

a. H_2O
b. NAD^+
c. O_2
d. Peroxide
e. NADPH

214. Nicotine addiction from cigarette smoking is related to rates of conversion of nicotine to cotinine, carried out by a member of the cytochrome P450 enzyme family called P450PB (formerly CYP2A3–MIM*122720). Individuals with variant alleles of the enzyme are predisposed toward nicotine addiction and the development of lung cancer. The P450 cytochromes are members of which family of oxidoreductases?

a. Catalase
b. Hydroperoxidase
c. Oxidase
d. Oxygenase
e. Dehydrogenase

215. Which of the following compounds is a high-energy phosphate donor to ATP during glycolysis?

a. Glucose 6-phosphate
b. Glucose 1-phosphate
c. Phosphoenolpyruvate
d. Phosphoglyceric acid
e. Fructose 6-phosphate

216. A 12-hour-old Caucasian boy is noted to maintain a frog-leg position with a weak cry and minimal spontaneous movement. A muscular dystrophy is suspected, and a serum enzyme is measured that reflects the abundance of a high energy storage molecule in muscle. Which of the following enzymes was measured?

a. Adenosine triphosphatase
b. Creatine phosphokinase
c. Glucose-1-phosphate dehydrogenase
d. Pyrophosphatase
e. ATP synthase

217. A 20-year-old Asian female is evaluated on her first prenatal visit and is found to have a hemoglobin of 10 g/dL (normal mean of 14). Prenatal vitamins with iron are prescribed but her anemia persists. Further evaluation shows an elevated reticulocyte count, and red cell enzyme levels are performed to find a cause for her hemolytic anemia. Partial deficiency of hexokinase (MIM*235700) is found, but the rare reports of this condition cause her physicians suspect an uncharacterized defect in red cell metabolism that depletes redox potential. This is because the conversion of glucose to glucose 6-phosphate requires coupling to ATP hydrolysis. Which of the following correctly explains the reason why?

a. The reaction has a positive free energy.
b. The reaction has a negative free energy.
c. Glucose 6-phosphate is unstable.
d. Glucose and other sugars are high-energy substrates.
e. Allosteric activation of hexokinase enzyme.

218. A 17-year-old Caucasian adolescent is evaluated for fainting spells and found to have a glucose level of 54 mg/dL (normal 75-105) 1 hour after eating. Her body mass index (BMI) is 17 (average 23-25) and physical examination reveals pallor, halitosis, discolored teeth with multiple caries. An eating disorder is suspected and she enlists in a research study that includes behavioral and dietary therapy along with metabolic studies. Administration of deuterium-labeled glucose shows initial rapid entry into liver and peripheral muscle followed by continued muscle but minimal liver intake. Which of the following accurately interprets these results?

a. Abnormal liver uptake reflecting starvation
b. Abnormal liver uptake reflecting latent diabetes mellitus
c. Abnormal liver uptake reflecting prior glycogen depletion
d. Normal liver uptake reflecting a lower K_m for liver hexokinase
e. Normal liver uptake reflecting a higher K_m for liver glucokinase

219. The figure below depicts the initial steps of glycolysis with enzyme reactions A and E, substrates B, C, and D. Which of the following options depicts the correct reaction sequence: 1—a reaction regulating glucose levels, 2—endergonic reaction(s) requiring ATP to ADP coupling, and 3—reaction(s) producing a substrate that will be reduced to produce NADH?

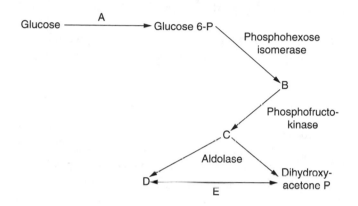

a. 1-reaction A, 2-reactions A and B to C, 3-reactions C to D and E
b. 1-reaction A, 2-reactions A and C to D, 3 reactions C to D and E
c. 1-reaction A, 2-reaction B to C, 3-reactions B to C and E
d. 1-reaction E, 2-reaction A, 3-reactions C to D and E
e. 1-reaction E, 2-reaction E, 3-reactions C to D and E

220. A 14-year-old African American adolescent competes well in short distance events as she tries out for the track team but does poorly at longer distances. Evaluation at a sports institute shows she has elevation of blood lactate after longer periods on a treadmill and suggests a defect in muscle energy metabolism. Although the girl's parents decline further expensive evaluation, which of the following reactions of muscle metabolism would be least affected after she has run a long distance?

a. Glucose 6-phosphate to fructose 6-phosphate
b. Glucose to glucose 6-phosphate
c. Fructose 6-phosphate to fructose 1,6-diphosphate
d. Phosphoenolpyruvate to pyruvate
e. Pyruvate to lactate

221. Which of the following enzymes catalyzes high-energy phosphorylation of substrates during glycolysis?

a. Pyruvate kinase
b. Phosphoglycerate kinase
c. Triose phosphate isomerase
d. Aldolase
e. Glyceraldehyde-3-phosphate dehydrogenase

222. Which of the following are products of triacylglycerol breakdown and subsequent β-oxidation that may undergo gluconeogenesis?

a. Propionyl-CoA
b. Acetyl-CoA
c. All ketone bodies
d. Some amino acids
e. β-Hydroxybutyrate

223. Which of the following regulates lipolysis in adipocytes?

a. Activation of fatty acid synthesis mediated by cyclic AMP
b. Activation of triglyceride lipase as a result of hormone-stimulated increases in cyclic AMP levels
c. Glycerol phosphorylation to prevent futile esterification of fatty acids
d. Activation of cyclic AMP production by insulin
e. Hormone-sensitive lipoprotein lipase

224. Oligomycin is an antibiotic derived from streptomyces, a genus of soil bacteria that has contributed over two-thirds of naturally derived antibiotics used in humans. Oligomycin is a macrolide antibiotic (containing a large macrolide ring like erythromycin or azithromycin) that inhibits ATP synthase required for oxidative phosphorylation. Which of the following options best explains the consequence of this inhibition?

a. Selective disruption of complex II function
b. Disruption of ubiquinone phosphorylation
c. Disruption of NADH entry into the respiratory chain
d. Disruption of proton flow across the inner mitochondrial membrane
e. Disruption of heme oxygen action

225. Patients with fatty acid oxidation disorders are particularly suscepti-ble to periods of fasting with disproportionate impact on muscular tissues. This is because, relative to energy from oxidation of glycogen (4 kcal/g or, when hydrated, 1.5 kcal/g), the yield from oxidation of triacylglyceride stores is which of the following?

a. 1 kcal/g
b. 2 kcal/g
c. 4 kcal/g
d. 9 kcal/g
e. 24 kcal/g

226. Which reaction in the figure below occurs in both muscle and liver but has substantially different qualities in the two?

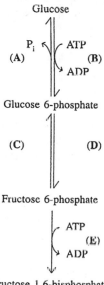

a. Reaction A
b. Reaction B
c. Reaction C
d. Reaction D
e. Reaction E

227. Nerve stimulation of skeletal muscle causes the release of calcium from sarcoplasmic reticulum and leads to muscle contraction. Simultaneously, the increased calcium concentration causes which of the following responses?

a. A dramatic rise in cyclic AMP levels
b. Inactivation of glycogen phosphorylase
c. Activation of phosphorylase kinase
d. Activation of cyclic AMP phosphodiesterase
e. Activation of protein phosphatase

228. A 16-year-old Caucasian adolescent presents for neurology evaluation because of fatigue that prevents participation in gym class. A consulting neurologist finds muscle weakness in the girl's arms and legs. Laboratory testing demonstrates elevated serum triacylglycerides and borderline low glucose. Muscle biopsy shows increased numbers of lipid vacuoles. Which of the following is the most likely diagnosis?

a. Fatty acid synthase deficiency
b. Tay-Sachs disease
c. Carnitine deficiency
d. Biotin deficiency
e. Lipoprotein lipase deficiency

229. A 24-hour-old Caucasian female infant has a rapid respiratory rate, often due to retained fluid from delivery (transient tachypnea of the newborn). The child then has feeding problems due to low muscle tone (hypotonia), and this seems to have central (nervous system) rather than peripheral origin, implying an encephalopathy. A liver biopsy reveals a very low level of acetyl-CoA carboxylase, but normal levels of the enzymes of glycolysis, gluconeogenesis, the citric acid cycle, and the pentose phosphate pathway. Which of the following is the most likely cause of the infant's respiratory problems?

a. Low levels of phosphatidyl choline
b. Excess adrenal fatty acids
c. Ketoacidosis
d. High levels of citrate
e. Glycogen depletion

230. Patients with riboflavin deficiency will have lower FAD levels, while those with niacin deficiency will have lower NAD levels. How do oxidations involving NAD compare with those involving FAD?

a. NAD-linked oxidations generate 3 mol ATP per half mole of O_2 consumed, whereas FAD-linked oxidations only generate 2 mol ATP per half mole of O_2 consumed.

b. FAD-linked oxidations generate 3 mol ATP per half mole of O_2 consumed, whereas NAD-linked oxidations only generate 2 mol ATP per half mole of O_2 consumed.

c. Both oxidations generate 2 mol ATP per half mole of O_2 consumed.

d. Both oxidations generate 3 mol ATP per half mole of O_2 consumed.

e. Both oxidations add hydrogens to substrates.

231. Individuals with disorders of the respiratory chain are often placed on supplements containing riboflavin and coenzyme Q. Which of the following is the role of coenzyme Q (ubiquinone) in the respiratory chain?

a. It links flavoproteins to cytochrome b, the cytochrome of lowest redox potential.

b. It links NAD-dependent dehydrogenases to cytochrome b.

c. It links each of the cytochromes in the respiratory chain to one another.

d. It is the first step in the respiratory chain.

e. It is a hydrogen receptor from NADH.

232. In the resting state, what is the primary condition that limits the rate of respiration?

a. Availability of ADP

b. Availability of oxygen

c. Availability of substrate

d. Availability of both ADP and substrate

e. Availability of oxygen and ATP

233. Oxidative phosphorylation couples generation of ATP with which of the following?

a. Proton translocation

b. Substrate level phosphorylation

c. Electron flow through cytochromes

d. Reduction of NADH

e. Reduction of water

234. In the past, the uncoupler 2,4-dinitrophenol was used as a weight-reducing drug until side effects like fatigue and breathlessness precluded its use. How could the use of this drug result in weight loss?

a. 2,4-dinitrophenol is an allosteric activator of ATP synthase and thus increases the rate of H^+ translocation and oxidation of fats and other fuels.
b. 2,4-dinitrophenol inhibits transport of pyruvate into the mitochondria. Fats are therefore metabolized to glycerol and subsequently to pyruvate, depleting fat stores.
c. 2,4-dinitrophenol allows oxidation of fats in adipose tissue without production of ATP. Fat oxidation can thus proceed continuously and fat stores will be used up.
d. 2,4-dinitrophenol causes ATP to be produced at a higher rate than normal, thus causing weight loss.
e. 2,4-dinitrophenol causes ADP to decrease and thus to increase rates of oxidative phosphorylation.

235. Many compounds poison the respiratory chain by inhibiting various steps of oxidation or phosphorylation. Which of the following steps is inhibited by carbon monoxide and cyanide?

a. Oxidation step between cytochrome and coenzyme Q and distal cytochromes
b. Oxidation step involving direct reduction of oxygen
c. Uncoupling of oxidation from phosphorylation
d. Oxidation step between cytochromes c and b
e. Oxidation step of flavin cytochromes to coenzyme Q

236. An important difference between respiratory chain inhibitors and uncouplers is which of the following?

a. The effect of respiratory chain inhibitors cannot be characterized spectroscopically, whereas that of uncouplers can.
b. Uncouplers do not inhibit electron transport, but respiratory chain inhibitors do.
c. Uncouplers are toxic substances, but respiratory chain inhibitors are not.
d. Respiratory chain inhibitors allow leakage of protons across the membrane but uncouplers do not.
e. Uncouplers accept protons from NADH before they can be transported across the mitochondrial membranes.

237. Hurricane survivors are evacuated from a back alley where they have been trapped for 4 days by flooding. Three adults have diarrhea with bloody stools, and a 5-month-old female infant is comatose with severe diarrhea and dehydration. Stool cultures reveal cholera and the adults treated with tetracycline, the infant with erythromycin to avoid injury to developing teeth. Cholera toxin causes massive and often fatal diarrhea by which of the following mechanisms?

a. Inactivating G_i protein
b. Irreversibly activating adenylate cyclase
c. Locking G_s protein into an inactive form
d. Rapidly hydrolyzing G protein GTP to GDP
e. Preventing GTP from interacting with G protein

238. Why is the yield of ATP from the complete oxidation of glucose lower in muscle and brain than in kidney, liver, and heart?

a. Different shuttle mechanisms operate to transfer electrons from the cytosol to the mitochondria in the two sets of tissues.
b. Muscle and brain cells have a lower requirement for ATP.
c. There are fewer mitochondria in muscle and brain cells.
d. There are fewer ATP synthases in muscle and brain cells.
e. Mitochondrial glycerophosphate dehydrogenase uses NAD rather than FAD.

239. A 2-year-old Caucasian girl presents to her pediatrician with a flu-like illness. She has sparse hair and a mild falloff in growth attributed to picky eating characteristic for this age. The pediatrician is concerned about her extreme lethargy with signs of dehydration and admits her to the hospital. Blood tests show a pH of 7.1, glucose of 40 mg/dL (normal 60-100), bicarbonate of 12 mEq/L (normal 16-24), and a white blood cell count of 4500 cells per cubic millimeter (normal 6-17,000). The metabolic acidosis and low white count raise concern for a metabolic disease, and a plasma acylcarnitine profile with total and free carnitine levels are ordered. Because children with organic acidemias or fatty acid oxidation disorder can have abnormal acylcarnitines that deplete free carnitine, intravenous carnitine is started at 100 mg/kg per day. Carnitine deficiency with decreased translocation of fatty acids into mitochondria will cause which of the following?

a. Inhibition of ATP synthase
b. Depletion of NADH needed for oxidation
c. Inhibition of cytochrome oxidase
d. Inhibition of electron transfer from cytochromes to coenzyme Q
e. Uncoupling of oxidation from phosphorylation

240. The problem of regenerating NAD^+ from NADH for cytoplasmic processes by using mitochondria is solved in the most energy-efficient manner by which of the following?

a. Reversing the direction of enzyme reactions like pyruvate dehydrogenase
b. Locating certain cytochromes in the cytoplasm
c. Shuttling of coupled reaction substrates like malate to aspartate
d. Reversing the direction of glycolysis
e. Direct oxidation of NADH by cytochromes P450

241. A certain class of disease is produced because of the tissue's lack of certain metabolic pathways. Which one of the following tissues can metabolize glucose, fatty acids, and ketone bodies for ATP production?

a. Liver
b. Muscle
c. Hepatocytes
d. Brain
e. Red blood cells

Bioenergetics and Energy Metabolism

Answers

208. The answer is c. (*Murray, pp 91-93. Scriver, pp 2261-2296.*) Mutations in nuclear or mitochondrial DNA may disrupt oxygen-coupled ATP energy generation (oxidative phosphorylation) in mitochondria and simulate anaerobic conditions. Although exercising muscle fibers can exceed respiratory chain capacity and generate lactic acid through cytosolic glycolysis (incorrect answers a, b), the lactate is quickly converted to glucose by the liver. Cytosolic glycogen breakdown (incorrect answers d, e) does have an energy advantage over glycolysis by yielding glucose 1-phosphate, interchangeable with glucose 6-phosphate, and avoiding the molecule of ATP consumed by hexokinase (which converts glucose to glucose 6-phosphate). When muscle energy deficits become severe, as with mitochondrial, muscle glycogen storage, or even coronary artery diseases with oxygen depletion, then lactate accumulates in cells and serum with muscle cell death, pain, and spasms (cramping).

Under conditions of plentiful oxygen (aerobic metabolism), pyruvate formed from glycolysis in the cytosol is metabolized to acetyl-CoA. Acetyl-CoA enters the mitochondria and the citric acid cycle in the conversion of oxaloacetate to citrate, generating NADH and $FADH_2$ reducing equivalents that generate ATP through oxidation in the mitochondrial respiratory chain. Mitochondria are called the powerhouses of the cell since they contain enzymes for the citric acid cycle, urea cycle, fatty acid oxidation, and the respiratory chain. Protein amino acids, fatty acids, and carbohydrates can be channeled through pyruvate, oxaloacetate, and the citric acid cycle to produce acetyl-CoA and NADH/$FADH_2$; coupling with respiratory chain cytochromes converts NADH from these catabolic reactions to ATP (oxidative phosphorylation) and regenerates NAD^+ for citric acid cycle conversions.

209. The answer is c. (*Murray, pp 143-148. Scriver, pp 2367-2424.*) In the citric acid cycle, the conversion of α-ketoglutarate to succinate results in decarboxylation, transfer of an H^+/e^- pair to $NADH^+$, H^+, and the substrate-level phosphorylation of GDP to GTP (incorrect answers a, b, d, e). The series of reactions involved is quite complex and analogous to those by which pyruvate dehydrogenase converts pyruvate to acetyl-CoA. First, α-ketoglutarate reacts with NAD^+ + CoA to yield succinyl-CoA + CO_2 + NADH + H^+. These reactions occur by the catalysis of the α-ketoglutarate dehydrogenase complex, which contains lipoamide, FAD^+, and thiamine pyrophosphate as prosthetic groups. Under the action of succinyl-CoA thiokinase (synthetase), succinyl CoA catalyzes the phosphorylation of GDP with inorganic phosphate coupled to the cleavage of the thioester bond of succinyl-CoA. Thus, the production of succinate from α-ketoglutarate yields one substrate-level phosphorylation and the production of 3 ATP equivalents from NADH via oxidative phosphorylation.

210. The answer is d. (*Murray, pp 108-112. Scriver, pp 2361-2374.*) The listed chemicals are inhibitors of the chain of oxidative reactions that couple oxidation of NADH to phosphorylation of ADP (respiratory chain that performs oxidative phosphorylation—see figure below Question 212). Barbiturates at high dosage including the common anticonvulsant phenobarbital (as well as piericidin A) inhibit complex I (incorrect answers a, b), antimycin A and dimercaprol inhibit complex III (incorrect answer c), and carbon monoxide or cyanide react with heme to block oxygenation at complex IV (incorrect answer e). Complex II connects the $FADH_2$ derived from succinate dehydrogenase to coenzyme Q and is inhibited by carboxin (incorrect answer b). Dinitrophenol is unique in that it disconnects the ordinarily tight coupling of electron transport and phosphorylation. In its presence, electron transport continues normally with no oxidative phosphorylation occurring. Instead, heat energy is generated. The same principle is utilized in a well-controlled way by brown fat to generate heat in newborn humans and cold-adapted mammals. The biological uncoupler in brown fat is a protein called thermogenin. Barbiturates, the antibiotic piericidin A, the fish poison rotenone, dimercaprol, and cyanide all act by inhibiting the electron transport chain at some point.

211. The answer is b. (*Murray, pp 174-183. Scriver, pp 4517-4554.*) NAD$^+$/NADH is a favored redox couple used in pathways such as the citric acid cycle and glycolysis, and the similar NADP/NADPH redox couple is used in the pentose phosphate pathway where glucose-6-phosphate dehydrogenase reduces glucose 6-phosphate to 6-phosphogluconate (answers a, c-e incorrect). The pentose phosphate steps generating NADPH are essential for reducing oxidized glutathione, also aided by the pyruvate/lactate redox couple in glycolysis. The fumarate/succinate and oxaloacetate/ malate couples in the citric acid cycle are not active in red blood cells since they lack mitochondria.

Since reduction involves the gain of electrons (loss of hydrogen protons) and oxidation the loss of electrons (gain of hydrogen protons), oxygen to water has the highest drive for oxidation in biological systems and thus the highest positive reduction (redox) potential of +0.82. The $NAD^+/NADP^+$ to NADH/NADPH couple has the highest redox potential with a negative value of −32, and other coupled reactions like those in the answer options will have intermediate redox potentials, allowing the oxygen to water potential to drive all metabolic reactions through the process of respiration.

212. The answer is e. (*Murray, pp 103-112. Scriver, pp 4517-4554.*) Cyanide and carbon monoxide displace oxygen from heme to form cyano- and carboxy-hemoglobin, respectively. No oxygen is available to drive oxidation of other respiratory chain complexes and thus all will be in the reduced state after cyanide or carbon monoxide poisoning (answers a-d incorrect). As electrons are received and passed down the electron transport chain (figure below Question 212), key molecules within the protein complexes are first reduced (electron added), then oxidized (electron lost), causing electrons to be shuttled from NADH/NADPH generated by redox couples, to the initial complexes (I, II, coenzyme Q), and then through complex III and IV to reduce oxygen to water. The high redox potential of this last step (E in the figure) drives the other reactions, causing all to fail when oxygen is blocked. The figure does not convey the mobility of electron carriers, coenzyme Q, and cytochrome c which link complexes I to IV located within the mitochondrial membrane. The complexes use energy from electron transfer to pump protons into the space between the two mitochondrial membranes, functioning as proton pumps. The proton movement creates energy that in turn drives a membrane ATP synthase to produce ATP from ADP and inorganic phosphate.

213. The answer is b. (*Murray, pp 103-112. Scriver, pp 4517-4554.*) Dehydrogenases are specific for their substrates but most use either NAD^+ or $NADP^+$ as the coenzyme (incorrect answers a-d). Some dehydrogenases use flavin coenzymes similar to FMN and FAD used by the oxidases. The final steps in the conversion of oxygen to water in the respiratory chain are carried out by cytochrome oxidase (cytochrome a3) as part of complex IV. This final enzyme is an oxidase, defined by its use of oxygen to oxidize metabolites and form water or hydrogen peroxide. The prior cytochromes of the respiratory chain (b, cl, c, a) can be described as dehydrogenases, transferring electrons (or H^+ protons in reverse) by oscillation between ferric (Fe^{+++}) and ferrous (Fe^{++}) ions.

214. The answer is d. (*Murray, pp 51-56, 609-615.*) Cytochrome P450 is a monooxygenase that can be reduced by NADH or NADPH and can in turn oxidize substrates by the hydroxylase cycle. In the liver, cytochrome P450 is found with cytochrome b_5 and plays an important role in detoxification. Other options have different mechanisms for adding hydrogen or electrons (incorrect answers a-c, e).

215. The answer is c. (*Murray, pp 92-97. Scriver, pp 2367-2424.*) In order to serve as a high-energy phosphate donor to ATP, the compound must have a more negative standard free energy of hydrolysis than ATP. ATP has a free energy of hydrolysis of −30.5 kJ/mol (−7.3 kcal/mol). Phosphoenolpyruvate has a standard free energy of hydrolysis of −61.9 kJ/mol (−14.8 kcal/mol). Thus, this compound can donate a high-energy phosphate to ATP. The other listed compounds have less negative standard free energies and thus cannot serve as phosphate donors to ATP (incorrect answers a-b, d-e) but may serve as phosphate acceptors.

216. The answer is b. (*Murray, pp 92-97. Scriver, pp 2367-2424.*) The enzyme creatine phosphokinase (CPK) transfers high energy phosphate from ATP to creatinine when energy levels are high in resting muscle and ATP is plentiful (incorrect answers a, c-e). The high concentration of CPK in muscle cells causes transfer to serum in various muscle disorders accompanied by muscle cell death (eg, muscular dystrophies with abnormal contractile protein structure, myopathies due to abnormal muscle growth, electrolytes, etc). Elevated serum CPK levels can provide a hint that muscle weakness is due to inherent muscle problems rather than innervation from the brain or peripheral nerves.

Creatine phosphate has a more negative standard free energy of hydrolysis than ATP, whereas ADP, glucose 1-phosphate, and pyrophosphate all have lower energy phosphate groups than ATP. When ATP is being utilized rapidly in skeletal muscle, creatine phosphate can be hydrolyzed and act as a phosphate donor to ADP to regenerate ATP. During resting periods when the ATP/ADP ratio is high, creatine can be phosphorylated to creatine phosphate to serve as storage for high-energy phosphate.

217. The answer is a. *(Murray, pp 92-97. Scriver, pp 2367-2424.)* The conversion of glucose to glucose 6-phophate is endergonic (requires energy, has a positive free energy—incorrect answer b) and must be coupled to an exergonic reaction that produces energy (negative free energy). The negative Gibbs free energy yield (ΔG) for the coupled reaction allows it to proceed rather than allosteric activation or instability of glucose 6-phosphate (incorrect answers c, e); glucose and other non-phosphorylated sugars are low energy substrates compared to their phosphorylated derivatives (incorrect answer d). Coupling of ATP hydrolysis with energetically unfavorable reactions cannot only allow the reaction to proceed in the forward direction, but can in some cases make the reaction irreversible if the free energy value is negative enough.

218. The answer is e. *(Murray, pp 131-142. Scriver, pp 2367-2424.)* Less glucose uptake by liver after postprandial glucose levels fall is normal (incorrect answers a-c) and does not reflect depleted glycogen or starvation from the patient's likely bulimia (thin tooth enamel and decay from frequent induced vomiting). Most peripheral tissues like muscle contain hexokinase with a low K_m and high affinity for glucose that brings it rapidly into cells. After a meal, glucose absorbed from the intestine will produce high levels in serum that decreases rapidly as extrahepatic tissues import and convert glucose to glucose 6-phophate with hexokinase. In contrast, liver has a different hexokinase enzyme called glucokinase (incorrect answer d) that has a high K_m and low affinity, removing glucose from the portal vein only when it is at high concentrations (shortly after a meal). This ensures that the liver will sequester glucose only when it is in excess and not needed by tissues like brain or heart, storing the excess glucose as glycogen for later use.

219. The answer is a. *(Murray, pp 92-97. Scriver, pp 2367-2424.)* Glucose is converted to glucose 6-phosphate (G6P) by hexokinase (reaction A in figure below Question 219) in most tissues. However, liver that has a glucokinase with higher K_m that ensures glucose import and conversion to glycogen occurs only during periods of glucose excess, that is after meals (incorrect answers d, e—see prior Answer 218 for more detail). Hexo- or glucokinase (reaction A in figure) and phosphofructokinase converting fructose 6-phosphate to fructose 1,6-bisphosphate (reaction B-C in figure) both are endergonic reactions that require energy and are coupled with exergonic ATP to ADP hydrolysis to allow conversion (incorrect answers b-e). This energy deficit is made up later in glycolysis by the exergonic phosphoglycerate kinase and pyruvate kinase reactions that generate ATP (4 per molecule of glucose entering glycolysis, giving a net yield of 2 ATP for each conversion of glucose to pyruvate. Glyceraldehyde 3-phosphate (substrate D in figure) is produced from fructose 1,6-diphosphate (substrate C) or from dihydroxyacetone phosphate by phosphotriose isomerase (reaction E) and reduced to yield NADH (incorrect answer c).

220. The answer is d. (*Murray, pp 92-97, 103-108. Scriver, pp 1471-1488.*) The indicated reactions are part of the glycolytic pathway and only the pyruvate kinase reaction (option d) is exergonic—produces energy that is coupled to produce ATP from ADP and P_i. Less effective energy production in muscle implied by the girl's fatigue would affect this reaction less than others that are endergonic or energy neutral (incorrect answers a-c, e). Major defects affecting muscle glycogen degradation or mitochondrial electron transport will produce weakness/developmental delay at young ages or exercise intolerance (muscle aches and spasms) at later ages. Milder defects produce more subtle symptoms that can manifest as early fatigue or poor performance in high intensity or endurance sports. It is interesting to speculate if mild mutations enhancing muscle energy pathways will be found in exceptional athletes, but the only supplements that are proven to work are those that increase muscle mass (steroids, growth hormone) rather than "energy drinks" or supplements like creatine.

221. The answer is e. (*Murray, pp 92-97. Scriver, pp 1471-1488.*) Using NAD^+ in an oxidation-reduction reaction, inorganic phosphate is added to glyceraldehyde 3-phosphate by the enzyme glyceraldehyde 3-phosphate dehydrogenase to form 1,3-diphosphoglycerate. Other enzymes (incorrect answers a, b, d) add high-energy phosphate bonds to substrates of glycolysis. Hexokinase—or, in the case of the liver, glucokinase—adds phosphate from ATP to glucose to form glucose 6-phosphate. Strictly speaking, this is not always considered a step of the glycolytic pathway. Phosphofructokinase uses ATP to convert fructose 6-phosphate to fructose 1,6-phosphate, while phosphoglycerate kinase and pyruvate kinase transfer substrate high-energy phosphate groups to ADP to form ATP. Triose phosphate isomerase interconverts dihydroxyacetone phosphate and glyceraldehyde 3-phosphate without phosphorylation (incorrect answer c).

222. The answer is a. *(Murray, pp 184-192. Scriver, pp 2327-2356.)* Lipolysis of triacylglycerols yields fatty acids and glycerol. The free glycerol is transported to the liver, where it can be phosphorylated to glycerol phosphate and enter the glycolysis or the gluconeogenesis pathways at the level of dihydroxyacetone phosphate. Acetyl-CoA and propionyl-CoA are produced in the final round of degradation of an odd chain fatty acid. Acetyl-CoA cannot be converted to glucose (incorrect answer b), but propionyl-CoA can. The three carbons of propionyl-CoA enter the citric acid cycle after being converted into succinyl-CoA. Succinyl-CoA can then be converted to oxaloacetate and enter the glycolytic scheme. Ketone bodies, including β-hydroxybutyrate, are produced from acetyl-CoA units derived from fatty acid β-oxidation. They may not be converted to glucose (incorrect answer c, d). Amino acids are not a product of triacylglycerol breakdown (incorrect answer d).

223. The answer is b. *(Murray, pp 184-192. Scriver, pp 2327-2356.)* Lipolysis is directly regulated by hormones in adipocytes. Epinephrine stimulates adenylate cyclase to produce cyclic AMP, which in turn stimulates a protein kinase. The kinase activates triglyceride lipase by phosphorylating it. Lipolysis then proceeds and results in the release of free fatty acids and glycerol. A futile re-esterification of free fatty acids is prevented, since adipocytes contain little glycerol kinase to phosphorylate the liberated glycerol (incorrect answer c), which must be processed in the liver. Inhibition of lipolysis occurs in the presence of insulin, which lowers cyclic AMP levels (incorrect answer d). Lipoprotein lipase is not an adipocyte enzyme (incorrect answer e) and fatty acid synthesis is the opposite of fatty acid breakdown/lipolysis (incorrect answer a).

224. The answer is d. *(Murray, pp 108-112. Scriver, pp 2367-2424.)* Oligomycin inhibits mitochondrial ATP synthase that is powered by the proton pumps of complex I to IV (see figure below Question 212). Accumulation of protons within the mitochondrial double membrane prevents electron transport and thus ablates phosphorylation and oxidation; inhibitors of terminal heme-oxygen/complex IV oxidation like cyanide will inhibit prior electron transfer reactions and keep all components in a reduced state (incorrect answer e). Selective complex inhibitors like carboxin for complex II or barbiturates for complex I where NADH enters the chain would cause partial disruption of electron transfer (incorrect answers a, b). Ubiquinone is one of three oxidation states of coenzyme Q (quinol to quinine to semiquinone) that cycle with forms of cytochrome c at the level of complex III; no coenzyme Q intermediates are phosphorylated (incorrect answer b). Oligomycin disrupts both phosphorylation and oxidation rather than uncoupling them like dinitrophenol.

225. The answer is d. (*Murray, pp 92-97, 184-192. Scriver, pp 2327-2356.*) Fats (triacylglycerols) are the most highly concentrated and efficient stores of metabolic energy in the body. This is because they are anhydrous and reduced. On a dry-weight basis, the yield from the complete oxidation of the fatty acids produced from triacylglycerols is approximately 9 kcal/g (answers a-c, e incorrect), compared with 4 kcal/g for glycogen and proteins. However, under physiologic conditions, glycogen and proteins become highly hydrated, whereas triacylglyceride stores remain relatively free of water. Therefore, although the energy yield from fat stores remains at approximately 9 kcal/g, the actual yields from the oxidation of glycogen and proteins are diluted considerably. Under physiologic conditions, fats yield three to four times the energy of glycogen stores. Patients with fatty acid oxidation disorders cannot switch to fat oxidation as efficiently when their glycogen is depleted by fasting, causing deficits in high energy requiring tissues like heart and skeletal muscle.

226. The answer is b. (*Murray, pp 149-156. Scriver, pp 2367-2424.*) The conversion of glucose to glucose 6-phosphate (reaction B in figure) is different in liver and muscle while others are similar (incorrect answers a, c-e). In muscle and most other tissues, hexokinase regulates the conversion of glucose to glucose 6-phosphate. When the major regulatory enzyme of glycolysis, phosphofructose kinase, is turned off, the level of fructose 6-phosphate increases and in turn the level of glucose 6-phosphate rises because it is in equilibrium with fructose 6-phosphate. Hexokinase is inhibited by glucose 6-phosphate. However, in the liver, glucose is phosphorylated even when glucose 6-phosphate levels are high because the enzyme regulating transformation of glucose into glucose 6-phosphate is glucokinase. Glucokinase is not inhibited by glucose 6-phosphate in the liver. Although hexokinase has a low K_m for glucose and is capable of acting on low levels of blood glucose, glucokinase has a high K_m for glucose and is effective only when glucose is abundant. Therefore, when blood glucose levels are low, muscle, brain, and other tissues are capable of taking up and phosphorylating glucose, whereas the liver is not. When blood glucose is abundant, glucokinase in the liver phosphorylates glucose and provides glucose 6-phosphate for the synthesis and storage of glucose as glycogen.

227. The answer is c. (*Murray, pp 545-565. Scriver, pp 2367-2424.*) Muscle contraction is caused by the release of calcium from the sarcoplasmic reticulum following nerve stimulation. In addition to stimulating contraction, the calcium released from the sarcoplasmic reticulum binds to a calmodulin subunit on phosphorylase kinase. This activates phosphorylase kinase, converting it from the D form to the A form (answers a-b, d-e incorrect). The activated phosphorylase then breaks down glycogen and provides glucose for energy metabolism during exercise. In this way, muscle contraction and glucose production from glycogen are coordinated by the transient increase of cytoplasmic calcium levels during muscle contraction.

228. The answer is c. (*Murray, pp 184-192. Scriver, pp 2297-2326.*) Carnitine acts as a Charon-like molecule that unites with organic and fatty acids as acylcarnitines and transports them across the mitochondrial membrane into the matrix that contains enzymes for fatty acid oxidation. Carnitine deficiency will reduce availability of fatty acids for oxidation and deplete energy to cause fatigue. Fatty acid synthase deficiency would be lethal and reduce muscle fat stores (incorrect answer a) while lipoprotein lipase deficiency would cause serum lipoprotein abnormalities (incorrect answer e), biotin deficiency diverse problems in carboxylation reactions (incorrect answer d), and Tay-Sachs disease neurologic symptoms from accumulation of abnormal brain lipids (incorrect answer b). Carnitine deficiency can result from mutations in a specific carnitine transporter (MIM*212140) or occur in preterm babies with liver problems and dialysis patients. Blockage of the transport of long chain fatty acids into mitochondria not only deprives the patient of energy production, but also disrupts the structure of the muscle cell with the accumulation of lipid droplets. Oral dietary supplementation usually can effect a cure.

229. The answer is a. (*Murray, pp 193-199. Scriver, pp 2297-2326.*) Acetyl-CoA carboxylase is the initial step in fatty acid synthesis, converting acetyl to malonyl CoA and, like other carboxylases, using biotin as a cofactor. Its deficiency has not been reported in humans and is embryolethal when created in mice. Deficiency would drastically impair fatty acid synthesis and therefore production of fatty acyl glycerol derivatives like phosphatidyl cholines that include surfactants for the lungs. Abnormalities described in answers b to e would not account for all of the clinical symptoms. Surfactant is a lipoprotein substance secreted by alveolar type II cells that lowers alveolar surface tension and facilitates gas exchange. Surfactant contains significant amounts of dipalmitoyl phosphatidylcholine, and palmitate is a major end product of de novo fatty acid synthesis.

230. The answer is a. (*Murray, pp 143-148. Scriver, pp 2297-2326.*) NAD-linked dehydrogenases generate one additional mole of ATP than flavoprotein-linked dehydrogenases (incorrect answers b-d). In the citric acid cycle, for example, three molecules of NADH and one molecule of $FADH_2$ are produced for each molecule of acetyl-CoA metabolized in one turn of the cycle. This leads to a total of 11 ATP produced by the respiratory chain for each turn of the citric acid cycle. An additional ATP is produced directly by substrate-level phosphorylation. Oxidation reactions may remove hydrogens from substrates to form water (incorrect answer e).

231. The answer is a. (*Murray, pp 103-112.*) Coenzyme Q collects reducing equivalents from flavoprotein complexes and passes them along the chain to the cytochromes (incorrect answers b-e). Reducing equivalents from a number of substrates are passed through coenzyme Q in the respiratory chain, including flavin adenine dinucleotide ($FADH_2$) that is produced from metabolic reactions. Supplements of riboflavin (to boost flavin levels), coenzyme Q (available from health food stores), and carnitine (to facilitate entry of metabolites into mitochondria) have produced mild improvements in patients with respiratory chain disorders. Commercial preparations often refer to coenzyme Q_{10}, where the 10 refers to the number of isoprene (5-carbon) unites attached to the ubiquinone ring.

232. The answer is a. (*Murray, pp 103-112.*) In the resting state, the level of ADP should be low and thus respiration will be slow (incorrect answers b-e). An increase in ADP indicates the cell is in the working state and respiration will increase. During heavy workloads, such as during exercise, respiration may be regulated by the availability of oxygen or the limit of the capacity of the respiratory chain itself.

233. The answer is a. *(Murray, pp 103-112. Scriver, pp 2261-2274.)* Proton translocation across the mitochondrial membrane generates an electrochemical potential difference composed of a pH gradient and an electrical potential (incorrect answers b-e). This electrochemical potential difference is used to drive ATP synthase to form ATP. During this process NADH and water are oxidized, not reduced, by coupling with oxygen as the ultimate electron donor.

234. The answer is c. *(Murray, pp 103-112. Scriver, pp 2261-2274.)* Uncouplers such as 2,4-dinitrophenol dissociate oxidation from phosphorylation. Thus, ADP is not phosphorylated to produce ATP and respiration becomes uncontrolled as it tries to replenish ATP supplies (incorrect answers a-b, d). This leads to increased metabolic turnover (as in fat oxidation) in the attempt to generate ATP. Less ADP will be converted to ATP, causing increased ADP and increased rates of oxidative phosphorylation (incorrect answer e). Prolonged energy deficits will lead to fatigue in energy-dependent tissues like muscle or heart (cardiomyopathy), the latter being potentially lethal.

235. The answer is b. *(Murray, pp 108-112. Scriver, pp 2261-2274.)* Carbon monoxide and cyanide inhibit cytochrome oxidase, the terminal step of the respiratory chain that is driven by oxygen reduction to water (incorrect answers a, c-e). Barbiturates block transfer from cytochrome to coenzyme Q, antimycin A, and dimercaprol the step between cytochromes c and b, and dinitrophenol is an uncoupler that releases the respiratory chain from regulation by energy (phosphorylation) needs. Oligomycin blocks phosphorylation by inhibiting ATP synthase, thus shutting down its coupled oxidation.

236. The answer is b. *(Murray, pp 108-112. Scriver, pp 2261-2274.)* Uncouplers such as 2,4-dinitrophenol increase the permeability of the inner mitochondrial membrane to protons, reduce the electrochemical potential, and inhibit ATP synthase (incorrect answers a, c-e). Respiratory chain inhibitors can include barbiturates, antibiotics such as antimycin A, and classic poisons such as cyanide and carbon monoxide. Barbiturates inhibit NAD-linked dehydrogenases by blocking the transfer of electrons from an iron-sulfur center to ubiquinone. Antimycin A inhibits the chain between cytochrome b and cytochrome c. Carbon monoxide and cyanide inhibit cytochrome oxidase and therefore totally arrest respiration.

237. The answer is b. (*Murray, pp 412-423. Scriver, pp 2367-2424.*) Cholera toxin is an 87-kDa protein produced by *Vibrio cholerae*, a gram-negative bacterium. The toxin enters intestinal mucosal cells by binding to G_{M1} ganglioside. It interacts with G_s protein, which stimulates adenylate cyclase. By ADP-ribosylation of G_s, the toxin blocks its capacity to hydrolyze bound GTP to GDP. Thus, the G protein is locked in an active form and adenylate cyclase stays irreversibly activated (incorrect answers a, c-e). Under normal conditions, inactivated G protein contains GDP, which is produced by a phosphatase catalyzing the hydrolysis of GTP to GDP. When GDP is so bound to the G protein, the adenylate cyclase is inactive. Upon hormone binding to the receptor, GTP is exchanged for GDP and the G protein is in an active state, allowing adenylate cyclase to produce cyclic AMP. Because cholera toxin prevents the hydrolysis of GTP to GDP, the adenylate cyclase remains in an irreversibly active state, continuously producing cyclic AMP in the intestinal mucosal cells. This leads to a massive loss of body fluid into the intestine within a few hours.

238. The answer is a. (*Murray, pp 412-423. Scriver, pp 2261-2274.*) Muscle and brain use the glycerophosphate shuttle to transfer reducing equivalents through the mitochondrial membrane. The glycerophosphate dehydrogenase inside the mitochondria utilizes FAD (incorrect answer e), whereas that in the cytosol uses NAD, resulting in only 2 mol of ATP produced instead of 3 ATP per atom of oxygen (incorrect answers b-d). In the malate shuttle used in the kidney, liver, and heart, the malate dehydrogenases on both sides of the mitochondrial membrane use NAD.

239. The answer is b. (*Murray, pp 184-192. Scriver, pp 2297-2326.*) The citric acid cycle and fatty acid oxidation are mitochondrial pathways that produce NADH (incorrect answers a, c-e) that is crucial for oxidative phosphorylation. Diminished production of ATP impacts tissues like heart and skeletal muscle with high-energy requirements. Children with organic acidemias like methylmalonic acidemia (MIM*251000) will tie up their carnitine as methylmalonyl carnitine, thus inhibiting transport of fatty acids into mitochondria (the medium and long chain fatty acids can only traverse the mitochondrial membrane as fatty acyl carnitines). Such children are often asymptomatic if well-fed, but can develop heart failure after fasting and glycogen depletion. Depletion of carnitine also causes accumulation of the organic acid with progressive metabolic acidosis.

240. The answer is c. *(Murray, pp 131-142. Scriver, pp 2367-2424.)* NADH generated from glycolysis must be relieved of an electron to form nicotinamide adenine dinucleotide (NAD⁺) so that glycolysis may continue. However, mitochondrial membranes are impermeable to both NADH and NAD⁺. The solution to this problem is the transfer of electrons from NADH to molecules that traverse the membrane (incorrect answers a-b, d-e). These shuttles include dihydroxyacetone phosphate (DHAP) to glycerol 3 phosphate—this shuttle regenerates NAD⁺ when the glycerol 3-phosphate diffuses into mitochondria, is oxidized by FAD back to DHAP, releasing DHAP back to the cytosol. In heart and liver, the more energy-efficient malate-aspartate shuttle moves electrons into mitochondria. Cytoplasmic oxaloacetate is reduced to malate, which diffuses into the mitochondria and is oxidized by NAD⁺ back to oxaloacetate. The mitochondrial oxaloacetate is converted to aspartate, which diffuses into the cytosol, where it is converted back into cytoplasmic oxaloacetate. The pyruvate dehydrogenase reaction may be reversed under anaerobic conditions when it generates NAD⁺ needed for glycolysis.

241. The answer is b. *(Murray, pp 184-192. Scriver, pp 4637-4664.)* Muscle cells are the only cells listed that are capable of utilizing all the energy sources available—glucose, fatty acids, and, during fasting, ketone bodies (incorrect answers a, c e). Mitochondria are required for metabolism of fatty acids and ketone bodies. Since red blood cells (erythrocytes) do not contain mitochondria, no utilization of these energy sources is possible. Red cells are thus extremely dependent on glycolysis, accounting for anemias caused by deficiency of glycolytic enzymes like hexokinase (MIM*235700). Although the brain may utilize glucose and ketone bodies, fatty acids cannot cross the blood-brain barrier. Hepatocytes (liver cells) are the sites of ketone body production, but the mitochondrial enzyme necessary for utilization of ketone bodies is not present in hepatocytes.

Lipid, Amino Acid, and Nucleotide Metabolism

Questions

242. A 1-year-old Hispanic boy is removed from parental care because of his second femoral fracture, both from falls that seemed insufficient to cause a severe break. Medical evaluation reveals a head size at the 90th percentile for age compared to a height at the 25th percentile for age, bluish-gray whites of the eyes (sclerae), and increased joint laxity. Skeletal radiographs show a healed right femoral fracture, recent left femoral fracture, and thin bones with several small fractures on both arms and lower legs. He is evaluated for osteogenesis imperfecta (MIM*166200) by taking a skin biopsy and examining the electrophoretic mobility of type I collagen proteins synthesized by cultured fibroblasts. Amino acids labeled with radioactive carbon 14 are added to the culture dishes in order to label the collagen. Which of the following amino acids would not result in labeled collagen?

a. Serine
b. Glycine
c. Aspartate
d. Glutamate
e. Hydroxyproline

243. A 65-year-old Caucasian male physician comes in for his annual physical examination and is noted to have palmar erythema, tremors, and a prominent abdomen with exaggerated superficial veins. Upon gentle inquiry, he admits to having three to four beers a night for most of his career except when on call, and discloses that his father died from cirrhosis. His family practitioner obtains a hepatic function panel that includes a serum aspartate aminotransferase level (AST also known as SGOT) of 350 U/L (normal 15-45) and a serum alanine aminotransferase (ALT also known as SGPT) of 280 U/L (normal 10-40). Which of the following best conveys the role transaminases like AST and ALT and the significance of their serum elevations?

a. Produce α-ketoglutarate, inhibit gluconeogenesis, reveal liver cell death
b. Produce glutamate, promote gluconeogenesis, reveal liver cancer
c. Produce urea, inhibit gluconeogenesis, reveal liver cancer
d. Remove ammonia, promote gluconeogenesis, reveal liver cell death
e. Remove ammonia, inhibit gluconeogenesis, reveal liver cancer

Questions 244 and 245

244. A 24-year-old Caucasian female is admitted for observation 3 days after contacting a flu-like illness. She has eaten little and says she is an adamant vegetarian because she got very sick eating hamburgers as a child. She has had lethargy and fatigue with progressive loss of coordination and memory; her speech is slurred. Laboratory studies include an ammonia level of 400 μmol/L (normal 0-35). With reference to the urea cycle diagram below, and given that ornithine transcarbamoylase is encoded on the X chromosome, select the option that indicates the compound deficient in this female and the compound derived from condensation of CO_2 and NH_4^+?

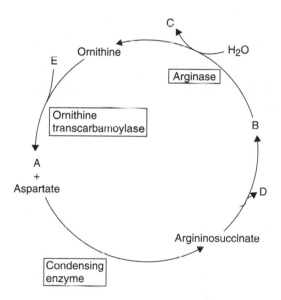

a. Compound A deficient, compound E from CO_2 and NH_4^+
b. Compound B deficient, compound E from CO_2 and NH_4^+
c. Compound C deficient, compound A from CO_2 and NH_4^+
d. Compound C deficient, compound B from CO_2 and NH_4^+
e. Compound E deficient, compound A from CO_2 and NH_4^+

245. A newborn Caucasian girl is the product of a normal gestation and delivery, feeding avidly until age 36 hours. Her mother reports less interest in breast-feeding and she becomes lethargic over a period of 4 to 6 hours, prompting transfer to intensive care, initiation of antibiotics for possible sepsis, and laboratory testing. An elevated serum ammonia is documented at 500 μmol/L (normal of 30-50). She is placed on glucose infusion plus a compound from the figure below Question 244 that "primes" the urea cycle. Which of the compounds in the figure would accomplish some removal of ammonia and increase substrate availability at the beginning of the cycle ("prime" the cycle)?

a. Compound A
b. Compound B
c. Compound C
d. Compound D
e. Compound E

246. Certain organic acidemias or fatty acid oxidation disorders will also involve elevated ammonia. This relates to the location of reactions of the urea cycle, occurring in which of the following?

a. In the cytosol
b. In lysosomes
c. In the mitochondrial matrix
d. In the mitochondrial matrix and the cytosol
e. In peroxisomes

247. A 2-day-old Caucasian boy becomes progressively lethargic after feeding and increases his respiratory rate. He becomes virtually comatose, responding only to painful stimuli, and exhibits mild respiratory alkalosis. Suspicion of a urea cycle disorder is aroused and evaluation of serum amino acid levels is initiated. In the presence of hyperammonemia, production of which of the following amino acids is always increased?

a. Glycine
b. Arginine
c. Proline
d. Histidine
e. Glutamine

248. A 23-year-old Caucasian female is found to have elevated blood pressure on her routine obstetric checkup at 8 months gestation, and testing by her obstetrician demonstrates anemia with hemolysis, elevated liver enzymes, and low platelets that are characteristic of disease represented by the acronym HELLP syndrome. The female is hospitalized and fetal maturity tests are performed that allow elective premature delivery. The female quickly recovers but the premature newborn has a dilated heart and elevated liver enzymes that are characteristic of a defect in long chain fatty acid oxidation. The potential enzyme deficiencies are those responsible for sequential oxidation of fatty acids, which include which of the following?

a. Dehydrogenase, hydratase, dehydrogenase, thiolase
b. Transacylase, synthase, reductase
c. Hydratase, reductase, thioesterase
d. Thioesterase, dehydrogenase, thiolase
e. Dehydrogenase, thiolase, thioesterase

249. A 2-year-old African American girl has been healthy until the past weekend when she contracted a viral illness at day care with vomiting, diarrhea, and progressive lethargy. She presents to the office on Monday having been unable to eat and drink much over the weekend; she is lethargic with signs of dehydration including cracked lips, sunken eyes, lack of tears, and flaccid skin with "tenting" on pinching. She also has a weak pulse with low blood pressure and increased deep tendon reflexes. Laboratory tests show low blood glucose, normal electrolytes, elevated liver enzymes, and (on chest x-ray) a dilated heart. Urinalysis reveals no infection and no ketones. The child is hospitalized and stabilized with 10% glucose infusion, and certain admission laboratories come back 1 week later showing elevated medium chain fatty acyl carnitines in blood and 6 to 8 carbon dicarboxylic acids in the urine. The most likely disorder in this child involves which of the following?

a. Defect of medium chain coenzyme A dehydrogenase
b. Defect of medium chain fatty acyl synthetase
c. Mitochondrial defect in the electron transport chain
d. Glycogen storage disease
e. Urea cycle disorder

250. A 30-year-old African American female is admitted with a diagnosis of diabetic ketoacidosis. She had onset of juvenile (type I) diabetes at age 16 and has done well until attendance at a destination wedding altered her diet and insulin habits. Which of the following would best apply to her liver metabolism upon admission?

a. Increased glucose uptake, increased fatty acid oxidation, decreased acetone synthesis
b. Increased glucose uptake, decreased fatty acid oxidation, increased β-hydroxy-butyrate synthesis
c. Decreased glucose uptake, increased fatty acid oxidation, increased acetone synthesis
d. Increased glucose uptake, increased fatty acid oxidation, increased acetoacetate synthesis
e. Increased glucose uptake, increased fatty acid oxidation, decreased acetoacetate synthesis

251. Which of the following enzymes is most important in regulating lipogenesis?

a. Acetyl-CoA carboxylase
b. Medium chain acetyl-CoA dehydrogenase
c. Short chain enoyl reductase
d. Long chain enoyl hydratase
e. 3-Ketoacyl reductase

252. A 13-year-old Caucasian adolescent of French Canadian descent develops hemiballismus (repetitive throwing motions of the arms) after anesthesia for a routine operation. She is tall and lanky, and it is noted that she and her sister both had previous operations for dislocated lenses of the eyes. The symptoms are suspicious for the disease homocystinuria (MIM*236300). Which of the following statements is descriptive of this disease?

a. Patients may be treated with dietary supplements of vitamin B_{12}.
b. Patients may be treated with dietary supplements of vitamin C.
c. There is deficient excretion of homocysteine.
d. There is deficient excretion of cysteine.
e. There is a defect in the ability to form cystathionine from homocysteine and serine.

253. An 8-year-old African boy from a Somali refugee camp presents with a red, scaly rash that is made worse by sunlight (photosensitive) and a poorly coordinated gait (ataxia). The rash resembles that of pellagra, a disease resulting from niacin (vitamin B_3) deficiency, and suggests malnutrition. However, his parents report that two siblings have had the same rash, and are affected with a disorder called Hartnup disease (MIM*234500). In this disorder, patients have a defect in neutral amino acid absorption from the intestine and become deficient in neutral amino acids (those with uncharged side chains). The physician reads about Hartnup disease and decides the rashes are likely to be pellagra, caused by deficiency of niacin. Which of the following abnormalities in Hartnup disease would account for the niacin deficiency?

a. Deficiency of lysine
b. Deficiency of arginine
c. Deficiency of taurine
d. Deficiency of aspartic acid
e. Deficiency of glutamic acid
f. Deficiency of ornithine
g. Deficiency of tryptophan

254. Which of the following is the important reactive group of glutathione in its role as an antioxidant?

a. Serine
b. Sulfhydryl
c. Tyrosine
d. Acetyl-CoA
e. Carboxyl

255. Which of the following processes generates the most ATP?

a. Citric acid cycle
b. Fatty acid oxidation
c. Glycolysis
d. Pentose phosphate pathway
e. Glycogenolysis

256. A 2-day-old Caucasian boy develops jaundice (yellow skin and yellow sclerae) that is greater than average at its usual peak at 3 days and requires laboratory evaluation. Which of the following porphyrin derivatives is conjugated, reacts directly, and is a major component of bile?

a. Bilirubin diglucuronide
b. Stercobilin
c. Biliverdin
d. Urobilinogen
e. Heme

257. A 40-year-old Caucasian female of fair complexion is admitted for evaluation of acute vomiting with abdominal pain. The episode began the night before after a fatty meal, and she has noted her stools are a peculiar gray white color. Abdominal examination is difficult because she is obese, but she exhibits acute tenderness in the right upper quadrant and has pain just below her left shoulder blade. Interference with which aspect of porphyrin metabolism best accounts for the white stools?

a. Sterile gut syndrome with defective bilirubin oxidation
b. Excess oxidation of bilirubin to urobilinogen
c. Heme synthesis defect causing increased bilirubin clearance
d. Bile duct excretion of bilirubin with oxidation to stercobilin
e. Excess reabsorption of urobilinogen with excess urobilin

258. A 35-year-old African American male has avoided health care but presents to his physician because his father recently died of a heart attack at age 55. The physician obtains a serum cholesterol of 320 mg/dL and a serum lipoprotein profile. Which of the following describes the order of lipoproteins from lowest to highest density along with the likely levels ($\uparrow$ = elevated, $\uparrow$ = decreased) in this patient if his blood is drawn 30 minutes after breakfast?

a. HDLs $\downarrow$ LDLs $\uparrow$, IDLs $\uparrow$, VLDLs $\uparrow$, chylomicrons $\downarrow$
b. Chylomicrons $\uparrow$, VLDLs $\uparrow$, IDLs $\uparrow$, LDLs $\uparrow$, HDLs $\downarrow$
c. VLDLs $\downarrow$, IDLs $\downarrow$, LDLs $\downarrow$, chylomicrons $\downarrow$, HDLs $\downarrow$
d. HDLs $\uparrow$, Chylomicrons $\uparrow$, IDLs $\uparrow$, VLDLs $\uparrow$, LDLs $\uparrow$
e. LDLs $\uparrow$, VLDLs $\uparrow$, IDLs $\uparrow$, chylomicrons $\uparrow$, HDLs $\uparrow$

259. A 3-year-old Caucasian girl is brought into the ER while you are on duty. She is cold and clammy and is breathing rapidly. She is obviously confused and lethargic. Her mother indicates she has accidentally ingested automobile antifreeze while playing in the garage. Following gastrointestinal lavage and activated charcoal administration, which of the following treatments should you immediately initiate?

a. Intravenous infusion of oxalic acid
b. Nasogastric tube for ethanol administration
c. Flushing out the bladder via a catheter
d. Intramuscular injection of epinephrine
e. Simply waiting and measuring vital signs

260. After finding that infants, particularly those with prematurity, are vulnerable to fatty acid deficiencies, major manufacturers began supplementing their infant formulas with these compounds. Which of the following is a nutritionally essential fatty acid along with its usual dietary source?

a. Eicosapentaenoic acid—plants
b. Linoleic acid—plants
c. Oleic acid—animals
d. Palmitoleic acid—animals
e. Linolenic acid—animals

261. A 62-year-old Caucasian male develops episodes of incoordination and slurred speech. His wife notes that he seems depressed and argumentative. His physician diagnoses multiple sclerosis, which is best described as which of the following?

a. Demyelinating disease with loss of phospholipids and ceramide from brain and spinal cord
b. Lipid storage disease with loss of sphingolipids and ceramide from brain and spinal cord
c. Lipid storage disease with loss of sphingolipids and gangliosides from brain and spinal cord.
d. Demyelinating disease with loss of phospholipids and sphingolipids from brain and spinal cord
e. Lipid storage disease with accumulation of sphingolipids in brain

262. A 2-year-old Caucasian girl with chronic diarrhea and anemia is evaluated and found to have abetalipoproteinemia (MIM*200100), a disorder caused by defective transport and deficiency of the apoB protein. Which of the following classes of serum lipids would be expected to be deficient in abetalipoproteinemia?

a. Lipoprotein (a)
b. High density lipoproteins (HDLs)
c. Chylomicrons
d. Triglycerides
e. Low density lipoprotein receptor

263. Children with very long or long chain fatty acid oxidation disorders are severely affected from birth, while those with short or medium chain oxidation defects may be asymptomatic until they have an intercurrent illness that causes prolonged fasting. The severe symptoms of longer chain diseases are best explained by which of the following statements?

a. Longer chain fatty acids inhibit gluconeogenesis and deplete serum glucose needed for brain metabolism.
b. Glycogen is the main fuel reserve of the body but is quickly depleted with fasting.
c. Starch is an important source of glucose and is inhibited by high fatty acid concentrations.
d. Triacylglycerols are the main fuel reserve of the body and are needed for energy production in actively metabolizing tissues.
e. Longer chain fatty acids form micelles and block synapses.

264. A 56-year-old Caucasian male with chronic alcoholism is admitted with hematochezia (bright red blood in stools) and hematemesis (bloody vomitus). Transfusions and esophageal tube pressure fail to maintain his blood pressure, and he dies from shock and cardiac failure. Autopsy would expect to show which of the following?

a. Normal liver with excess chylomicrons
b. Cirrhotic liver with excess HDL
c. Fatty liver with excess LDL
d. Fatty liver with VLDL
e. Cirrhotic and fatty liver with excess triacylglycerol

265. It has been noted that infants placed on extremely low-fat diets for a variety of reasons often develop skin problems and other symptoms. This is most often due to which of the following?

a. Lactose intolerance
b. Glycogen storage diseases
c. Antibody abnormalities
d. Deficiency of fatty acid desaturase greater than Δ^9
e. Deficiency of chylomicron and VLDL production

266. Which of the following best explains why statin therapy is effective for individuals with hypercholesterolemia?

a. Statins inhibit HMG-CoA reductase, a key regulator of cholesterol synthesis.
b. Statins inhibit HMG-CoA synthase, key step for synthesis of mevalonate that inhibits fatty acid synthesis.
c. Stains stimulate thiolase, thus making more malonyl-CoA for inhibition of the tricarboxylic acid cycle.
d. Statins bind to LDL receptor, displacing cholesterol and inhibiting cholesterol synthesis.
e. Statins stimulate synthesis of trans-unsaturated fatty acids.

267. A 15-month-old boy from Nigeria is evaluated for developmental delay. His coloring seems much lighter than that of his family background, and his physician orders a blood amino acid test that demonstrates elevated phenylalanine. A special low phenylalanine formula is begun (Lofenalac) as treatment for phenylketonuria (MIM*261600), but the parents refuse to come in for follow-up appointments. A public health evaluation reports that the child is failing to thrive despite apparent adherence to the diet by his parents. The symptoms of decreased skin pigment and later failure to thrive in this child are most likely related to which of the following?

a. Deficiency of alanine
b. Deficiency of tyrosine and melanin
c. Deficiency of tryptophan and niacin
d. Deficiency of leucine and isoleucine
e. Deficiency of phenylalanine

268. Niemann-Pick disease (MIM*257220), like other neurolipidoses, presents in infancy or childhood with plateauing of development and neurologic regression. The accumulating substance is a phospholipid made in which of the following steps in the figure below?

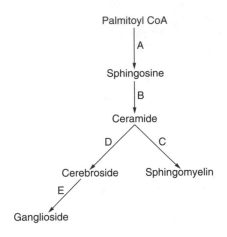

a. Step A
b. Step B
c. Step C
d. Step D
e. Step E

269. A 10-year-old Caucasian girl presents with chest pain and unusual skin patches over her elbows and knees. Her father died of a heart attack at age 35 and her mother is known to have high cholesterol. Her physician suspects familial hypercholesterolemia (MIM*144010) in the parents with homozygous severe disease in the daughter. This disease results from mutations in the receptor for low density lipoprotein (LDL) or the ligand portion of its apoprotein coat, which is which of the following?

a. A-I
b. B-48
c. C-II
d. B-100
e. E

270. A 45-year-old Caucasian male is found to have a serum cholesterol of 300 mg/dL (normal <200 depending on criteria) after a 12-hour fast. Which of the following lipoproteins would contribute to plasma cholesterol following a 12-hour fast?

a. Very low density lipoproteins (VLDLs) and low density lipoproteins (LDLs)
b. High density lipoproteins (HDLs) and low density lipoproteins (LDLs)
c. Chylomicrons and very low density lipoproteins (VLDLs)
d. Chylomicron remnants and very low density lipoproteins (VLDLs)
e. Low density lipoproteins (LDLs) and adipocyte lipid droplets

271. A 2-day-old Caucasian male neonate with meconium ileus (plugging of the small intestine with meconium or fetal stool) is found to have air in the bowel wall (pneumatosis intestinalis) and free air in the abdomen. Antibiotics are begun for suspected peritonitis, and emergency surgery is performed to remove the diseased intestinal segment and heal the intestinal perforation that led to air in the abdomen. Because the gut must be kept at rest for healing, meconium peritonitis was usually fatal until parenteral alimentation solutions were developed. Hyperalimentation consists of essential amino acids and other metabolites that provide a positive calorie balance while keeping the bowel at rest. The alimentation solution must be kept to a minimum of metabolites because of its high osmotic load that necessitates frequent changing of intravenous sites or catherization of a large vein. Which of the following amino acids could be excluded from the alimentation solution?

a. Cysteine
b. Phenylalanine
c. Histidine
d. Methionine
e. Tryptophan

272. A 15-year-old Caucasian adolescent has a long history of school problems and is labeled as hyperactive. His tissues are puffy, giving his face a "coarse" appearance. His IQ tests have declined recently and are now markedly below normal. Laboratory studies demonstrate normal amounts of sphingolipids in fibroblast cultures with increased amounts of glycosaminoglycans in urine. Which of the following enzyme deficiencies might explain the intellectual deterioration?

a. Hexosaminidase A
b. Glucocerebrosidase
c. α-L-iduronidase
d. α-Galactocerebrosidase
e. β-Galactosidase

273. Leukocyte samples isolated from the blood of a newborn Caucasian boy are homogenized and incubated with ganglioside GM_2. Approximately 47% of the expected normal amount of N-acetylgalactosamine is liberated during the incubation period. These results indicate which of the following regarding this infant?

a. He is a heterozygote (carrier) for Tay-Sachs disease.
b. He is homozygous for Tay-Sachs disease.
c. He has Tay-Sachs syndrome.
d. He will most likely have mental deficiency.
e. He has relatively normal β-N-acetylhexosaminidase activity.

274. A 4-year-old boy of Middle-Eastern ancestry is known to have inherited favism, a sensitivity to fava beans due to glucose-6-phosphate dehydrogenase deficiency (MIM*305900). Which of the following indicates the primary pathway affected by this deficiency and the pathway secondarily affected because one of its energy substrates will be deficient?

a. Pentose phosphate pathway, fatty acid synthesis
b. Pentose phosphate pathway, fatty acid oxidation
c. Citric acid cycle, fatty acid oxidation
d. Citric acid cycle, glycolysis
e. Glycolysis, citric acid cycle

275. Which enzyme catalyzes the only step of fatty acid oxidation that requires energy?

a. Acyl-CoA dehydrogenase
b. Acyl-CoA synthetase
c. Δ2-Enoyl-CoA hydratase
d. L(+)-3-Hydroxyacyl-CoA dehydrogenase
e. Thiolase

276. A 16-month-old Caucasian girl is admitted for evaluation of failure to thrive with weight below the third percentile for age despite apparent normal food intake. She is extremely pale and fair-haired, and laboratory studies include a creatinine level of 2.1 mg/dL (normal for age 0.3-0.7). An ophthalmology consult discovers unusual crystals in the lens of her eye by slit-lamp examination. Her physician suspects an amino acid disorder in which the accumulating amino acid (1) is the product of reduction from another amino acid and (2) can be transaminated to pyruvate. Which of the following amino acids would fulfill these characteristics?

a. Alanine
b. Cysteine
c. Serine
d. Glycine
e. Hydroxyproline

277. Adults with liver disease or milder urea cycle defects often exhibit neurologic symptoms (confusion, memory loss, motor incoordination) when interval high-protein meals or anorexia with protein catabolism elevates their serum ammonia. Ammonia intoxication is most obvious in neonates with severe urea cycle defects, manifest by lethargy and coma. Given that the cerebral cortex is a very active tissue with high-energy requirements, which of the following consequences of hyperammonemia are most likely responsible for cerebral symptoms?

a. Decreased glutamine, increased carboymal phosphate synthase activity
b. Increased α-ketoglutarate, increased arginase activity
c. Decreased glutamine, increased arginase activity
d. Increased glutamine, increased carbamoyl phosphate synthase activity
e. Decreased α-ketoglutarate, increased arginase activity

278. Which of the following transamination reactions produces an intermediate that will directly facilitate oxidative phosphorylation as well as gluconeogenesis?

a. Asparagine to aspartate to oxaloacetate
b. Cystine to cysteine
c. Lysine to glutaryl-CoA
d. Serine to glycine
e. Methionine to cystine

279. Which of the following is not used in the synthesis of fatty acids?

a. ATP
b. Cobalamin (vitamin B_{12})
c. $FADH_2$
d. HCO_3^-
e. NADPH

280. Hormones like insulin or glucagon act at cell membranes to stimulate release of "second messengers" like cyclic AMP that effect cellular responses. Which of the following options best describes their mechanism of action?

a. Soluble hormones enter channels within symmetric membranes Structure A
b. Soluble hormones react with surface receptors on asymmetric membranes
c. Soluble hormones within micelles fuse with symmetric membranes
d. Insoluble hormones diffuse through membranes to the cytosol
e. Insoluble hormones adhere to desmosomes between cells

281. Which of the diagrammatic structures below models the configuration of lipids emulsified prior to hydrolysis during digestion?

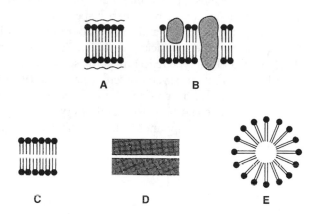

A   B

C   D   E

a. Structure A
b. Structure B
c. Structure C
d. Structure D
e. Structure E

282. Coronary artery disease is a multifactorial disorder involving occlusion of the coronary artery with atherosclerotic plaques. Several Mendelian disorders affecting lipid metabolism increase susceptibility for heart attacks, while environmental factors include smoking and high-fat diets. A 45-year-old Caucasian male has a mild heart attack and is placed on diet and mevastatin therapy. Which of the following will be the most likely result of this therapy?

a. Low blood glucose
b. Low blood LDLs
c. High blood cholesterol
d. High blood glucose
e. Low oxidation of fatty acids

283. A 36-hour-old African American boy is evaluated because of inability to breast-feed and found to have severe hypotonia (low muscle tone). The child lays in a frog leg posture with minimal spontaneous movements, and the head and legs dangle to the bed when suspended by his stomach. A large anterior fontanel is noted, and initial laboratory tests indicate elevated liver enzymes. The physician suspects Zellweger syndrome (MIM*214100), an end phenotype reflecting peroxisome dysfunction that may be caused by mutations in several different peroxisomal membrane protein genes. The diagnosis is confirmed by demonstrating elevated plasma levels of very long chain fatty acids and of erythrocyte plasmalogens. Which of the following compounds is the starting point of ether lipid and plasmalogen synthesis?

a. Acetyl-CoA
b. Pyruvate
c. Dihydroxyacetone phosphate
d. Malonyl-CoA
e. Palmitoyl-CoA

284. A 5-year-old Caucasian girl presents to the emergency room for evaluation of respiratory distress. She has seemed tired for the past week in that she does not play after school and goes to bed without prompting. The presiding physician obtains a basic metabolic panel that shows glucose of 250 mg/dL (normal 70-100) and a pH of 7.1. Urinalysis using a standard reagent strip is negative for nitrites and white blood cells that indicate infection but is strongly positive for the presence of ketones. The physician concludes that the child has likely diabetic ketoacidosis and that the respiratory distress is due to Kussmaul breathing—reflexive deep respirations that attempt to compensate for the acidosis by lowering carbon dioxide. Which of the following are "ketone bodies" that registered positive on the urine reagent strip for ketones in this child?

a. Acetone and ethanol
b. β-Hydroxybutyrate and acetoacetate
c. Pyruvate and lactate
d. Fumarate and succinate
e. Oxaloacetate and pyruvate

285. Gangliosides and receptors for hormones such as glucagon can be found in which of the following structures?

a. Plasma membrane
b. Mitochondria
c. Lysosomes
d. Endoplasmic reticulum
e. Ribosomes

286. Folic acid deficiency may present with megaloblastic anemia or be diagnosed by its effect on certain metabolic pathways. Which of the following amino acids and their catabolic products require folate along with an intermediate that, when elevated in serum, indicates folate deficiency?

a. Serine, glycine, carbon dioxide
b. Cystine, cysteine, mercaptopyruvate
c. Glycine, alanine, pyruvate
d. Threonine, acetaldehyde, acetate
e. Histidine, formiminoglutamate, glutamate

287. Which of the following is the major source of extracellular cholesterol for human tissues?

a. Very low density lipoproteins (VLDLs)
b. Low density lipoproteins (LDLs)
c. High density lipoproteins (HDLs)
d. Albumin
e. γ-Globulin

288. Which amino acid can be converted to an intermediate of the citric acid cycle and can be directly converted to urea?

a. Ornithine
b. Lysine
c. Arginine
d. Glutamate
e. Tyrosine

289. When the liver is actively synthesizing fatty acids, a concomitant decrease in β-oxidation of fatty acids is due to which of the following?

a. Inhibition of a translocation between cellular compartments
b. Inhibition by an end product
c. Activation of an enzyme
d. Detergent effects
e. Decreases in adipocyte lipolysis

290. A 4-year-old African American girl presents in the clinic with megaloblastic anemia (fewer red blood cells that are larger than normal) and failure to thrive. Blood chemistries reveal orotic aciduria (MIM*258900). Enzyme measurements of white blood cells reveal a deficiency of the pyrimidine biosynthesis enzyme orotate phosphoribosyltransferase and abnormally high activity of the enzyme aspartate transcarbamoylase. Which of the following treatments will reverse all symptoms if carried out chronically?

a. Blood transfusion
b. White blood cell transfusion
c. Dietary supplements of phosphoribosylpyrophosphate (PRPP)
d. Oral thymidine
e. Oral uridine

291. A 1-year-old Hispanic boy has a normal birth and infantile history except for delay in sitting up, crawling, and standing (delayed motor milestones). He begins the unusual habit of chewing on his fingers and lips, and in one instance bites through the lip and leaves a large wound. His physician documents an elevated serum uric acid and suspects Lesch-Nyhan syndrome (MIM*300322). In considering potential therapy, the physician reads that purines are overproduced in gout and Lesch-Nyhan syndrome, causing hyperuricemia, yet the hypoxanthine analogue allopurinol is only effective in gout. Allopurinol does not treat the neurologic symptoms of Lesch-Nyhan syndrome because it does not do which the following?

a. Decrease de novo purine synthesis
b. Decrease de novo pyrimidine synthesis
c. Diminish urate synthesis
d. Increase phosphoribosylpyrophosphate (PRPP) levels
e. Inhibit xanthine oxidase

292. Which of the following would make hyperuricemia very unlikely in a patient?

a. Lesch-Nyhan syndrome
b. Gout
c. Xanthine oxidase hyperactivity
d. Carbamoyl phosphate synthase deficiency
e. Purine overproduction secondary to von Gierke disease

293. A 45-year-old Caucasian female seeks evaluation for vague complaints of "tired blood" and "rheumatism." Her physician first considers chronic fatigue syndrome or depression, but performs a complete blood count (CBC) showing a hemoglobin of 9.0 g/dL (normal mean 14), white blood cell count of 3000/mm³ (normal mean 7 4), and platelet count of 30,000/mm³ (normal 150-350). A diagnosis of aplastic anemia is made and bone marrow chromosome studies initiated with knowledge that aplastic anemia can be a preleukemic state. A previously unreported chromosome translocation is found that suggests the female has a very unusual leukemia. The hematology-oncology consultant has no protocols gleaned from experience with like patients to rely on, but wishes to try a metabolic treatment that will inhibit leukemic cell division without using harsh chemotherapy poisons that could further damage the bone marrow. Which of the following strategies would cause the greatest inhibition of DNA synthesis?

a. Lowering aspartate
b. Lowering carbamoyl phosphate
c. Increasing uric acid
d. Increasing glutamine
e. Increasing orotic acid

294. A 23-year-old Caucasian female consults her physician because of occasional periods of confusion and lethargy, usually after a meal. The physician suspects a deficiency in an enzyme of the urea cycle, which in this case would most likely be which of the following?

a. Arginase
b. Argininosuccinase
c. Argininosuccinic acid synthase
d. Carbamoyl phosphate synthase I
e. Ornithine transcarbamylase

295. A 35-year-old Caucasian male presents to the emergency room with an acute abdomen (severe abdominal pain with tightness of muscles, decreased bowel sounds, and vomiting and/or diarrhea). He has been drinking, and a urine sample is unusual because it has a port-wine color. Past history indicates several prior evaluations for abdominal pain, including an appendectomy. The physician notes unusual neurologic symptoms with partial paralysis of his arms and legs. At first concerned about food poisons like botulism, the physician recalls that acute intermittent porphyria may cause these symptoms (MIM*176000) and consults a gastroenterologist. Elevation of which of the following urinary metabolites would support a diagnosis of porphyria?

a. Urobilinogen and bilirubin
b. Delta-aminolevulinic acid and porphobilinogen
c. Biliverdin and stercobilin
d. Urobilin and urobilinogen
e. Delta-aminolevulinic acid and urobilinogen

296. A 52-year-old Caucasian male seeks evaluation for sleeplessness because his great toes become swollen, red, and painful each night. Examination reveals small, moveable lumps (nodules) on his ears, fingers, and toes. His physician makes a diagnosis of gout and is informed that two of the man's six siblings are affected with the disease. Which of the following enzyme defects might be responsible for hereditary gout in this family?

a. Adenylosuccinase
b. Formyltransferase
c. IMP cyclohydrolase
d. PRPP glutamyl amidotransferase
e. PRPP synthetase

297. Hyperuricemia in Lesch-Nyhan syndrome is due to a defect in which of the following pathways?

a. Purine biosynthesis
b. Pyrimidine biosynthesis
c. Purine salvage
d. Pyrimidine salvage
e. Urea cycle

298. Which of the following is the rate-controlling step of pyrimidine synthesis that exhibits allosteric inhibition by cytidine triphosphate (CTP)?

a. Aspartate transcarbamoylase
b. Hypoxanthine-guanine phosphoribosyl transferase (HGPRT)
c. Thymidylate synthase
d. Ribose-phosphate pyrophosphokinase
e. Xanthine oxidase

299. Which of the following compounds is a required substrate for purine biosynthesis?

a. 5-Methyl thymidine
b. Ara C
c. Ribose phosphate
d. 5-Phosphoribosylpyrophosphate (PRPP)
e. 5-FU

300. Which of the following compounds is an analogue of hypoxanthine?

a. Ara C
b. Allopurinol
c. Ribose phosphate
d. 5-Phosphoribosylpyrophosphate (PRPP)
e. 5-FU

301. Which of the following compounds is joined with nicotinamide to form NAD and NADP, components that are deficient in niacin deficiency?

a. Cytosine monophosphate
b. Inosine diphosphate
c. Thymidine monophosphate
d. Hypoxanthine monophosphate
e. Adenosine diphosphate

302. A hitherto unknown disease is suggested by a 28-year-old male who has reducing substances in his urine, mild liver disease, and decreased liver glycogen upon liver biopsy. Which of the following metabolites would be the best candidate for measurement as a clue to the cause of disease?

a. Glucose 1-phosphate
b. Fructose 6-phosphate
c. Fructose 1,6-bisphosphate
d. Cytosine diphosphate
e. Uridine diphosphate

Lipid, Amino Acid, and Nucleotide Metabolism

Answers

242. The answer is e. (*Murray, pp 31-42, 527-544. Scriver, pp 5241-5286.*) Proline and lysine are encoded by collagen mRNAs and then hydroxylated during assembly of collagen peptides and formation of the triple helix (amino acids in choices a-d are incorporated during translation and could be labeled). In addition to large amounts of glycine and proline, the unusual amino acids 4-hydroxyproline and 5-hydroxylysine are modified after translation using a reducing agent such as ascorbate (vitamin C). Vitamin C deficiency (scurvy) produces weaker collagen and skeletal changes analogous to genetic alterations of collagens in osteogenesis imperfecta (MIM*166200).

243. The answer is d. (*Murray, pp 248-261. Scriver, pp 1667-1724.*) Enzymes specific for a few tissues can reveal injury to that tissue by leaking into the bloodstream, illustrated by increased serum aspartate aminotransferase level (AST also known as SGOT) and serum alanine aminotransferase (ALT also known as SGPT) in liver diseases (hepatitis, alcoholic cirrhosis) that destroy hepatic tissue. Cancers derived from normal tissues (eg, hepatocarcinoma from hepatic cells) usually have their own marker proteins (eg, α-fetoprotein for hepatocarcinoma—the liver cancer portion makes answers b, c, e incorrect). Aminotransferases have several roles including control of toxic ammonium ion (NH_4^+); they transfer the amino groups of amino acids to α-ketoglutarate and then to glutamate, followed by oxidative deamination to produce ammonium ion. The ammonium ion can enter the urea cycle to form urea or be excreted to balance acidosis (the first parts of answers a-e are all correct). Several transamination reactions (eg, alanine to pyruvate) provide substrates for gluconeogenesis (middle parts of answers a, c, e incorrect) and most are reversible and able to provide amino acids for protein synthesis.

244. The answer is a. (*Murray, pp 239-247. Scriver, pp 1909-1964.*) The female is likely a heterozygote (carrier) for a mutation in ornithine transcarbamoylase, giving her sufficient enzyme to avoid symptoms unless she ingests large amounts of protein or has illness with anorexia and endogenous protein catabolism. She will thus have excess ornithine and deficient citrulline (compound A—answers b-e incorrect). The initial and rate-limiting step for the urea cycle forms carbamoyl phosphate (compound E—answers c-e incorrect) from ammonium ion and carbon dioxide; this synthase is activated by acetylglutamate. Urea cycle disorders are generally severe and present in the newborn period with ammonia levels progressing to the 500 to 3000 µmol/L range shortly after initiation of feeding with progression to lethargy and coma. Severe urea cycle disorders exhibit X-linked or autosomal recessive inheritance with affected children being homozygotes or male hemizygotes with minimal enzyme activity. Female heterozygotes will have half-normal enzyme amounts and avoid symptoms except when ingesting or degrading protein.

245. The answer is b. (*Murray, pp 239-247. Scriver, pp 1909-1964.*) In humans and other land mammals, excess NH_4^+ is converted into urea (compound C in the urea cycle diagram below Question 244) in the liver for excretion by the kidneys. Urea is cleaved from compound B (arginine), so providing arginine will allow removal of urea by arginase and provide ornithine for another round of the cycle. Arginine bypasses the most severe urea cycle defects—carbamoyl phosphate synthetase deficiency (formation of compound E, MIM*237300), ornithine transcarbamylase deficiency (ornithine and compound E to citrulline [compound A, MIM*311250]), citrullinemia (A to argininosuccinate, MIM*215700), argininosuccinic aciduria (MIM*209700—argininosuccinate to arginine with release of fumarate, compound D)—and increases the substrate concentration for the last enzyme defect, argininemia (MIM*208700). Note that nitrogen is excreted in the form of urea with its two nitrogen and one carbonyl group (see Figure 18 of the High-Yield Facts). The first nitrogen is derived from free NH_4^+ (condensed with CO_2 to form carbamoyl phosphate—compound E) and the second nitrogen from the amino group of aspartate.

246. The answer is d. (*Murray, pp 239-247. Scriver, pp 1909-1964.*) The steps of the urea cycle are divided between the mitochondrial matrix and cytosol of liver cells in mammals. The formation of ammonia, its reaction with carbon dioxide to produce carbamoyl phosphate, and the conversion to citrulline occur in the matrix of mitochondria. Citrulline diffuses out of the mitochondria, and the next three steps of the cycle, which result in the formation of urea, all take place in the cytosol. Fatty acid oxidation and some reactions of organic acid degradation also occur in the mitochondria. Peroxisomes have single membranes, in contrast to the double membranes of mitochondria. They house catalase and enzymes for medium to long chain fatty acid oxidation.

247. The answer is e. *(Murray, pp 239-247. Scriver, pp 1909-1964.)* A major reason for the toxicity of ammonia is the severe depletion of ATP levels caused by the siphoning off of α-ketoglutarate from the citric acid cycle to form glutamine (incorrect answers a-d). Glutamate dehydrogenase and glutamine synthetase, respectively, catalyze the following reaction:

$$\alpha\text{-ketoglutarate} + NH_4^+ \rightarrow \text{glutamate} + NH_4^+ \rightarrow \text{glutamine}$$

As can be seen, this is the reverse order of steps whereby glutamine is successively deaminated first to glutamate and then to α-ketoglutarate by the enzymes glutaminase and glutamate dehydrogenase, respectively. It is thought that the high level of ammonia ions shifts the equilibrium of the dehydrogenase in favor of the formation of glutamate. Depending on the step in the urea cycle that is blocked, levels of arginine may be decreased.

248. The answer is a. *(Murray, pp 184-192. Scriver, pp 2297-2326.)* Fatty acids are bound to coenzyme A as thiol esters for synthesis or degradation, each proceeding in two-carbon steps. The serially repeated steps in fatty acid oxidation involve (a) removal of two hydrogens to form a double bond between the carbons adjacent to the acid group (acyl-CoA dehydrogenase), (b) addition of water to the double bond so that a hydroxyl is on the second carbon (enoyl-CoA hydratase), (c) oxidation of the hydroxyl group to a ketone (3-hydroxyacyl-CoA dehydrogenase), and (d) removal of acetyl-CoA (thiolase) to leave a fatty acyl-CoA that is two carbons shorter (other sequence options incorrect). At least three groups of these sequentially acting enzymes are present in the mitochondrion, specific for very long or long chain, medium chain, or short chain fatty acids. Children with very long or long chain oxidation enzyme deficiencies, for example, very long chain fatty acyl-CoA dehydrogenase deficiency (VLCAD, MIM*201475) accumulate fat in their heart and liver and have energy deficits in heart and muscle due to inadequate fat oxidation. Severely affected children often die of cardiac failure in the newborn period, and their enzyme deficiency combined with the maternal heterozygote state may cause HELLP syndrome in the last trimester of pregnancy, a variant of toxemia or preeclampsia that can be fatal. Premature delivery may be necessary for maternal health, and therapy with low-fat diets, frequent feeding (to minimize need for fat oxidation), and carnitine (to maximize transport of fatty acyl-CoAs into mitochondria) may be attempted with the affected child.

249. The answer is a. (*Murray, pp 184-192. Scriver, pp 2297-2326.*) Fatty acid oxidation is a major source of energy after serum glucose wanes and glycogen is depleted 3 to 4 hours after a meal. Severe exacerbation of a routine illness by poor feeding is typical of fatty acid oxidation disorders (incorrect answers b-e). The medium chain fatty acyl carnitines are diagnostic, reflecting the coupling of fatty acids with coenzyme A with transfer to carnitine for mitochondrial import for oxidation in steps that remove two carbons. The fatty acyl-CoA dehydrogenases, enoyl hydratases, hydroyacyl-CoA dehydrogenases, and thiolases that carry out each oxidation step are present in three groups with specifities for very long/long, medium, and short chain fatty acyl esters.

Lack of acetyl-CoA from fatty acid oxidation defects will decrease gluconeogenesis and produce hypoglycemia; the energy deficit leads to heart, liver, and muscle disease that may be lethal. Unlike other alterations in glucose metabolism (hypoglycemia, diabetes mellitus) that increase normal fat oxidation, defective fatty acid oxidation may not produce 4-carbon ketones (acetoacetate, β-hydroxybutyrate) measured by ketostix reagent strips—those ketones formed will have longer chains and lower effective concentration of the ketone group—thus the term "nonketotic hypoglycemia" as a red flag for fatty acid disorders.

Medium chain coenzyme A dehydrogenase (MCAD) deficiency (MIM*201450) can be fatal if not recognized, and sometimes presents as Sudden Unexplained Death Syndrome (SUDS—usually at older ages than Sudden Infant Death Syndrome —SIDS) that presents before age 6 months due to altered respiration. A child like that described in the question died before MCAD deficiency was recognized and treated by the simple strategy of frequent feeding; the child's parents were politically active and helped promote expanded newborn screening that now recognizes some 30 disorders in addition to phenylketonuria.

250. The answer is d. (*Murray, pp 131-142. Scriver, pp 2327-2356.*) Deficiency of insulin in diabetes mellitus causes decreased glucose uptake in extrahepatic tissues, but the special hexokinase (glucokinase with high K_m) in liver cells renders glucose import less sensitive to insulin (incorrect answer c). Unavailability of glucose in other tissues causes an increase in fatty acid oxidation with transport of free fatty acids to liver; these fatty acids plus increased gluconeogenesis and fatty acid oxidation in liver stimulate formation of acetoacetate (which degrades to acetone) and β-hydroxybutyrate—the "ketone bodies" (answers a, b, e incorrect). Their designation as "ketones" is not strictly correct since only acetone has a ketone group.

251. The answer is a. (*Murray, pp 193-199. Scriver, pp 2327-2356.*) Acetyl-CoA carboxylase catalyzes the first step of lipogenesis in which acetyl-CoA is linked to malonyl-CoA (answers b-e concern fatty acid oxidation). This enzyme is activated by citrate. Acetyl-CoA does not readily cross the mitochondrial membrane. Instead, citrate translocates to the cytosol where it is cleaved to acetyl-CoA and oxaloacetate by ATP-citrate lyase. Citrate increases in the fed state and indicates an abundant supply of acetyl-CoA for lipogenesis.

The acetyl- and malonyl-CoA groups are added to sulfydryl groups of fatty acid synthase multienzyme complex (one on each subunit) through transacylation reactions. Condensation forms acetoacetyl-S-enzyme on one subunit and a free sulfydryl group of the other subunit—a sequence of enzyme reactions then converts the acetoacetyl-S-enzyme to acyl (acetyl) enzyme. A second round of two-carbon addition begins as another malonyl-CoA residue displaces the acyl-S-enzyme to the other sulfhydryl group, then condenses to extend the acyl group by two carbons. Fatty acid synthesis then proceeds by successive addition of malonyl-CoA residues with condensation, causing the acyl chain to grow by two carbons with each cycle.

252. The answer is e. (*Murray, pp 248-261. Scriver, pp 2007-2056.*) In the synthesis of cysteine, the following sequence of steps occurs, where SAM is S-adenosylmethionine, cys is cysteine, and α-KG is α-ketoglutarate:

$$\text{methionine} \rightarrow \text{SAM} \rightarrow \text{homocysteine} + \text{adenosine}$$

$$\text{homocysteine} + \text{serine} \rightarrow \text{cystathionine} \rightarrow \text{cys} + \alpha\text{-KG} + \text{NH}_4^+$$

A defect in cystathionine synthetase will thus cause increased homocysteine and related metabolites like homocystine and methionine (incorrect answers c, d), and some defects are improved by adding pyridoxine (vitamin B_6), the precursor to enzyme cofactor pyridoxal-5′-phosphate (incorrect answers a and b). If cy represents $-CH_2CH(NH_2)COOH$, then methionine is CH_3-S-CH_2-cy, cysteine is $HS-cy$, homocysteine $HS-CH_2-cy$ (homo- = extra methyl group), cystathionine $cy-SCH_2-cy$, and homocystine $cyCH_2-S-S-CH_2-cy$. The conversions of methionine and cysteine can thus be seen as adding/subtracting activated methyl groups using SAM and transfer of sulfhydryl groups (transsulfuration). Deficiency of cystathionine synthase leads to a buildup of methionine (CH_3-S-CH_2-cy) and homocysteine ($HS-CH_2-cy$) which dimerizes to form homocystine ($cyCH_2-S-S-CH_2-cy$) that gives the disease its name. Affected patients may have mild mental retardation and symptoms of lax connective tissue including dislocated lenses, tall, asthenic build, and a clotting diathesis that, if unanticipated, may cause strokes and neurologic symptoms during periods of low fluid intake as when under anesthesia.

253. The answer is g. *(Murray, pp 248-261. Scriver, pp 2079-2108.)* Hartnup disease (MIM*234500) is caused by defective neutral amino acid transport in the intestinal and/or kidney—neutral meaning uncharged side chains like the phenyl group of phenylalanine, the methyl group of alanine, the indole ring of tryptophan. Answers a to f are incorrect because of negatively charged carboxyl groups (aspartate, glutamate) or positively charged amino groups (lysine, taurine, ornithine). Neutral aminoaciduria is observed as well as increased fecal excretion of indole derivations due to bacterial conversion of unabsorbed dietary tryptophan. The disorder is very rare in industrialized countries with good diets, since deficiency of tryptophan as a precursor for niacin synthesis causes the most severe symptoms. Niacin deficiency is called pellagra and produces skin rashes, psychiatric symptoms, and neurologic problems like ataxia (wobbly gait) or diplopia (double vision). Many individuals with Hartnup disease are asymptomatic and detected by screening programs, so the pellagra in some patients likely reflects gene-environmental interaction with suboptimal nutrition.

254. The answer is b. *(Murray, pp 593-615. Scriver, pp 2205-2216.)* The antioxidant activity of glutathione is dependent on maintenance of its reduced state. The enzyme glutathione reductase transfers electrons from NADPH via FAD to oxidized glutathione. Oxidized glutathione is composed of two glutathione molecules held together by a disulfide bridge. Reduced glutathione is a tripeptide with a free sulfhydryl group. It is the presence of the free sulfhydryl group that is of importance to the antioxidant activity of glutathione. In red blood cells, the function of cysteine residues of hemoglobin and other proteins is maintained by the reducing power of glutathione.

255. The answer is b. (*Murray, pp 92-97, 174-183. Scriver, pp 4517-4554.*) The pentose phosphate pathway does not generate any ATP but instead forms NADPH and ribose phosphate (incorrect answer d). Glycolysis produces a net two ATP molecules per glucose (incorrect answer c) while glycogenolysis yields glucose (incorrect answer e). The citric acid cycle produces a net 12 ATP per turn of the cycle (incorrect answer a). Fatty acid oxidation of palmitate results in a total of 129 ATP. Electron transport in the respiratory chain results in 5 ATP for each of the first 7 acetyl-CoA produced by the oxidation of palmitate for a total of 35 ATP. Each of the 8 acetyl-CoA molecules produced from palmitate results in 12 ATP from the citric-acid cycle for 96 total ATP. This gives a total of 131 ATP per palmitate oxidized, minus 2 ATP for the initial activation of palmitate for a grand total of 129 ATP per palmitate.

256. The answer is a. (*Murray, pp 271-284. Scriver, pp 2961-3104.*) Bilirubin, which is quite insoluble, is transported to the liver attached to albumin. In the liver, bilirubin is conjugated to two glucuronic acid molecules to form bilirubin diglucuronide. Urobilinogen (urine) and stercobilin (stool) are bilirubin compounds in tissues while heme is its precursor and biliverdin the immediate cleavage product of heme porphyrin (incorrect answers b-e). Bilirubin diglucuronide is transported against a concentration gradient into the bile. If bilirubin is not conjugated, it is not excreted.

Jaundice refers to the yellow color of the skin and eyes caused by increased levels of bilirubin in the blood. It has many causes, including increased production of bilirubin due to hemolytic anemia or malaria, blockage in the excretion of bilirubin due to liver damage, or obstruction of the bile duct. In newborns, jaundice is normal (physiologic) because of liver immaturity. Only excess jaundice is evaluated (bilirubin over 10-12 at age 3-4 days) based on the age of the infant. High levels of bilirubin in serum (indirect bilirubin) points toward hemolysis from materno-fetal blood group incompatibility, whereas high levels of bilirubin diglucuronide (one of several conjugated bilirubins tested as direct bilirubin) suggest liver/gastrointestinal disease.

Reticuloendothelial cells degrade red blood cells following approximately 120 days in the circulation. The steps in the degradation of heme include (1) formation of the green pigment biliverdin by the cleavage of the porphyrin ring of heme, (2) formation of the red-orange pigment bilirubin by the reduction of biliverdin, (3) uptake of bilirubin by the liver and the formation of bilirubin diglucuronide, and (4) active excretion of bilirubin into bile and eventually into the stool. The change in color of a bruise from bluish-green to reddish-orange reflects the heme degradation and the change in color of the bile pigments biliverdin and bilirubin.

257. The answer is d. *(Murray, pp 271-284. Scriver, pp 2961-3104.)* Once bile is excreted into the gut, bilirubin diglucuronide is hydrolyzed and reduced by bacteria to form urobilinogen, which is colorless. Much of the urobilinogen of the stools is further oxidized by intestinal bacteria to stercobilin, which gives stools their characteristic brown color. Some urobilinogen is reabsorbed by the gut into the portal blood, transported to the kidney, and converted and excreted as urobilin, which gives urine its characteristic yellow color. The female has usual risk factors for cholecystitis (inflammation of the gall bladder) remembered as four Fs—female, fair, fat, and forty. The inflammation can block excretion of conjugated bilirubin into the intestine, reducing oxidation to stercobilin and producing white (acholic) stools.

258. The answer is b. *(Murray, pp 212-223. Scriver, pp 2705-2716.)* Serum lipoproteins bind lipids and transport various lipid components from intestine and liver to peripheral tissues. Chylomicrons have the highest fat content and thus the lowest density, followed by very low density (VLDL), intermediate density (IDL), low density (LDL), and several high/very high density (HDL/VHDL) lipoproteins (incorrect answers a, c-e). Chylomicrons transport triglycerides and other lipids absorbed from the intestine and thus are elevated after a meal (incorrect answers a, c). Very low density lipoproteins (VLDLs) are triglyceride- and cholesterol-containing particles from the liver; removal of triglycerides from VLDLs leads to formation of intermediate forms (IDLs) and finally to a cholesterol-enriched small particle, the low density lipoprotein (LDL). VLDL, IDL, and LDL fractions all contain cholesterol and will be elevated in patients with hypercholesterolemia (incorrect answer c). Table 8 in the High-Yield Facts summarizes the characteristics of these plasma lipoproteins.

259. The answer is b. *(Scriver, pp 2297-2326, 121-138, 287-320. Murray pp 212-223.)* Untreated ethylene glycol of antifreeze can be oxidized to produce oxalic acid that can crystallize in the renal tubules and destroy renal function; flushing out the bladder (incorrect answer c) or observation (incorrect answer e) would not prevent renal damage. The first committed step in this process is the oxidation of ethylene glycol to an aldehyde by alcohol dehydrogenase. This is normally the route for converting ethanol (drinking alcohol) to acetate. Patients who have ingested ethylene glycol or wood alcohol (methanol) are placed on a nearly intoxicating dose of ethanol by a nasogastric tube together with intravenous saline and sodium bicarbonate (incorrect answers a, d). This treatment is carried out intermittently along with hemodialysis until no traces of ethylene glycol are seen in the blood. Ethanol acts as a competitive inhibitor of alcohol dehydrogenase with respect to ethylene glycol or methanol metabolism.

260. The answer is b. *(Murray, pp 200-202.)* Linoleic and α-linolenic acid are nutritionally essential in that they cannot be made by most animals and are instead made only by plants. Oleic acid and palmitoleic acid can be produced by introduction of a double bond at the Δ^9 position of a saturated fatty acid. These essential unsaturated fatty acids are required for synthesis of prostaglandin, thromboxane, leukotriene, and lipoxin.

261. The answer is d. *(Murray, pp 506-526. Scriver, pp 5875-5902.)* Multiple sclerosis (MIM*126200) is a demyelinating disease in which both phospholipid and sphingolipid levels are decreased, while lipid storage diseases exhibit accumulation of lipid substances (sphingolipid, ceramide) in brain (incorrect answers b, c, e). Multiple sclerosis exhibits multifactorial determination with autoimmune characteristics with susceptibility influenced by DNA and HLA markers. Ceramide is an important signaling molecule for apoptosis and is a precursor for glycosphingolipids and gangliosides; it does not form a major component of myelin (incorrect answer a). Sphingolipids and phospholipids are structural lipids in membranes and myelin that insulate the nervous system; patchy loss of this insulation in multiple sclerosis causes variable, episodic symptoms in vision, hearing, bladder control, sensation, and behavior.

262. The answer is c. *(Murray, pp 212-223. Scriver, pp 2705-2716.)* ApoB is the major protein of chylomicrons, very low density lipoproteins

(VLDLs), and low density lipoproteins (LDLs); these serum lipids are reduced in the lipoprotein electrophoretic patterns of children with abetal-ipoproteinemia (MIM*200100). The disorder is benefited by administration of fat-soluble vitamins like E that are malabsorbed. Chylomicrons are one of four major groups of lipoproteins and are responsible for transport of lipids from digestion and absorption. The other groups of lipoproteins are very low density lipoproteins (VLDLs), which are responsible for transport of triacylglycerol from the liver, low density lipoproteins (LDLs), which deliver cholesterol, and high density lipoproteins (HDLs), which remove cholesterol from tissues.

263. The answer is d. (*Murray, pp 184-192.*) Longer chain fatty acids will contain many more two-carbon units for oxidation than shorter chains, accounting for disproportionate energy depletion and severe cardiac and skeletal disease in children with longer chain enzyme deficiencies (incorrect answers a-c, e). Triacylglycerol is the major fuel reserve in the body and is mainly stored and hydrolyzed in adipose tissue. Triglyceride and fatty acid metabolism become active during fasting after glycogen stores are depleted in 3 to 4 hours. However, stores of triglycerides in heart and muscle are needed for energy even with adequate feeding. Glucose is important as a brain nutrient but will not be depleted by fatty acid oxidation. Glycogen (in animals) and starch (in plants) are glucose storage molecules. Glycogen is depleted with fasting but is not the major fuel reserve in mammals.

264. The answer is e. (*Murray, pp 212-223.*) Fatty liver is associated with a buildup of triacylglycerol either due to an inability to produce enough VLDL or an inability to produce plasma lipoproteins (incorrect answer a). Under normal conditions, VLDL is responsible for the transport of triacylglycerol from the liver to extrahepatic tissues. Alcoholism causes chronic injury to liver cells, producing increased fat retention in early stages and scarring due to cell death (cirrhosis) at later stages (incorrect answers b-d).

265. The answer is d. (*Murray, pp 203-207. Scriver, pp 2705-2716.*) Infants placed on chronic low-fat formula diets often develop skin problems, impaired lipid transport, and eventually poor growth. This can be overcome by including linoleic acid to make up 1% to 2% of the total caloric requirement. Essential fatty acids are required because humans have only Δ^4, Δ^5, Δ^6, and Δ^9 fatty acid desaturase. Only plants have desaturase greater than Δ^9. Consequently, certain fatty acids such as arachidonic acid cannot be made "from scratch" (de novo) in humans and other mammals. However, linoleic acid, which plants make, can be converted to arachidonic acid. Arachidonate and eicosapentaenoate are 20-carbon prostanoic acids that are the starting point of the synthesis of prostaglandins, thromboxanes, and leukotrienes.

266. The answer is a. (*Murray, pp 224-233. Scriver, pp 2863-2914.*) Cholesterol is formed in five steps. The first step, biosynthesis of mevalonate, is catalyzed by three enzymes—acetyl-CoA thiolase, HMG-CoA synthase, and HMG-CoA reductase. Thiolase catalyzes the condensation of two molecules of acetyl-CoA to form acetoacetyl-CoA. HMG-CoA synthase catalyzes the addition of a third molecule of acetyl-CoA to form HMG-CoA. This compound is reduced to mevalonate by HMG-CoA reductase. This enzyme is the rate-limiting and thus principal regulatory step in the pathway. In the second step of cholesterol synthesis, mevalonate is phosphorylated and decarboxylated to produce isopentyl diphosphate. Six of these isoprenoid units are condensed to form squalene in the third step. Lanosterol is formed in the fourth step and is subsequently converted to cholesterol.

Malonyl-CoA is a 3-carbon acyl-CoA that condenses with acetyl-CoA to initiate fatty acid synthesis. Malonate does inhibit the Krebs tricarboxylic acid cycle at the step from succinate to fumarate and may have an important role in diabetes mellitus.

267. The answer is b. (*Murray, pp 248-261. Scriver, pp 1667-1724.*) Phenylalanine is an essential amino acid that is converted to tyrosine by phenylalanine hydroxylase. Tyrosine is metabolized to various dopamine metabolites as well as melanin. Children with phenylketonuria (PKU-MIM*261600) have deficiency of phenylalanine hydroxylase or its tetrahydrobiopterin cofactor, causing elevated phenylalanine with severe mental deficiency that is perhaps related to brain dopamine pathways. Dietary treatment of PKU is effective if begun before age 2 to 3 months (hence neonatal screening that may not be done in underdeveloped countries), but it must be monitored because phenylalanine cannot be completely excluded from the diet. Complete absence of phenylalanine will cause protein malnutrition and failure to grow. Tyrosine is a precursor to melanin, so deficient tyrosine synthesis in children with PKU often causes a lighter hair and skin color than usual for their family. Phenylalanine and tyrosine levels must be monitored every 3 to 4 months in children on low phenylalanine diets to ensure balance between accumulation and deficiency.

268. The answer is c. (*Murray, pp 506-526. Scriver, pp 2297-2326.*) Ceramide is the basic unit composing all sphingolipids, which include sphingomyelin and gangliosides. Sphingomyelin, which usually contains phosphocholine as a polar head group, is the only phospholipid that does not have a glycerol backbone. In contrast, gangliosides have complex oligosaccharide head groups. The defect in Niemann-Pick disease is in the enzyme sphingomyelinase, resulting in accumulation of ceramide-phosphocholine (sphingomyelin).

269. The answer is d. (*Murray, pp 212-223. Scriver, pp 2863-2914.*) The shell of apoproteins coating blood transport lipoproteins is important in the physiologic function of the lipoproteins. Some of the apoproteins contain signals that target the movement of the lipoproteins in and out of specific tissues. B-48 and E seem to be important in targeting chylomicron remnants to be taken up by liver. B-100 is synthesized as the coat protein of VLDLs and marks their end product, LDLs, for uptake by peripheral tissues. Other apoproteins are important for the solubilization and movement of lipids and cholesterol in and out of the particles. C-II is a lipoprotein lipase activator that VLDLs and chylomicrons receive from HDLs. The A apoproteins are found in HDLs and are involved in lecithin–cholesterol acyl transferase (LCAT) regulation. Familial hypercholesterolemia (MIM*144010) causes early heart attacks in heterozygotes, particularly in males, and childhood disease in rare homozygotes. The daughter's chest pain was likely angina due to coronary artery occlusion and her skin patches were fatty deposits known as xanthomata.

270. The answer is b. (*Murray, pp 212-223. Scriver, pp 2863-2914.*) In the postabsorptional (postprandial) state, plasma contains all the lipoproteins: chylomicrons derived from dietary lipids packaged in the intestinal epithelial cells and their remnants; very low density lipoproteins (VLDLs), which contain endogenous lipids and cholesterol packaged in the liver; low density lipoproteins (LDLs), which are end products of delipidation of VLDLs; and high density lipoproteins (HDLs), which are synthesized in the liver. HDLs are in part catalytic, since transfer of their C-II apolipoprotein to VLDLs or chylomicrons activates lipoprotein lipase. In normal patients, only LDLs and HDLs remain in plasma following a 12-hour fast, since both chylomicrons and VLDLs have been delipidated. Most of the cholesterol measured in blood plasma at this time is present in the cholesterol-rich LDLs. However, HDL cholesterol also contributes to the measurement. In addition to total plasma cholesterol, the ratio of HDL (good) to LDL (bad) cholesterol is also useful for predicting heart attack risks.

271. The answer is a. (*Murray, pp 248-261. Scriver, pp 1667-2108.*) Cysteine can be formed from the essential amino acid methionine, one of nine essential amino acids (histidine, isoleucine, luecine, lysine, methionine, phenylalanine, threonine, tryptophan, valine) and one semiessential amino acid (arginine) that is needed for growth. Tyrosine can be made from phenylalanine, proline or glutamine from glutamate, asparagines from aspartate. Other metabolites like 3-phosphoglycerate (serine), glyoxylate (glycine), pyruvate (alanine) can be converted to amino acids at reasonable rates, rendering them nonessential. Hydroxylysine, hydroxyproline, and selenocysteine are converted from parent amino acids after incorporation into protein. Hyperalimentation solutions required years of research to define essential nutrients, which include unsaturated fatty acids, vitamins, and trace elements. Though effective for healing and growth, hyperalimentation still has unexplained side effects like liver disease that can arise during or after therapy.

272. The answer is c. (*Murray, pp 506-526. Scriver, pp 3421-3452.*) The two major groups of lysosomal storage disease are sphingolipidoses and mucopolysaccharidoses. An absence of α-L-iduronidase, as in Hurler syndrome (MIM*252800) and Scheie syndrome (MIM*252800), leads to accumulations of dermatan sulfate and heparan sulfate. Scheie syndrome is less severe, with corneal clouding, joint degeneration, and increased heart disease. Hurler syndrome has the same symptoms plus mental and physical retardation leading to early death. The later onset in this child is compatible with a diagnosis of Scheie syndrome. Note that Hurler and Scheie syndromes result from mutations at the same locus—hence their identical McKusick numbers. The reasons for the differences in disease severity are unknown. All of the other enzyme deficiencies listed lead to the lack of proper breakdown of sphingolipids and their accumulation as gangliosides, glucocerebrosides, and sphingomyelins. Symptoms of lipidoses may include organ enlargement, mental retardation, and early death.

273. The answer is a. (*Murray, pp 506-526. Scriver, pp 121-138, 287-320, 3827-3876.*) Gangliosides are continually synthesized and broken down. The specific hydrolases that degrade gangliosides by sequentially removing terminal sugars are found in lysosomes. In the lipid storage disease known as Tay-Sachs disease (MIM*272800), ganglioside GM_2 accumulates because of a deficiency of β-N-acetylhexosaminidase, a lysosomal enzyme that removes the terminal N-acetylgalactosamine residue. Homozygotes produce virtually no functional enzyme and suffer weakness, retardation, and blindness. Death usually occurs before infants are 3 years old. Carriers (heterozygotes) of the autosomal recessive disease produce approximately 50% of the normal levels of enzyme but show no ill effects. In high-risk populations, such as Ashkenazi Jews or French Canadians, screening for carrier status may be performed.

274. The answer is a. (*Murray, pp 193-199. Scriver, pp 2297-2326.*) Fatty acid synthesis requires NADPH that is provided by the pentose phosphate pathway plus malate formed by reduction of oxaloacetate (answers b-e incorrect). Citrate is split by citrate lyase into acetyl-CoA and oxaloacetate, and the latter reduced to pyruvate and carbon dioxide using NADP-linked malate enzyme Thus, the diffusion of excess citrate from the mitochondria to the cytoplasm of cells not only provides acetyl-CoA for synthesis of fatty acids but NADPH as well. One NADPH is produced for each acetyl-CoA produced. However, most of the NADPHs needed for synthesis of fatty acids are derived from the pentose phosphate pathway. For this reason, adipose tissue has an extremely active pentose phosphate pathway.

275. The answer is b. (*Murray, pp 184-192.*) The first step of fatty acid oxidation requires activation of the fatty acid to an acyl-CoA. This reaction is catalyzed by the enzyme acyl-CoA synthetase and requires 1 ATP. In subsequent reactions, two carbons are removed at a time from the carboxyl end to form acetyl-CoA.

276. The answer is b. (*Murray, pp 248-261, 432-441.*) Cysteine can be made from cystine (essentially a cysteine dimer with disulfide linkage) by cystine reductase, and is converted by transamination to 3-mercaptopyruvate and then pyruvate (eliminates answers c, e since alanine serine, and glycine can be converted to pyruvate [then acetyl-CoA] and glycine can be made from serine). The inborn error cystinosis (MIM*219800) results from mutations in a lysosomal membrane transporter, causing cystine accumulation in lysosomes with crystals in the lens of the eye and renal proximal tubules (eliminates answers a, d). Children with cystinosis present in early childhood with short stature, photophobia, and progressive renal disease. The synthetic compound cysteamine can complex with cystine and allow egress from lysosomes, slowing the progression of renal failure.

Most amino acids except lysine, threonine, proline, and hydroxyproline can undergo transamination to convert α-amino acids into α-keto acids. Transamination reactions can contribute amino groups to the urea cycle for urea biosynthesis or initiate catabolism of the amino acid. Six amino acids (listed as answer options) are degraded to pyruvate, joining another six (tyrosine, phenylalanine, lysine, hydroxylysine, tryptophan, methionine) that are in part converted to acetyl-CoA.

277. The answer is d. *(Murray, pp 239-247. Scriver, pp 1909-1964.)* Major mechanisms for removal of ammonia include transfer of amino acid amino groups to α-ketoglutarate to form glutamate, adding ammonia to glutamate to form glutamine (coupled to ATP hydrolysis), and conversion of ammonia to urea via the urea cycle. Among urea cycle enzymes, the initial carbamoyl phosphate synthase reaction requires 2 ATPs, one as a phosphate donor and the other to drive the raction. Depletion of α-ketoglutarate to form glutamate and glutamine (incorrect answers a, c) may interfere with citric acid cycle energy NADH production, and the decreased ATP from oxidative phosphorylation may be further reduced by the glutamate to glutamine reaction and the greater ATP needs for carbamoyl phosphate synthesis relative to other steps of the urea cycle (incorrect answers b, c, e). Conversion of aspartate to argininosuccinate by its synthase is the other urea cycle reaction that requires ATP.

278. The answer is a. *(Murray, pp 239-247.)* Asparagine is converted to aspartate by the enzyme asparaginase and then to oxaloacetate by transamination. The other amino acid conversions do not directly yield components of citric acid cycle or gluconeogenesis although glycine, cysteine/cystine—and thus methionine—ultimately are catabolized to pyruvate. Oxaloacetate combines with acetyl-CoA from pyruvate to form citrate and initiate the citric acid cycle with NADH for oxidative phosphorylation: oxaloacetate is regenerated by the citric acid cycle and can form phosphoenolpyruvate through its carboxykinase on the path to glucose by gluconeogenesis. The phosphoenolpyruvate carboxykinase consumes a GTP while the α-ketoglutarate to succinate reaction generates a GTP, providing a link between cycles to ensure gluconeogenesis does not deplete oxaloacetate and deplete energy from citric acid cycle-oxidative phosphorylation.

279. The answer is c. *(Murray, pp 193-199. Scriver, pp 2297-2326.)* Two major enzyme complexes are involved in the synthesis of fatty acids. The first is acetyl-CoA carboxylase, which synthesizes malonyl-CoA by the steps shown below for the synthesis of palmitate:

$$7 \text{ acetyl-CoA} + 7 \text{ HCO}_3^- + 7 \text{ ATP} \rightarrow 7 \text{ malonyl-CoA} + 7 \text{ ADP} + 7 \text{ P}_i$$

Using the malonyl-CoA, palmitate is then synthesized by seven cycles of the fatty acid synthetase complex, whose stoichiometry is summarized below:

$$\text{acetyl-CoA} + 7 \text{ malonyl-CoA} + 14 \text{ NADPH} \rightarrow \text{palmitate} + 7 \text{ CO}_2 \\ + 14 \text{ NAD}^+ + 8 \text{ CoA} + 6 \text{ H}_2\text{O}$$

As can be seen from the equations above, the necessary amount of malonyl-CoA is synthesized. Palmitate is subsequently synthesized from malonyl-CoA and one initial acetyl-CoA. Thus, acetyl-CoA, NADPH, ATP, and HCO_3^- are all necessary in this process. In contrast, $FADH_2$ is not utilized in fatty acid synthesis, but is one of the products of fatty acid oxidation. Vitamin B_{12} is required for conversion of propionic acid to methylmalonic acid, a step in the β-oxidation of odd-numbered fatty acid chains.

280. The answer is b. *(Murray, pp 407-412. Scriver, pp 2297-2326.)* Plasma membranes are mosaics of globular proteins distributed asymmetrically in a phospholipid bilayer (incorrect answers a, c). Small peptide hormones like insulin or glucagon are water-soluble, circulating in plasma to reach receptors on the surfaces of target cell membranes (incorrect answers d, e). Action with receptors triggers second messenger release (cAMP in this case) that alters proteins (eg, phosphate addition/removal from glycogen phosphorylase) and/or patterns of transcription.

The lipids and proteins in plasma membranes are in a fluid and dynamic state capable of translational (side-to-side) movement within the lipid bilayer. The phospholipid and protein components are amphipathic with polar (water-binding) regions exposed to the aqueous phases (outer extracellular fluid, inner cytosol) and nonpolar (hydrophobic) regions buried within the membrane. The glycerol-phosphate "heads" of acylglycerols are polar regions facing the bilayer surface while the fatty acid "tails" align within the hydrophobic membrane interior. Membrane proteins may extend through the membrane with polar amino acid regions at each surface and nonpolar amino acids forming channels within the membrane interior (integral membrane proteins). Other proteins may be localized to one membrane surface and serve as receptors for hormones. The lateral or translational motion allows some surface receptors to aggregate on special membrane surface structures, illustrated by the caveolae that contain low density lipoprotein receptors.

281. The answer is e. (*Murray, pp 212-223. Scriver, pp 2297-2326.*) During digestion, hydrophobic fat globules are emulsified by the detergent action of phospholipids and bile acids in the gut. Hydrophilic glycerol molecules (circles in diagram E of the figure) are on the outside of the micelles with hydrophobic fatty acid chains on the inside, thus increasing the surface area available for the action of hydrolytic lipases (other diagrams show linear membrane structures with similar outside glycerols and inside fatty acid chains; incorrect answers a-d). Mixed micelle formation is dependent on the amphipathic (polar/nonpolar) properties of bile acids and phospholipids that act as detergents. The formation of micelles solves the fundamental problem of transporting and incorporating insoluble lipids into the high water content of most biological structures (including the transport of blood lipoproteins).

282. The answer is b. (*Murray, pp 224-233. Scriver, pp 2863-2914.*) The lowering of cholesterol by mevastatin lowers amounts of the lipoprotein that transports cholesterol to the peripheral tissues, low density lipoprotein (LDL). Mevastatin, an analogue of mevalonic acid, acts as a feedback inhibitor of 3′-hydroxy-3′-methylglutaryl-CoA (HMG-CoA) reductase, the regulated enzyme of cholesterol synthesis. Effective treatment with mevastatin, along with a low-fat diet, decreases levels of blood cholesterol and will not have immediate effects on glucose levels or fatty acid oxidation (incorrect answers a, c-e). Because lipids like cholesterol and triglycerides are insoluble in water, they must be associated with lipoproteins for transport and salvage between their major site of synthesis (liver) and the peripheral tissues. Those lipoproteins associated with more insoluble lipids thus have lower density during centrifugation (see Table 8 in the High-Yield Facts), a technique that separates the lowest-density chylomicrons from very low density lipoproteins (VLDLs with pre-β-lipoproteins), low density lipoproteins (LDLs with β-lipoproteins), intermediate density lipoproteins (IDLs), and high density lipoproteins (HDLs with α-lipoproteins). Each type of lipoprotein has typical apolipoproteins such as the apo B-100 and apo B-48 (translated from the same messenger RNA) in LDL. LDL is involved in transporting cholesterol from the liver to peripheral tissues, whereas HDL is a scavenger of cholesterol. The ratio of HDL to LDL is thus a predictor of cholesterol deposition in blood vessels, the cause of myocardial infarctions (heart attacks). The higher the HDL/LDL ratio, the lower the rate of heart attacks.

283. The answer is c. *(Murray, pp 193-199. Scriver, pp 3181-3218.)* Triacylglycerols are assembled from glycerol and saturated fatty acids that are synthesized from condensation of malonyl and acetyl-CoA through the fatty acyl synthase complex. Plasmalogens and certain signaling agents like platelet activating factor are ether lipids, distinguished by an ether (C-O-C) bond at carbon 1 of glycerol. Ether lipid synthesis is initiated by placing an acyl group on carbon 1 of dihydroxyacetone phosphate (DHAP) using DHAP acyltransferase. The acyl side chain is then exchanged with an alcohol to form an ether linkage by an acyl-DHAP synthase—the acyltransferase and synthase plus other enzymes of ether lipid synthesis are localized in peroxisomes. Subsequent additions of phosphocholine yield ether/acyl glycerols analogous to lecithins (including platelet activating factor), and addition of a phosphoethanolamine to carbon 3 of ether (alkyl) glycerols forms plasmalogens. Acetyl and palmitoyl-CoA can contribute to these ether lipid modifications after the core carbon 1 ether linkage has produced an alkylglycerol. Disruption of peroxisome structure by mutations in various peroxisomal membrane proteins ablates DHAP acyltransferase and other enzymes for ether lipid/plasmalogen synthesis, causing deficiency of brain lipids, severe neurologic disease, hypotonia, and liver failure—the most severe phenotype of which is Zellweger syndrome (MIM*214100).

284. The answer is b. *(Murray, pp 184-192. Scriver, pp 1471-1488, 2327-2356.)* The "ketone bodies," β-hydroxybutyrate and acetoacetate (plus acetone made from acetoacetate that is the only chemical with a true ketone group), are synthesized in liver mitochondria from acetyl-CoA. The liver produces ketone bodies under conditions of fasting associated with high rates of fatty acid oxidation. The inability to get glucose into extrahepatic cells because of insulin deficiency in diabetes also increases fatty acid oxidation and ketogenesis. The acid groups of β-hydroxybutyrate and acetoacetate cause acidosis and an anion gap (sum of serum sodium and potassium minus the sum of chloride and bicarbonate) that is greater than normal (over 8-15). In the case of diabetes, the "hidden anions" that add to bicarbonate in balancing the cations can be recognized as ketones through urine reagent strip testing. (Special ketostix strips that measure only ketones are available and used in low-carbohydrate diets to ensure a state of fat oxidation.) In metabolic disorders like methylmalonic aciduria (MIM*251000) or fatty acid oxidation defects, there are scanty abnormal or no ketones (if fat cannot be oxidized) so the hidden anions must be identified by plasma acylcarnitine or urine organic acid profiles. Acetone is a ketone body produced in diabetes that produces an acrid breath during ketoacidosis.

285. The answer is a. (*Murray, pp 406-424. Scriver, pp 2297-2326.*) Plasma membranes are unique as compared to intracellular membranes in that their composition contains cholesterol, glycoproteins, and glycolipids known as gangliosides. Plasma membranes of the cells of different tissues are distinguished from each other because of the properties that make them unique. Hormone receptors allow each cell type to respond to systemic stimulation appropriately. All chronic hormone receptors are localized to plasma membranes and upon stimulation release a second messenger into the interior of the cell. Glucagon, like epinephrine and norepinephrine, stimulates adenylate cyclase to produce cyclic AMP. Glucagon is found on the plasma membranes of liver and adipose tissue cells.

286. The answer is e. (*Murray, pp 406-424. Scriver, pp 3897-3944.*) Of the indicated amino acids and catabolic intermediates—the serine to glycine, glycine to carbon dioxide and ammonia, and formiminoglutamate (from histidine) to glutamate reactions—all require tetrahydrofolate as a cofactor. In folate deficiency, the figlu accumulates abnormally and is an unusual metabolite that serves as a diagnostic marker. Methyltetrahydrofolate and vitamin B_{12} (cobalamin) are required for conversion of homocysteine to methionine (with accompanying conversion of methyl- to tetrahydrofolate), so vitamin B_{12} deficiency can "trap" folate reserves as methyltetrahydrofolate and cause secondary folate deficiency. Mutations in the converting enzyme methionine synthase can cause one form of homocystinuria (MIM*236200) with connective tissue disease resembling Marfan syndrome. Certain of these mutations can be ameliorated by folate and B_{12} supplementation to augment residual enzyme activity.

287. The answer is b. *(Murray, pp 224-233. Scriver, pp 2705-2716.)* The uptake of exogenous cholesterol by cells results in a marked suppression of endogenous cholesterol synthesis. Low density human lipoprotein not only contains the greatest ratio of bound cholesterol to protein but also has the greatest potency in suppressing endogenous cholesterogenesis. LDLs normally suppress cholesterol synthesis by binding to a specific membrane receptor that mediates inhibition of hydroxymethylglutaryl (HMG) coenzyme A reductase. In autosomal dominant familial hypercholesterolemia (MIM*143890), where the abnormal allele encodes a dysfunctional LDL receptor, cholesterol synthesis is less responsive to plasma cholesterol levels. Treatment was pioneered through suppression of HMG-CoA reductase using inhibitors (statins) that mimic the structure of mevalonic acid that is the first substrate for cholesterol synthesis and is a feedback inhibitor of the enzyme. In multifactorial hypercholesterolemia involving interaction of environmental factors (diet, cigarettes) and genetic factors (influencing glucose, lipoprotein, homocysteine metabolism, etc), statins are used to keep serum cholesterol below recommended limits (below 200 mg/dL although criteria vary by sex, age, and practitioner) and maximize levels of low-cholesterol, high density lipoprotein (HDL). Cholesterol is found in arterial plaques that block coronary arteries to cause heart attacks or cerebral arteries that cause strokes, but the pathogenesis of such atherosclerosis is extremely complex.

288. The answer is c. *(Murray, pp 239-247. Scriver, pp 1909-1964.)* Arginase catalyzes the conversion of arginine to ornithine with liberation of urea (answers a, b, d, e incorrect). Ornithine and glutamate can be converted to α-ketoglutarate as can asparagine (through asparaginase to aspartate) and glutamine (through glutaminase). Tyrosine yields acetyl-CoA through transamination to hydroxyphenylpyruvate, homogentisic acid, fumarylacetoacetate, and acetoacetate; lysine also yields acetyl-CoA through glutaryl-CoA and propionyl-CoA. As with arginase deficiency, each of the latter reaction steps is deficient in a specific inborn error of metabolism.

289. The answer is a. (*Murray, pp 193-199. Scriver, pp 2297-2326.*) Under conditions of active synthesis of fatty acids in the cytosol of hepatocytes, levels of malonyl-CoA are high. Malonyl-CoA is the activated source of 2 carbon units for fatty acid synthesis. Malonyl-CoA inhibits carnitine acyltransferase I, which is located on the cytosolic face of the inner mitochondrial membrane. Thus, long-chain fatty acyl-CoA units cannot be transported into mitochondria where β-oxidation occurs, and translocation from cytosol to mitochondrial matrix is prevented. In this situation compartmentalization of membranes as well as inhibition of enzymes comes into play.

290. The answer is e. (*Murray, pp 292-301. Scriver, pp 2663-2704.*) Orotic aciduria (MIM*258900) is the buildup of orotic acid due to a deficiency in one or both of the enzymes that convert it to UMP. Either orotate phosphoribosyltransferase and orotidylate decarboxylase are both defective, or the decarboxylase alone is defective. UMP is the precursor of UTP, CTP, and TMP. All of these end products normally act in some way to feedback inhibit the initial reactions of pyrimidine synthesis. Specifically, the lack of CTP inhibition allows aspartate transcarbamoylase to remain highly active and ultimately results in a buildup of orotic acid and the resultant orotic aciduria. The lack of CTP, TMP, and UTP leads to decreased DNA synthesis in bone marrow erythroblasts, slower cell division, more cytoplasm per daughter cell, and thus larger erythrocytes once the erythroblast nucleus is lost. Uridine treatment is effective because uridine can easily be converted to UMP by omnipresent tissue kinases, thus allowing UTP, CTP, and TMP to be synthesized and feedback inhibit further orotic acid production.

291. The answer is a. (*Murray, pp 292-301. Scriver, pp 2537-2570.*) Some forms of gout derive from deficiency of phosphoribosyl pyrophosphate (PRPP) synthase, the first step of purine synthesis (eg, MIM*311850). Other patients may have a partial deficiency of hypoxanthine-guanine phosphoribosyl transferase (HGPRTase), which salvages hypoxanthine and guanine by transferring the purine ribonucleotide of PRPP to the bases and forming inosinate and guanylate, respectively. In all of these patients, the hypoxanthine analogue allopurinol has two actions: (1) it inhibits xanthine oxidase, which catalyzes the oxidation of hypoxanthine to xanthine and then to uric acid stones and tissue deposits; and (2) it forms an inactive allopurinol ribonucleotide from PRPP in a reaction catalyzed by HGPRTase, thereby decreasing the rate of purine synthesis. In contrast, because of the total loss of HGPRTase activity in Lesch-Nyhan patients, the allopurinol ribonucleotide cannot be formed. Thus, PRPP levels are not decreased and de novo purine synthesis continues unabated. The gouty arthritis caused by urate crystal formation is relieved in Lesch-Nyhan patients, but their neurological symptoms (mental deficiency, self-mutilation with compulsive chewing of fingers and lips) are not.

292. The answer is d. (*Murray, pp 239-247, 292-301. Scriver, pp 2513-2570.*) Carbamoyl phosphate (CAP) synthase I is found in mitochondrial matrix and is the first step in urea synthesis, condensing CO_2 and NH_4^+. Hyperammonemia occurs when CAP is deficient. CAP synthase II forms CAP as the first step in pyrimidine synthesis. Its complete deficiency would probably be a lethal mutation. When its activity is decreased, purine catabolism to uric acid is decreased, decreasing the possibility of hyperuricemia. In contrast, gout, Lesch-Nyhan syndrome, high xanthine oxidase activity, and von Gierke disease (glycogen storage disease type Ia [MIM*232200]) all lead to increased urate production and excretion.

293. The answer is a. (*Murray, pp 292-301. Scriver, pp 2513-2570.*) Glutamine and aspartate participate in both purine and pyrimidine synthesis, so increasing glutamine would not inhibit DNA synthesis (incorrect answer d). Carbamoyl phosphate synthase II (as opposed to CPS I in the urea cycle) initiates pyrimidine synthesis by producing carbamoyl phosphate that adds to aspartic acid and eventually forms orotic acid (incorrect answer e). Purine synthesis begins with ribose 5-phosphate and phosphoribosyl pyrophosphate (PRPP) via PRPP synthase, so decreasing CPS II would not effect purine synthesis (incorrect answer b). Uric acid is formed from purines through xanthine and xanthine oxidase, and its excess might produce some feedback inhibition for PRPP synthase that is inhibited by both purines and pyrimidines to help coordinate their synthesis and equivalent incorporation into DNA. However, the main effect of uric acid excess is deposit of the chemical in joint spaces to cause the severe pain of gout (incorrect answer c).

During purine ring biosynthesis, the amino acid glycine is completely incorporated to provide C4, C5, and N7. Glutamine contributes N3 and N9, aspartate provides N1, and derivatives of tetrahydrofolate furnish C2 and C8. Carbon dioxide is the source of C6. In pyrimidine ring synthesis,

C2 and N3 are derived from carbamoyl phosphate, while N1, C4, C5, and C6 come from aspartate.

294. The answer is e. *(Murray, pp 239-247. Scriver, pp 2513-2570.)* Although defects in any of these enzymes will result in a buildup of ammonia in the bloodstream and ammonia intoxication, blocks at carbamoyl phosphate synthase I and ornithine transcarbamylase are usually more severe. Ornithine transcarbamylase deficiency (MIM*300461) is an X-linked recessive disorder, allowing for mild manifestations in female carriers; deficiencies in the other four enzymes are autosomal recessive traits. Gene therapy approaches to treatment are being tested, but resulted in the death of one patient due to suspected reaction to the adenovirus vector.

295. The answer is b. *(Murray, pp 271-284. Scriver, pp 2961-3062.)* The porphyrias are a group of inborn errors that affect synthesis of porphyrins, the precursors of heme in hemoglobin. Defective synthesis of heme would not elevate heme breakdown products of the heme catabolic pathway, including bilirubin to conjugated bilirubin diglucuronide (in liver), bilirubin diglucuronide to urobilinogen and stercobilin (by bacteria in stool), and reabsorption of urobilinogen to be excreted in urine as urobilin. Delta-aminolevulinic acid (ALA) is synthesized from succinyl-CoA and glycine followed by condensation of two ALA molecules to form porphobilinogen (PBG) with a 5-member pyrrole ring. Four molecules of PBG are converted to the four-ring uroporphyrin by hydroxymethylbilane synthase, the primary defect in acute intermittent porphyria (MIM*176000). Deficiencies in other enzymes of the pathway from ALA to heme cause symptoms varying from anemia to photosensitivity to the well known but rarely encountered presentation with abdominal pain and neuropsychiatric symptoms.

296. The answer is e. *(Murray, pp 292-301.)* PRPP synthetase catalyzes the first reaction in purine biosynthesis from ribose 5-phosphate. This enzyme is normally subject to feedback inhibition by purines or pyrimidines, and is part of the mechanism to ensure coordinated purine and pyrimidine synthesis appropriate to their equal amounts in DNA. Defects in this enzyme or its regulation can result in overproduction and overexcretion of purine catabolites including uric acid that causes gout. The excess uric acid exceeds its solubility in certain bodily fluids like those of the subcutaneous tissues and joint spaces. The resulting solid crystals evoke an inflammatory reaction, causing sore nodules (tophi) beneath the skin and joint/tissue pain so exquisite that covering bedsheets are avoided.

297. The answer is c. (*Murray, pp 292-301. Scriver, pp 2537-2570.*) Uric acid is a purine derivative, increased by purine salvage reactions that convert purines, purine ribonucleosides, and purine deoxyribonucleoside to mononucleotides (incorrect answer d). Such salvage reactions require much less energy than de novo synthesis (incorrect answers a, b). The liver is the major site of purine nucleotide biosynthesis and provides excess purines for other tissues that cannot synthesize purines. A defect in hypoxanthine-guanine phosphoribosyl transferase, one of the enzymes of purine salvage, is responsible for purine overproduction and subsequent hyperuricemia observed in Lesch-Nyhan syndrome. Carbamoyl phosphate involved in pyrimidine synthesis is also an intermediate of the urea cycle, but different enzymes convert this substrate in the two pathways (incorrect answer e).

298. The answer is a. (*Murray, pp 292-301. Scriver, pp 2513-2570.*) Aspartate transcarbamoylase catalyzes the first reaction unique to pyrimidine biosynthesis. This enzyme is inhibited by CTP but activated by ATP. Both ATP and CTP bind at a different site from either substrate. Aspartate transcarbamoylase consists of multiple catalytic and regulatory subunits. Each regulatory subunit contains at least two CTP binding sites.

299. The answer is d. (*Murray, pp 292-301. Scriver, pp 2513-2570.*) 5'-Phosphoribosyl-1-pyrophosphate (PRPP) donates the ribose phosphate unit of nucleotides and is absolutely required for the beginning of the synthesis of purines. In fact, the enzymes regulating the synthesis of PRPP and the subsequent synthesis of phosphoribosylamine from PRPP are all end product–inhibited by inosine monophosphate (IMP), adenosine monophosphate (AMP), and guanosine monophosphate (GMP), the products of this reaction pathway.

300. The answer is b. (*Murray, pp 292-301. Scriver, pp 2513-2570.*) The degradation of purines to urate can lead to gout when an elevated level of urate is present in serum, causing the precipitation of sodium urate crystals in joints. The excessive production of urate in many patients seems to be connected to a partial deficiency of hypoxanthine-guanine phosphoribosyl transferase (HGPRT). Allopurinol, an analogue of hypoxanthine, is a drug used to correct gout. It accomplishes this by inhibiting the production of urate from hypoxanthine and in doing so undergoes suicide inhibition of xanthine oxidase. Ribose phosphate and PRPP are required for purine synthesis. 5-Fluorouracil (5-FU) and cytosine arabinoside (Ara C) are cancer chemotherapy agents, the former being an analogue of thymine that inhibits thymidylate synthetase and the latter an inhibitor of RNA synthesis.

301. The answer is e. (*Murray, pp 292-301, 489-505. Scriver, pp 2513-2570.*) Adenosine diphosphate (adenylate) is joined to nicotinamide to form nicotinamide adenine dinucleotide (NAD), further phosphorylated at the 3' position of ribose to form NADP. Niacin can be synthesized from tryptophan and is not strictly a vitamin. Deficiency of tryptophan and niacin can occur from diet or with diseases that increase requirements, causing pellagra (photosensitivity, dermatitis, psychosis).

Ribonucleosides consist of a base at the 1' position of ribose, while ribonucleotides have 5'-phosphate groups. Guanosine (G) and adenosine (A) contain purine bases, cytosine (C), uridine (U), and thymidine (T) pyrimidine bases. Ribonucleotides (adenylate, guanidylate, cytidylate, uridylate) have a phosphate ester on the 5'-hydroxyl of ribose (note that the ribo- prefix is usually omitted). Deoxyribonucleotides have a phosphate ester on the 5'-hydroxyl of deoxyribose (deoxyadenylate, deoxyguanidylate, deoxycytidylate, and thymidylate). The ribonucleosides A, G, C, and U can be incorporated into RNA, while the deoxyribonucleosides A, G, C, and T join with deoxyribose (lacking a hydroxyl at the 2' carbon) and are incorporated into DNA. Uridine occurs only as the ribonucleoside, thymidine as the deoxyribonucleotide (actually as thymidylate deoxyribonucleotide) synthesized from uridylate by thymidylate synthetase. Hypoxanthine and inosine are precursors of purine A, G synthesis.

302. The answer is e. (*Murray, pp 292-301. Scriver, pp 2513-2536.*) The activated form of glucose utilized for the synthesis of glycogen and galactose is UDP-glucose, which is formed from the reaction of glucose 1-phosphate and UTP. The indicated glucose or fructose phosphates could regulate glycogen stores but would not prevent synthesis of glycogen or block galactose metabolism (answers a-c incorrect). Cytidine diphosphate is important for the synthesis of phospholipids, forming high energy CDP-diacylglycerol that transfers diacylglycerol to form phosphatidylinositols (important signal transducers) and cardiolipin that is abundant in the mitochondrial membrane and elicits antibodies in certain autoimmune disorders. The conversion of galactose to glucose is at the UDP-sugar level, and is deficient in galactosemia (MIM*230400). UDP derivatives of glucose and galactose and of sugar amines (glucosamine, N-acetylmannosamine or neuraminic/sialic acids) are key precursors for synthesis of derivative polysaccharide chains including cerebrosides and gangliosides. A group of neurolipidoses with developmental regression and neurodegeneration result from deficiencies in enzymes that degrade complex polysaccharides (glycosphingolipids).

Vitamins and Minerals

Questions

303. A 48-year-old Caucasian male presents with congestive heart failure with elevated liver enzymes. His skin has a grayish pigmentation. The levels of liver enzymes are higher than those usually seen in congestive heart failure, suggesting an inflammatory process (hepatitis) with scarring (cirrhosis) of the liver. A liver biopsy discloses a marked increase in iron storage. In humans, molecular iron (Fe) is which of the following?

a. Stored primarily in the spleen
b. Stored in combination with ferritin
c. Excreted in the urine as Fe^{2+}
d. Absorbed in the intestine by albumin
e. Absorbed in the ferric (Fe^{3+}) form

304. Intestinal bowel resections are necessary for autoimmune inflammatory diseases like Crohn disease and for congenital anomalies like malrotation or volvulus (twisted intestine with impaired blood supply). Once the absorptive intestinal mucosa falls below a certain length, oral or parenteral alimentation must be instituted to maintain nutrition. In such solutions, which of the following nutrients is most dispensable?

a. Protein
b. Iodine
c. Carbohydrates
d. Lipids
e. Calcium

305. Which of the following disorders or symptoms are typical of cobalamin deficiency?

a. Pellagra
b. Beriberi
c. Pernicious anemia
d. Scurvy
e. Rickets

306. In adults, a severe deficiency of vitamin D causes which of the following disorders?

a. Night blindness
b. Osteomalacia
c. Rickets
d. Osteogenesis imperfecta
e. Osteopetrosis

307. A 40-year-old African American male is concerned about weight gain acquired during his stressful schedule as a small business executive. He embarks on a low-carbohydrate diet consisting of packaged or dried meats that are convenient for travel and office meals. Which of the following vitamins would most likely become deficient on this diet?

a. Thiamine
b. Niacin
c. Cobalamin
d. Pantothenic acid
e. Vitamin C

308. Children with autism and other disorders with mental disability are often put on megavitamin supplements despite no scientific evidence of benefit. Although most vitamins are harmless in excess, merely being excreted in urine, vitamin A can be toxic. Which of the following accurately describes vitamin A?

a. It is not an essential vitamin.
b. It is related to tocopherol.
c. It is a component of rhodopsin.
d. It is derived from ethanol.
e. It is also known as opsin.

309. A 12-year-old Caucasian girl is hospitalized for evaluation of a possible seizure disorder because she has staring spells, lethargy, and irritability (not herself) once or twice per day. A 24-hour electroencephalogram shows diffuse epileptic foci that develop some 4 to 6 hours after feeding, and low serum glucose is noted during these periods. Which of the following dietary supplements might help this child?

a. Malate and niacin
b. Acetyl-CoA and biotin
c. Acetyl-CoA and thiamine pyrophosphate
d. Oxaloacetate and pyridoxine
e. Oxaloacetate and niacin

310. A group of neurodegenerative diseases with onset ranging from neonates to adults have been found to involve deficiency of pantothenic acid kinase (eg, Hallervorden-Spatz disease, MIM*234200). The correlation between defective pantothenic acid activation and loss of myelin to cause neurodegenerative disease relates to its role in which of the following?

a. Decarboxylation reactions
b. Acetylation and acyl group metabolism
c. Dehydrogenation and redox reactions
d. Phosphorylation reactions
e. Methyl transfer reactions

311. Mothers taking warfarin for anticoagulation during pregnancy may have children with fetal warfarin syndrome involving very short nose and skeletal changes. Studies of the actions of the anticoagulants dicumarol and warfarin (the latter also a hemorrhagic rat poison) have revealed which of the following?

a. Vitamin C is necessary for the synthesis of fibrinogen.
b. Vitamin C activates fibrinogen.
c. Vitamin K is a clotting factor.
d. Vitamin K is essential for γ-carboxylation of glutamate.
e. The action of vitamin E is antagonized by these compounds.

312. A 2-year-old Caucasian girl presents with hair loss, a scaly red skin rash, and exaggerated acidosis after infections. The child is found to have deficiency of biotinidase (MIM*253260), and improves dramatically with biotin therapy. Biotin is involved in which of the following types of reactions?

a. Hydroxylations
b. Carboxylations
c. Decarboxylations
d. Dehydrations
e. Deaminations

313. Which of the following vitamins is the precursor of CoA?

a. Riboflavin
b. Pantothenate
c. Thiamine
d. Cobalamin
e. Pyridoxamine

314. A 5-year-old girl immigrant from India has had a falloff in growth with arm and leg pains. Her parents attributed this to "growing pains," but seek evaluation for her growth delay. Examination reveals some wasting of her lower limb muscles with slow fading of pits made by thumb pressure on her shins (pitting edema). Blood tests reveal mild elevations of lactate and pyruvate. The girl is diagnosed with beriberi. Beriberi is caused by a deficiency of which of the following vitamins?

a. Choline
b. Ethanolamine
c. Thiamine
d. Serine
e. Glycine

315. A 14-year-old Caucasian girl has been dieting to maximize her performance on the mile run with her track team. Although her lower weight initially improves her performance, she begins to fade in the last quarter-mile despite the exhortations of her trainer. She reports increasing muscle cramps and fatigue and undergoes stress testing that shows a progressive inefficiency of oxygen to energy conversion accompanied by increased blood lactate levels. Her sports medicine subspecialist attributes this to deficient fat stores and suggests a particular supplement. Which of the following would be most likely to benefit this patient?

a. Glycine and tyrosine
b. Thymidine
c. Pantothenic acid
d. Uridine
e. Folate

316. Chronic alcoholics are at risk to develop lactic acidosis and neuro logic symptoms, one example of which is the Wernicke-Korsakoff syndrome (MIM*277730). This complex of symptoms includes nerve problems like nystagmus (oscillating eyes), ophthalmoplegia (deviated or weak eye), peripheral numbness/tingling and cerebral problems like confusion, delirium, coma, and memory loss in survivors. Explanation of why certain alcoholics get Wernicke-Korsakoff encephalopathy was suggested when altered transketolase (an important enzyme in the pentose phosphate pathway) was found in these individuals. Which of the following is most likely to be important in the development of lactic acidosis and/or Wernicke-Korsakoff susceptibility in alcoholics?

a. Thiamine pyrophosphate
b. Lipoamide
c. ATP
d. NADH
e. FADH

317. Which of the following cofactors must be utilized during the conversion of acetyl-CoA to malonyl-CoA?

a. Thiamine pyrophosphate
b. Acyl carrier protein (ACP)
c. NAD_1
d. Biotin
e. FAD

318. Tryptophan deficiency in diet or disease can cause pellagra, a condition with skin rash on sunlight exposure (photosensitivity), diarrhea, and death. Tryptophan can be a precursor for one part of a compound that is an enzyme cofactor and donor of ADP-ribose that is added to certain histones and DNA repair enzymes (topoisomerases). Which of the following components can be derived from tryptophan, along with its active compound?

a. Biotin, carboxybiotin
b. Intrinsic factor, cobalamin
c. Pantothenic acid, coenzyme A
d. Nicotinamide, nicotinamide adenine dinucleotide
e. Pyridoxine, pyridoxal phosphate

319. One of the first chemotherapeutic agents was methotrexate, a compound that was effective in killing rapidly dividing cells like those of leukemias. This compound would be expected to elevate concentrations of which of the following compounds?

a. Homocysteine and dUMP
b. Thymine and choline
c. Serine and methionine
d. Glycine and methionine
e. Homocysteine and thymine

320. One of many roles for vitamins is their use as a reactive agent at the active sites of enzymes. Since these are catalytic reactions, the vitamin is not consumed in the reaction and is required in small amounts. Knowledge of this common mechanism should discourage use of megavitamin supplements that are promoted as cures for autism, cancer, and colds, but an unfortunate 30% of the American public admit to taking such supplements. Which of the following enzymes uses a vitamin-derived cofactor that is reoxidized by but different from NAD^+?

a. Lactate dehydrogenase
b. Glutamate dehydrogenase
c. Pyruvate dehydrogenase
d. Malate dehydrogenase
e. Glyceraldehyde-3-phosphate dehydrogenase

321. Which of the following foods should be emphasized for individuals with peripheral neuritis, insomnia, mouth and skin irritation, and diarrhea?

a. Human and cow (not goat) milk, uncooked fruits, vegetables
b. Milk, eggs, meats, fruits
c. Vegetables, cereals, fruits
d. Liver, poultry, eggs
e. Egg yolks, fish oils, leafy vegetables

322. Which of the following foods should be emphasized for individuals with dry eyes and decreased vision in dim light?

a. Human and cow (not goat) milk, uncooked fruits, vegetables
b. Milk, eggs, meats, fruits
c. Vegetables, cereals, fruits
d. Liver, poultry, eggs
e. Egg yolks, fish oils, leafy vegetables

323. A 5-year-old African American girl complains that she is always tired and refuses to play with her friends. Evaluation reveals that she has mild elevations of lactic acid and mitochondrial DNA studies reveal a mutation in the mitochondrial gamma polymerase (POLG-MIM*174763). POLG deficiencies lead to depletion of DNA in a proportion of the patient's mitochondria with less efficient oxidative phosphorylation. Which of the following compounds would be most effective in improving the girl's energy metabolism?

a. Glucose 6-phosphate, xylitol
b. Glucose 1-phosphate, UDP-glucose
c. Ornithine, arginine
d. Lipoic acid, thiamine
e. Creatine, lactate

324. A 15-month-old Caucasian girl is hospitalized for failure to gain weight and a chronic rash which is thought due to yeast infection. Evaluation shows the rash is not typical of yeast in that it is distributed beyond the genital area and is worst on the extremities. She also has swelling of the hands and feet (edema) and has lost her hair. Which one of the following is likely to be deficient?

a. Arsenic
b. Lead
c. Zinc
d. Antimony
e. Vanadium

325. A 10-day-old male Sudanese infant is evaluated in a refugee camp and found to have large areas of bruising on the skin (purpura) with oozing of blood from his umbilicus. Which of the following statements best describes his likely vitamin deficiency and its mechanism?

a. The vitamin is broken down by intestinal bacteria and facilitates synthesis of clotting factors.
b. The vitamin is antagonized by heparin and facilitates glycosylation of clotting factors.
c. The vitamin is obtained by eating egg yolk and liver but not green vegetables.
d. The vitamin is antagonized by a rat poison, is active in glutamate carboxylation, and facilitates calcium chelation.
e. The vitamin was discovered by studying hemorrhagic disease of the newborn.

326. A 1-year-old African boy has recently emigrated from Africa and exhibits intermittent diarrhea, pallor (pale skin), extreme tenderness of the bones, "rosary" of lumps along the ribs, nose bleeds, bruising over the eyelids, and blood in the urine. Which of the following is the most likely cause?

a. Deficiency of vitamin C due to a meat-deficient diet during pregnancy.
b. Hypervitaminosis A due to ingestion of beef liver during pregnancy.
c. Deficiency of vitamin C because of reliance on a milk only diet.
d. Deficiency of vitamin K because of neonatal deficiency and continued poor nutrition.
e. Deficiency of vitamin D due to darker skin pigmentation and poor sun exposure.

327. Which of the following statements best describes vitamin A?

a. Vitamin A promotes maintenance of epithelial tissue.
b. Vitamin A is necessary for hearing but not for vision.
c. Vitamin A is synthesized in skin.
d. All vitamin A derivatives are safe to use during pregnancy.
e. Vitamin A is a form of calciferol.

328. Which of the following conditions most rapidly produces a functional deficiency of vitamin K?

a. Coumadin therapy to prevent thrombosis in patients prone to clot formation
b. Broad-spectrum antibiotic therapy
c. Lack of red meat in the diet
d. Lack of citrus fruits in the diet
e. Premature birth

329. A 3-month-old African American boy presents with poor feeding and growth, low muscle tone (hypotonia), elevation of blood lactic acid (lactic acidemia), and mild acidosis (blood pH 7.3-7.35). The ratio of pyruvate to lactate in serum is elevated, and there is decreased conversion of pyruvate to acetyl coenzyme A in fibroblasts. Which of the following compounds should be considered for therapy?

a. Pyridoxine
b. Thiamine
c. Free fatty acids
d. Biotin
e. Ascorbic acid

330. A homeless 22-year-old Caucasian male is brought into the emergency room with psychotic imagery and alcohol on his breath. Which of the following compounds is most important to administer?

a. Glucose
b. Niacin
c. Nicotinic acid
d. Thiamine
e. Riboflavin

331. Which of the following vitamins becomes a major electron acceptor, aiding in the oxidation of numerous substrates?

a. Vitamin B_6
b. Niacin
c. Riboflavin
d. Thiamine
e. Vitamin B_1

332. Your patient is an adult who avoids bright light; has sore eyes, mouth, and tongue; plus feels tired and confused. Which of the following vitamins would most likely be deficient in this patient?

a. Riboflavin
b. Retinol
c. Niacin
d. Thiamine
e. Pyridoxine

333. A 2-year-old Caucasian boy presents with neonatal meconium ileus, chronic cough and bronchitis, growth failure, and chronic diarrhea with light-colored, foul-smelling stools. A deficiency of which of the following vitamins should be considered?

a. Vitamin A
b. Vitamin C
c. Vitamin B_1
d. Vitamin B_2
e. Vitamin B_6

334. Pantothenic acid is important for which of the following steps or pathways?

a. Pyruvate carboxylase
b. Fatty acid synthesis
c. Pyruvate carboxykinase
d. Gluconeogenesis
e. Glycolysis

335. Which of the following enzymes requires a vitamin that is rarely deficient except in those eating fad diets with excess raw egg white?

a. Pyruvate carboxylase
b. Pyruvate dehydrogenase
c. Phosphoenolpyruvate carboxykinase
d. Glucokinase
e. Fructokinase

336. Neural tube defects such as anencephaly and spina bifida have higher frequencies in certain populations like those of Celtic origin and in certain regions like South Texas. This suggestion of environmental cause produced research showing that deficiency of which of the following vitamins is associated with the occurrence of neural tube defects (anencephaly and spina bifida)?

a. Ascorbic acid (vitamin C)
b. Thiamine (vitamin B_1)
c. Riboflavin (vitamin B_2)
d. Niacin (vitamin B_3)
e. Folic acid

337. A 15-month-old African American boy presents with prominent forehead, bowing of the limbs, broad and tender wrists, swellings at the costochondral junctions of the ribs, and irritability. The head is deformable, able to be depressed like a ping-pong ball, while palpation of the joints is very painful. Which of the following treatments is recommended?

a. Lotions containing retinoic acid
b. Diet of baby food containing leafy vegetables
c. Diet of baby food containing liver and ground beef
d. Milk and sunlight exposure
e. Removal of eggs from diet

Vitamins and Minerals

Answers

303. The answer is b. (*Murray, pp 467-481. Scriver, pp 3127-3162.*) Ferrous iron (Fe^{2+}) is the form absorbed in the intestine by ferritin, transported in plasma by transferrin, and stored in the liver in combination with ferritin or as hemosiderin (incorrect answers a, d, e). There is no known excretory pathway for iron, either in the ferric or ferrous form (incorrect answer c). For this reason, excessive iron uptake over a period of many years may cause hemochromatosis (MIM*235200), the likely diagnosis for this male. This is a condition of extensive hemosiderin deposition in the liver, myocardium, pancreas, and adrenals. The resulting symptoms include liver cirrhosis, congestive heart failure, diabetes mellitus, and changes in skin pigmentation.

304. The answer is c. (*Murray, pp 435-438. Scriver, pp 1623-1650.*) Certain amino acids and lipids are dietary necessities because humans cannot synthesize them. The energy usually obtained from carbohydrates can be obtained from lipids and the conversion of some amino acids to intermediates of the citric acid cycle (incorrect answers a, d). These alternative substrates can thus provide fuel for oxidation and energy plus reduce equivalents for biosynthesis. Iodine is important for thyroid hormone synthesis, whereas calcium is essential for muscle contraction and bone metabolism (incorrect answers b, e).

305. The answer is c. (*Murray, pp 467-481. Scriver, pp 3897-3964.*) Inability to absorb cobalamin (vitamin B_{12}) from the gastrointestinal tract and its deficiency in vegetarian diets causes megaloblastic anemia and neurologic symptoms (numbness, extremity weakness, poor coordination, and dementia—incorrect answers a, b and d, e). The presence of neurologic symptoms led to the term "pernicious anemia" because they are progressive and eventually irreversible. The absorption of vitamin B_{12} from the intestine requires a binding protein called intrinsic factor that is secreted by the gastric mucosa and absorbed in the ileum; Pernicious anemia can result from gastric atrophy at older ages or, more rarely, from mutations affecting the intrinsic factor itself that present in childhood (eg, MIM*261000). Inability to absorb vitamin B_{12} from the gastrointestinal tract causes more severe deficiency than nutritional deprivation in vegetarian diets. Intrinsic factor may also be diminished by autoantibodies in autoimmune diseases like diabetes mellitus or Graves disease (hyperthyroidism). Clinical signs of pernicious anemia may not appear until 3 to 5 years following the onset of vitamin B_{12} deficiency and the neurologic signs may occur without obvious anemia.

Pellagra is caused by niacin (vitamin B_3) and tryptophan deficiency, leading to photosensitive dermatitis and neurologic symptoms. Scurvy is caused by vitamin C deficiency and is characterized by bleeding gums and bone disease. Rickets is softening and deformation of the bones due to vitamin D deficiency or defects in vitamin D processing. Beriberi (neurologic and/or cardiac symptoms) is caused by thiamine (vitamin B_1) deficiency and is common in Asians who eat polished white rice minus the thiamine-rich husk.

306. The answer is b. *(Murray, pp 467-481. Scriver, pp 3897-3964.)* Osteomalacia is the name given to the disease of bone seen in adults with vitamin D deficiency. It is analogous to rickets, which is seen in children with the same deficiency. Both disorders are manifestations of defective bone formation. The osteogenesis imperfectas are a group of genetic bone disorders caused by collagen gene mutations. Osteopetrosis is a hardening of the bones that occurs in certain hereditary conditions. Night blindness is associated with vitamin A deficiency.

307. The answer is e. *(Murray, pp 467-481. Scriver, pp 3897-3964.)* Ascorbic acid (vitamin C) is found in fresh fruits (citrus, strawberries, tomatoes) and vegetables (broccoli, potatoes, cabbage, spinach). Pantothenic acid (vitamin B_5) is found in most foods including meat and whole grains (incorrect answer d), as are niacin (vitamin B_3—not strictly a vitamin since it can be synthesized—incorrect answer b), thiamine (vitamin B_1—incorrect answer a), and cobalamin (vitamin B_{12}—found in meat, milk, and eggs—incorrect answer c). Deficiency of ascorbic acid produces scurvy, the "sailor's disease." Ascorbic acid is necessary for the hydroxylation of proline to hydroxyproline in collagen, a process required in the formation and maintenance of connective tissue. The failure of mesenchymal cells to form collagen causes the skeletal, dental, and connective tissue deterioration seen in scurvy. Thiamine, niacin, cobalamin, and pantothenic acid can all be obtained from fish or meat products. The nomenclature of vitamins began by classifying fat-soluble vitamins as A (followed by subsequent letters of the alphabet such as D, E, and K) and water-soluble vitamins as B. Components of the B vitamin fraction were then given subscripts, eg, thiamine (B_1), riboflavin (B_2), niacin (nicotinic acid [B_3]), pantothenic acid (B_5), pyridoxine (B_6), and cobalamin (B_{12}). The water-soluble vitamins C, biotin, and folic acid do not follow the B nomenclature.

308. The answer is c. (*Murray, pp 467-481. Scriver, pp 3897-3964.*) The retinal pigment rhodopsin is composed of the 11-cis-retinal form of vitamin A coupled to opsin. Light isomerizes 11-cis-retinal to all-trans-retinal, which is hydrolyzed to free all-trans-retinal and opsin. In order for regeneration of rhodopsin to occur, 11-cis-retinal must be regenerated. This dark reaction involves the isomerization of all-trans-retinal to 11-cis-retinal, which combines with opsin to reform rhodopsin. A deficiency of vitamin A, which is often derived from the β-carotene of plants, results in night blindness. Excess of vitamin A (hypervitaminosis A) can cause cerebral edema and other problems postnatally and severe birth defects when retinoids are taken prenatally (eg, women taking Accutane for acne).

309. The answer is b. (*Murray, pp 131-142. Scriver, pp 3897-3964.*) Hypoglycemia during fasting suggests a disorder of gluconeogenesis, which involves the enzymes pyruvate carboxylase, phosphoenolpyruvate carboxykinase, fructose-1,6-bisphosphatase, and glucose-6-phosphatase to reverse key reaction steps in glycolysis. Pyruvate carboxylase catalyzes the conversion of pyruvate to oxaloacetate (incorrect answers d, e) and requires biotin with allosteric activation by acetyl-CoA. Biotin is a cofactor in several carboxylation reactions, while niacin is a source for NAD and NADH reactions (incorrect answers a, e) and pyridoxine for pyridoxal phosphate that is important in amino acid transferase reactions and steroid hormone action (incorrect answer d). Thiamine is important for pyruvate dehydrogenase, a first step in oxidative phosphorylation (incorrect answer c). High levels of acetyl-CoA indicate a fed state with oxidative breakdown of foods and high energy (ATP) levels. When ATP levels are high, oxaloacetate is consumed in gluconeogenesis and when ATP levels are low oxaloacetate enters the citric acid cycle. Gluconeogenesis only occurs in the liver and kidneys.

310. The answer is b. *(Murray, pp 467-481. Scriver, pp 121-138, 287-320, 3897-3964.)* Pantothenic acid combines with the amino acid cysteine to become the pantetheine sulfhydryl component of coenzyme A (CoA) and acyl carrier protein (important for fatty acid synthesis). Acetyl-CoA is the activated form of acetate employed in acetylation reactions, including the citric acid cycle and lipid metabolism. Loss of myelin in Hallervorden-Spatz disease correlates with a role for activated pantothenic acid as a cofactor for fatty acid synthesis and as a carrier of acyl chains (which must be added to glycerol to form triacylglycerols), alkylacylglycerols (ether lipids), and (by acyl addition to sphingosine) cerebrosides, sphingomyelin, and gangliosides.

Mutations with severe impact on pantothenic acid kinase (mediating activation by its phosphorylation) present with neurologic signs in infancy (eg, infantile neuroaxonal dystrophy—MIM*256600) while those with less impact present in the second or third decades with cognitive decline, dementia, and psychiatric symptoms (eg, Hallervorden-Spatz disease, MIM*234200). Nutritional deficiencies of pantothenic acid have not been described except in artificial studies, perhaps because they would limit CoA and have deadly consequences in mammals. However, because it is common in foodstuffs, there is little evidence of pantothenic acid deficiency in humans.

311. The answer is d. *(Murray, pp 467-481. Scriver, pp 3897-3964.)* The most active forms of vitamin K appear to be phylloquinones from green vegetables since menaquinones synthesized by intestinal bacteria will not counteract dietary deficiency. Vitamin K acts to catalyze γ-carboxylation of glutamic acid residues in key proteins like mediate coagulation (prothrombin and other factors) or bone formation (osteocalcin—incorrect answers a-c, e). The anticoagulants warfarin and dicumarol are structural analogues that block the γ-carboxylation of prothrombin by substituting for vitamin K. Hence, the prothrombin produced has a weak affinity for Ca^{2+} and cannot properly bind to platelet membranes in order to be converted to thrombin. Exposure of the fetus to warfarin during maternal therapy can produce a syndrome involving small, "fleur-de-lys" nose and skeletal defects.

In order to be converted to thrombin during clot formation, prothrombin must bind Ca^{2+}, which allows it to anchor to platelet membranes produced by injury. Prothrombin's affinity for Ca^{2+} is dependent on the presence of 10 γ-carboxyglutamate residues found in the first 35 amino acid residues of its amino terminal region. Vitamin K–dependent γ-carboxylation of prothrombin is added after prothrombin is synthesized and passes into the lumen of the endoplasmic reticulum and passes into the lumen of the reticulum.

312. The answer is b. (*Murray, pp 467-481. Scriver, pp 3935-3964.*) The vitamin biotin is the cofactor required by carboxylating enzymes such as acetyl-CoA, pyruvate, and propionyl-CoA carboxylases. The fixation of CO_2 by these biotin-dependent enzymes occurs in two stages. In the first, bicarbonate ion reacts with adenosine triphosphate (ATP) and the biotin carrier protein moiety of the enzyme; in the second, the "active CO_2" reacts with the substrate—for example, acetyl-CoA. The other reactions are catalyzed by diverse groups of enzymes with no common cofactor.

313. The answer is b. (*Murray, pp 467-481. Scriver, pp 3897-3964.*) Pantothenate is the precursor of CoA, which participates in numerous reactions throughout the metabolic scheme. CoA is a central molecule of metabolism involved in acetylation reactions. Thus a deficiency of pantothenic acid would have severe consequences. There is no documented deficiency state for pantothenate, however, because this vitamin is common in foodstuffs. Other choices are vitamins concerned with several metabolic pathways including electron transport (riboflavin, thiamine), organic acid conversion (cobalamin), and sulfhydryl group transfer (pyridoxamine).

314. The answer is c. (*Murray, pp 467-481. Scriver, pp 3897-3964.*) Polished white rice that removes the husk and vitamin B_1 (thiamine) is a common staple of East Asian diets, causing thiamine deficiency disease (beriberi—incorrect answers a, b and d, e). Thiamine pyrophosphate is the necessary prosthetic group of enzymes transferring activated aldehyde units, including transketolase, pyruvate dehydrogenase, and α-ketoglutarate dehydrogenase. Beriberi is a wasting disease named from a Sinhalese phrase meaning "I cannot, I cannot" and has weight loss with neurologic symptoms (extremity pain, muscle weakness, numbness, emotional changes—"dry" beriberi) and/or symptoms of cardiac failure (arrhythmias, heart enlargement, peripheral edema—"wet" beriberi). Yeast products, whole grains, nuts, and pork are rich in thiamine. Choline, ethanolamine, and serine are polar head groups of phospholipids while glycine is a common amino acid.

315. The answer is c. *(Murray, pp 193-199, 467-481. Scriver, pp 2297-2356.)* Pantothenic acid (vitamin B_5) is a component of coenzyme A (CoA) and acyl carrier protein (ACP). These proteins carry acyl groups with acetyl-CoA being important for fatty acid oxidation and many other metabolic reactions while ACP functions in fatty acid synthesis. Folic acid is made from glycine, serine, and choline and is important for methyl (one carbon) reactions such as the conversion of deoxyuridine monophosphate to thymidine (incorrect answers a, b and d, e). Stable forms of folate (folinic acid, synthetic leucovorin) can be used as part of a supplement mixture (thiamine, riboflavin, coenzyme Q, lipoic acid) for mitochondrial dysfunction. The reactive prosthetic group of both ACP and CoA is a phosphopantetheine sulfhydryl. In ACP, the phosphopantetheine group is attached to the 77-residue polypeptide chain via a serine hydroxyl. In CoA, the phosphopantetheine is linked to the 5' phosphate of adenosine that is phosphorylated in its 3' hydroxyl.

316. The answer is a. *(Murray, pp 467-481. Scriver, pp 3897-3964.)* Thiamine (vitamin B_1) activated as its pyrophosphate is a cofactor for pyruvate dehydrogenase, α-ketoglutarate dehydrogenase of the citric acid cycle, branched chain ketoacid dehydrogenase that metabolizes leucine/isoleucine/valine, and transketolase of the pentose phosphate pathway. Deficiency of thiamine causes beriberi and exacerbates encephalopathy in alcoholics, having impact on the nervous system in both diseases. Since pyruvate dehydrogenase commits pyruvate from glycolysis to acetyl-CoA in the citric acid cycle, its impairment will increase lactate (lactic acidosis), deplete energy (by impacting the citric acid cycle and the first steps of oxidative phosphorylation), and impair glucose metabolism—all key to neural function. Impairment of transketolase and the pentose phosphate shunt would reduce NADPH production, key to glutathione maintenance and reduction of oxidants in brain. Certain mutations in transketolase may thus increase susceptibility to Wernicke-Korsakoff syndrome (MIM*277730), a nice example of a Mendelian enzyme alteration brought out by environment (alcohol dependency) to cause a multifactorial disease (encephalopathy).

Lipoamide is also a cofactor in pyruvate dehydrogenase, transferring the acetyl group in pyruvate to coenzyme A. Lipoamide becomes acetyl-lipoamide and then dihydrolipoamide as it first accepts and then transfers an acyl group. This reaction and the regeneration of lipoamide are catalyzed by different parts of the dehydrogenase enzyme complex. ATP transfers phosphoryl groups, thiamine pyrophosphate transfers aldehyde groups, NADH and FADH transfer protons. Mutations in the multipeptide pyruvate dehydrogenase complex occur in Leigh disease (MIM*256000), an end phenotype of many mutations that simulate the lactic acidosis and encephalopathy accompanying acute forms of thiamine deficiency (beriberi).

317. The answer is d. *(Murray, pp 193-199, 467-481. Scriver, pp 2297-2326.)* The key enzymatic step of fatty acid synthesis is the carboxylation of acetyl-CoA to form malonyl-CoA; again there is the correlation of a carboxylation reaction and biotin (incorrect answers a-c, e). The carboxyl of biotin is covalently attached to an epsilon amino group of a lysine residue of acetyl-CoA carboxylase. The reaction occurs in two stages. In the first step, a carboxybiotin is formed:

$$HCO_3^- + \text{biotin-enzyme} + ATP \rightarrow CO_2\text{-biotin-enzyme} + ADP + P_i$$

In the second step, the CO_2 is transferred to acetyl-CoA to produce malonyl-CoA:

$$CO_2\text{-biotin-enzyme} + \text{acetyl-CoA} \rightarrow \text{malonyl-CoA} + \text{biotin-enzyme}$$

None of the other cofactors listed are involved in this reaction.

318. The answer is d. *(Murray, pp 467-481. Scriver, pp 3897-3964.)* The component that can be produced from tryptophan is nicotinamide, which is joined with adenosine diphosphate to form the important cofactor and ADP-ribose donor, nicotinamide adenine dinucleotide (NAD). Nicotinamide and nicotinic acid were discovered as the essential nutrient niacin that could be used to treat pellagra. Niacin is not strictly a vitamin because it can be derived from tryptophan, but its dietary deficiency contributes to pellagra along with deficiencies of riboflavin (vitamin B_2) and pyridoxine (vitamin B_6) that are involved in the biosynthesis of niacin from tryptophan. NAD^+ is a cofactor required by all dehydrogenases and NADPH, produced by the pentose phosphate shunt is utilized in reductive synthesis of compounds such as fatty acids. Since photosensitivity is common in DNA repair disorders like xeroderma pigmentosum (MIM*278730), it is possible that deficient ADP-ribosylation of DNA repair topoisomerases relates to the photosensitivity of pellagra.

Pantothenic acid and coenzyme A are involved in acetylation and acyl-transfer reactions important in fatty acid metabolism, biotin and carboxy-biotin in carboxylation reactions like those deficient in multiple carboxylase deficiency (MIM*253270). Intrinsic factor is a protein secreted by the gastric mucosa that is important for binding and absorption of cobalamin (vitamin B_{12}). Pyridoxal phosphate also is involved in amino acid metabolism (transamination), muscle glycogen breakdown (glycogen phosphorylase), and steroid hormone action (removes hormone-receptor complexes from DNA, terminating their action).

319. The answer is a. (*Murray, pp 467-481. Scriver, pp 3897-3964.*) The vitamin folic acid is provided commercially and pharmaceutically as the stable 5-formyltetrahydrofolate known as folinic acid or its synthetic analogue leu-covorin. Addition of folate to foods (bread) and encouragement of precon-ceptional vitamins with folate was prompted by its ability to lower the incidence of neural tube defects by two- to threefold. Folic acid is biologically active as the interconvertible forms tetrahydrofolate (THF), methyl THF, and other methylated forms (methylene THF, N5, N10-methylene THF) that are important for one-carbon (methyl) transfers and interconversions (glycine-serine, formate-formylmethionine, formate-CO_2 homocysteine-methionine, uracil-thymine). THF is required in two steps of purine synthesis and thus required in the de novo synthesis of ATP and GTP. Although de novo synthesis of the pyrimidine ring does not require tetrahydrofolate, the methyla-tion of deoxyuridine monophosphate (dUMP) to form thymine from uracil does. In this thymidylate synthetase reaction, methylene THF donates a methyl group and is converted to dihydrofolate which requires action of dihydrofolate reductase to regenerate THF. Methotrexate inhibits dihydrofo-late reductase, depletes THF pools, and thus would elevate substrates of enzymes dependent on this cofactor like dUMP. THF is also a cofactor for methionine synthase that converts homocysteine to methionine, an enzyme deficient in one form of homocystinuria (MIM*236200).

320. The answer is c. (*Murray, pp 467-481. Scriver, pp 3897-3964.*) The vitamin riboflavin (vitamin B_2) is a precursor of two cofactors involved in electron transport systems, riboflavin 5'-phosphate, also known as flavin mononucleotide (FMN), and flavin adenine dinucleotide (FAD). Strictly speaking, these compounds are not nucleotides, as they contain the sugar alcohol ribitol, not ribose. The cofactors are strongly bound to their apoenzymes and function as dehydrogenation catalysts. Pyruvate dehydrogenase is a multienzyme complex and contains the enzyme dihydrolipoyl dehydrogenase, which has as its prosthetic group two molecules of FAD per molecule of enzyme. In the overall reaction, the reduced FAD is reoxidized by NAD$^+$. Mutations at several loci encoding the components of pyruvate dehydrogenase cause the clinical phenotype of Leigh syndrome (MIM*256000) with seizures, low muscle tone, neurodegeneration, and lactic acidosis. Succinate dehydrogenase also contains tightly bound FAD, one molecule per molecule of enzyme. Glutamate, lactate, malate, and glyceraldehyde-3-phosphate dehydrogenases all use nicotinamide dinucleotide cofactors and do not contain FAD as a prosthetic group.

321. The answer is c. (*Murray, pp 467-481. Scriver, pp 3897-3964.*) Pyridoxine (vitamin B$_6$) deficiency usually occurs concurrently with deficiency of other B vitamins or in association with drug therapy in individuals who are slow metabolizers for the antituberculosis drug isoniazid and others like penicillamine or sulfa antibiotics (MIM*243400). Pyridoxine is present in many foods, particularly vegetables, cereals, and fruits. Niacin (precursor to nicotinamide adenine dinucleotide) is abundant in liver, poultry, and eggs; tetrahydrofolate in human and cow (not goat) milk, uncooked fruits, and vegetables; riboflavin (vitamin B$_2$—precursor to flavin adenine mononucleotide) in milk, eggs, meats, and fruits; retinoic acid (vitamin A) in animal tissues like egg yolks, fish oils with other carotenoids in leafy vegetables.

The coenzyme pyridoxal phosphate is a versatile compound that aids in amino acid transaminations, deaminations, decarboxylations, and transulfurations. It is also important for operation of glycogen phosphorylase. A common feature of these reactions is formation of a Schiff-base intermediate with a specific lysine group at the active site of the appropriate enzymes.

322. The answer is e. (*Murray, pp 467-481. Scriver, pp 3897-3964.*) Vitamin A is a fat-soluble vitamin that can be deficient in combination with thiamine and riboflavin deficiencies in dry climates with food shortages, with other fat-soluble vitamins (D, E, K) in disorders associated with intestinal malabsorption, and in hypothyroidism where there is defective conversion of carotene to vitamin A. Carotenes and carotenoids in plants (yellow corn, carrots, sweet potatoes, leafy vegetables, green peas) are converted to retinaldehyde in the intestinal mucosa (then to retinol), while retinol is found in animal tissues like egg yolks, fish oils, butter, liver, kidney. The first symptoms of vitamin A deficiency are dryness of the eyes (xerophthalmia) with decreased vision in dim light (night blindness), followed by photophobia, corneal irritation, ulceration, and destruction of the eye. Dry skin and rashes also occur. The importance of eggs in people with restricted diets was vividly portrayed in James Clavell's novel, *King Rat*, where they were prized for prevention of blindness.

Pyridoxine is present in vegetables, cereals, and fruits, niacin in liver, poultry, and eggs; tetrahydrofolate in milk, uncooked fruits, and vegetables; and riboflavin in milk, eggs, meats, and fruits.

323. The answer is d. (*Murray, pp 75-83, 143-148. Scriver, pp 3897-3964.*) Lipoic acid is a short-chain fatty acid with two sulfhydryl groups that is a coenzyme for the pyruvate dehydrogenase reaction that converts pyruvate to acetyl-CoA. This reaction also requires the vitamin thiamine and commits pyruvate to the citric acid cycle with generation of NADH, then ATP through mitochondrial oxidative phosphorylation. Mutations affecting the pyruvate dehydrogenase enzyme complex cause Leigh syndrome of lactic acidosis and neurologic disease (MIM*256000), one of many mitochondrial disorders that are treated by supplementing with lipoic acid, thiamine, carnitine, and coenzyme Q. The other choices include glucose 1-phosphate or glucose 6-phosphate that can generate energy through glycolysis (incorrect answers a, b), ornithine and arginine that dispose of ammonia through the urea cycle (incorrect answer c), and creatine, lactate that are generated in muscle (creatine cycles with creatine-phosphate to supplement oxidative phosphorylation in muscle, and lactate also accumulates during exercise when limiting oxygen causes muscle to use glycolysis (incorrect answer e).

324. The answer is c. (*Murray, pp 467-481. Scriver, pp 3897-3964.*) Zinc deficiency causes a clinical syndrome called acrodermatitis enteropathica (MIM*201100) with growth failure, diarrhea, loss of hair, eyelashes, and eyebrows, and skin rashes with redness and scaling on the extremities (incorrect answers a, b and d, e). Minerals are important cofactors for enzyme reactions (cofactors are distinguished from coenzymes that function in group transfer and undergo chemical reaction), including cobalt, copper, iron, molybdenum, selenium, and zinc. Examples include copper in cytochrome oxidase, iron in all the cytochromes, magnesium for all enzymes utilizing ATP, and zinc in lactate dehydrogenase. Arsenic, lead, and antimony cause disease when present in excess while vanadium (along with silicon, nickel, and tin) is known to be essential from experimental nutrition studies although its role is not defined. Fluoride (preventing dental caries) and lithium (a therapy for depression) have effects on humans but are not known to be essential nutrients.

325. The answer is d. (*Murray, pp 467-481, 583-592. Scriver, pp 4293-4326.*) The major role of vitamin K is in the synthesis of prothrombin and other clotting factors (eg, VII, IX, and X). Vitamin K acts on the inactive precursor molecules of these proteins, allowing carboxylation of glutamic acid residues to γ-carboxyglutamate. Once carboxylated, the factors bind calcium through these groups and are able to attach to cell membranes as part of clot formation. A true vitamin K deficiency in adults is unusual because vitamin K is found in a variety of foods and can be produced by intestinal bacteria. Liver, egg yolk, spinach, cauliflower, and cabbage are some of the sources of vitamin K. Poor fat metabolism, decreased liver function (reduced clotting factor synthesis), and sterile gut that reduces menadiones from bacterial metabolism are chronic causes of vitamin K deficiency. Decreased bile excretion in newborns renders them susceptible to vitamin K deficiency and hemorrhagic disease of the newborn; this is prevented by routine vitamin K injection in industrialized countries. Disorders with increased coagulation are treated with analogues of vitamin K that inhibit its conversion from dietary phylloquinone to hydroquine, epoxide, and quinone. Such inhibitors include coumadin and warfarin, a substance used as rat poison. Heparin is a complex polysaccharide that potentiates antithrombin III and inhibits clotting without effects on vitamin K.

326. The answer is c. (*Murray, pp 467-481. Scriver, pp 3897-3964.*) Prolonged vitamin C deficiency (scurvy) often reflects severe malnutrition associated with famine, prisoners of war, alcoholism, or extreme food faddism (answers b, d, e incorrect). Vitamin C is abundant in citrus fruits (hence the term "limey" for British sailors) and certain vegetables (peppers, broccoli, cabbage, spinach—incorrect answer a). Exclusive feeding of cow's milk, as may occur in areas of famine with poor supplies of maternal milk, can result in infantile scurvy with the symptoms described in the question. Pasteurization destroys vitamin C so it is added to commercially prepared milk. X-rays of the limbs are helpful in diagnosing scurvy, with a white line at the metaphysis and occasional subperiosteal hemorrhage. These radiologic features may be seen in copper deficiency associated with hyperalimentation, emphasizing the role of ascorbic acid (vitamin C) as a coenzyme for proline/lysine hydroxylases that modify collagen and also require copper.

Vitamin K deficiency is rare due to its presence in diverse foods and deficiencies of the fat-soluble vitamins A, E, and D can occur with intestinal malabsorption but would cause different symptoms. Vitamin D deficiency (rickets) can also cause a series of rib lumps (rosary) but would have soft bones and skeletal deformities. Hypervitaminosis A can cause liver toxicity but not bleeding; deficiency of vitamin E can be associated with anemia in premature infants but is unknown in older children and adults.

327. The answer is a. (*Murray, pp 467-481. Scriver, pp 3897-3964.*) Vitamin A is essential for the normal differentiation of epithelial tissue as well as normal reproduction. Yellow and dark green vegetables as well as fruits are good sources of carotenes, which serve as precursors of vitamin A. However, egg yolk, butter, cream, and liver and kidneys are good sources of preformed vitamin A. Vitamin A is necessary for vision, not hearing. The visual pigment rhodopsin is formed from the protein opsin and 11-cis-retinal. During the photobleaching of rhodopsin, all-trans-retinal plus opsin is formed from dissociated rhodopsin, causing an impulse that is transmitted by the optic nerve to the brain. Isomerized form trans-retinal, 11-cis-retinal combines with opsin to reform rhodospin, making it ready for another photochemical cycle. All-trans-retinoic acid (tretinoin) has been found to be effective for topical treatment of psoriasis. Another form of vitamin A is 13-cis-retinoic acid (Accutane), which has been found to be effective in the treatment of severe cases of acne. Accutane causes birth defects of the face and brain if taken during the first trimester of pregnancy. Vitamin A is not synthesized in the skin. Vitamin D (derivatives of calciferol) can be synthesized in the skin under the influence of sunlight from 7-dehydrocholesterol, an intermediate in cholesterol synthesis.

328. The answer is a. (*Murray, pp 467-481. Scriver, pp 121-138, 287-320, 3897-3964.*) Vitamin K is essential for the posttranscriptional modification of prothrombin by γ-carboxylation of glutamate residues. A functional deficiency exists in patients treated with analogues of vitamin K such as the Coumadin derivatives. The analogues act as anticoagulants by competing with vitamin K and preventing the production of functional prothrombin. By administration of vitamin K, hemorrhage can be prevented in such patients. Vitamin K is normally obtained from green, leafy vegetables in the diet (not from citrus fruits or red meat). Intestinal bacteria also synthesize the vitamin, but even broad-spectrum antibiotic therapy does not completely sterilize the intestine. A deficiency of vitamin K can cause hemorrhagic disease in newborn infants because their intestines do not have the bacteria that produce vitamin K and because vitamin K does not cross the placenta. The neonatal deficiency occurs in term or premature infants.

329. The answer is b. *(Murray, pp 467-481. Scriver, pp 2275-2296.)* An elevation of pyruvate and a deficiency of acetyl-CoA suggest a deficiency of pyruvate dehydrogenase (PDH). This multisubunit enzyme assembly contains pyruvate dehydrogenase, dihydrolipoyl transacetylase, dihydrolipoyl dehydrogenase, and two enzymes involved in regulation of the overall enzymatic activity of the complex. PDH requires thiamine pyrophosphate as a coenzyme, dihydrolipoyl transacetylase requires lipoic acid and CoA, and dihydrolipoyl dehydrogenase has an FAD prosthetic group that is reoxidized by NAD^+. Biotin, pyridoxine, and ascorbic acid are not coenzymes for PDH. An ATP-dependent protein kinase can phosphorylate PDH to decrease activity, and a phosphatase can activate PDH. Increases of ATP, acetyl-CoA, or NADH (increased energy charge) and of fatty acid oxidation increase phosphorylation of PDH and decrease its activity. PDH is less active during starvation, increasing pyruvate, decreasing glycolysis, and sparing carbohydrates. Free fatty acids decrease PDH activity and would not be appropriate therapy for PDH deficiency. PDH deficiency (MIM*246900 and MIM*312170) exhibits genetic heterogeneity, as would be expected from its multiple subunits, with autosomal and X-linked recessive forms. The infant also could be classified as having Leigh's disease (MIM*266150), a heterogenous group of disorders with hypotonia and lactic acidemia that can include PDH deficiency.

330. The answer is d. *(Murray, pp 467-481. Scriver, pp 3897-3964.)* Chronic alcoholics are at risk for thiamine deficiency, which is thought to play a role in the incoordination (ataxia) and psychosis that can become chronic (Wernicke-Korsakoff syndrome). The thiamine deficiency produces relative deficiency of the pyruvate dehydrogenase complex. The administration of glucose without checking glucose levels can therefore be dangerous, since excess glucose is converted to pyruvate by glycolysis. The low rate of pyruvate dehydrogenase conversion of pyruvate to coenzyme A (and entry into the citric acid cycle) causes pyruvate to be converted to lactate (through lactate dehydrogenase). Lactic acidosis can be fatal. Chronic alcoholics can be deficient in the other vitamins mentioned, but thiamine is most likely to help the neurologic symptoms.

331. The answer is b. (*Murray, pp 467-481. Scriver, pp 3897-3964.*) Nicotinamide adenine dinucleotide (NAD^+) is the functional coenzyme derivative of niacin. It is the major electron acceptor in the oxidation of molecules, generating NADH, which is the major electron donor for reduction reactions. Thiamine (also known as vitamin B_1) occurs functionally as thiamine pyrophosphate and is a coenzyme for enzymes such as pyruvate dehydrogenase. Riboflavin (vitamin B_2) functions in the coenzyme forms of flavin mononucleotide (FMN) or flavin adenine dinucleotide (FAD). When concentrated, both have a yellow color due to the riboflavin they contain. Both function as prosthetic groups of oxidation-reduction enzymes or flavoproteins. Flavoproteins are active in selected oxidation reactions and in electron transport, but they do not have the ubiquitous role of NAD^+.

332. The answer is a. (*Murray, pp 467-481. Scriver, pp 3897-3964.*) Riboflavin deficiency involves the insidious onset of photophobia, a burning sensation in the eyes, sore mouth (stomatitis) and tongue (glossitis), oily skin with rash (seborrheic dermatitis), and weight loss, confusion, dizziness, headache, and weakness. Retinol deficiency would cause night blindness and dry eyes that could be part of the described disorder, niacin deficiency rash (pellagra) with neurologic symptoms, thiamine deficiency heart failure and neurologic symptoms if acute (beriberi) or more chronic neuritis, pyridoxine deficiency infantile convulsions or peripheral neuritis (numbness and tingling, more common in slow metabolizers of drugs like isoniazid).

333. The answer is a. (*Murray, pp 467-481. Scriver, pp 5121-5138.*) Vitamins A, D, E, and K are all fat-soluble. The physical characteristics of fat-soluble vitamins derive from the hydrophobic nature of the aliphatic chains composing them. The other vitamins listed are water-soluble, efficiently administered orally, and rapidly absorbed from the intestine. Fat-soluble vitamins must be administered intramuscularly or as oral emulsions (mixtures of oil and water). In intestinal disorders such as chronic diarrhea or malabsorption due to deficient digestive enzymes, fat-soluble vitamins are poorly absorbed and can become deficient. Supplementation of fat-soluble vitamins is thus routine in disorders like cystic fibrosis (MIM*219700), a cause of respiratory and intestinal disease that is the likely diagnosis in this child.

334. The answer is b. (*Murray, pp 467-481. Scriver, pp 3897-3964.*) Pantothenic acid is phosphorylated and complexed with the amino acid cysteine to form 4-phosphopantetheine, the precursor for coenzyme A (CoA) and the acyl carrier protein (ACP) that participates in fatty acid synthesis. The thiol group of 4-phosphopantetheine is a carrier of acyl groups in CoA (A stands for acetylation or acetyl group) and ACP (fatty acyl groups). CoA is one of the major molecules in metabolism, carrying a pantetheine group bound to adenosine ribonucleotide-3'-phosphate via a 5' diphosphate (pyrophosphate). Acetyl groups are linked to the reactive terminal sulfhydryl group to produce acetyl-CoA, which has a high acetyl transfer potential. CoA carries and transfers acetyl groups in much the same way as ATP transfers activated phosphoryl groups. CoA is involved in fatty acid synthesis, fatty acid β-oxidation, and the citric acid cycle; it is not involved in glycolysis or gluconeogenesis, where acetyl transfer does not occur.

Gluconeogenesis generates glucose by converting pyruvate to oxaloacetate (via pyruvate carboxylase) to phosphoenopyruvate (via phosphoenopyruvate carboxykinase) to fructose-1,6-bisphosphate (through reversal of glycolytic enzymes) to fructose 6-phosphate (via fructose-1,6-bisphosphatase) to glucose 6-phosphate (through reversal of phosphohexose isomerase) to glucose (through glucose-6-phosphatase). Special enzymes are required at steps where reversal of glycolysis is not energetically feasible.

335. The answer is a. (*Murray, pp 467-481. Scriver, pp 3935-3964.*) Biotin functions to transfer carbon dioxide to substrates, adding a carboxyl group. Pyruvate carboxylase and enzymes of the holocarboxylase complex that degrade organic acids (propionate, metabolites of leucine) require biotin to transfer an activated carbonyl group. Biotin may be depleted by a deficiency of the enzyme biotinidase (MIM*253260), rendering the mentioned carboxylases less active and producing accumulation of the mentioned organic acids with severe acidosis. Nutritional deficiency of biotin is virtually unknown, but can be induced with raw egg white which contains avidin, a biotin-binding protein. Biotin deficiency causes skin rashes and hair loss, symptoms also seen in biotinidase enzyme deficiency. Thiamine is required for the reactions catalyzed by pyruvate dehydrogenase, transketolases, and α-ketoglutarate dehydrogenase. Kinases such as those in glycolysis require ATP as a cofactor.

336. The answer is e. *(Murray, pp 467-481. Scriver, pp 3897-3964.)* Spina bifida, or myelomeningocele, is a defect of the lower neural tube that produces an exposed spinal cord in the thoracic or sacral regions. Exposure of the spinal cord usually causes nerve damage and results in paralysis of the lower limbs and urinary bladder. Anencephaly is a defect of the anterior neural tube that results in lethal brain anomalies and skull defects. Folic acid is necessary for the development of the neural tube in the first few weeks of embryonic life, and the children of women with nutritional deficiencies have higher rates of neural tube defects. Because neural tube closure occurs at a time when many women are not aware that they are pregnant, it is essential that all women of childbearing age take a folic acid supplement of approximately 0.4 mg per day. Frank folic acid deficiency can also cause megaloblastic anemia because of a decreased synthesis of the purines and pyrimidines needed for cells to make DNA and divide. Deficiencies of thiamine in chronic alcoholics are related to Wernicke-Korsakoff syndrome, which is characterized by loss of memory, lackadaisical behavior, and a continuous rhythmic movement of the eyeballs. Thiamine dietary deficiency from excess of polished rice can cause beriberi. Niacin deficiency leads to pellagra, a disorder that produces skin rash (dermatitis), weight loss, and neurologic changes including depression and dementia. Riboflavin deficiency leads to mouth ulcers (stomatitis), cheilosis (dry, scaly lips), scaly skin (seborrhea), and photophobia. Because biotin is widely distributed in foods and is synthesized by intestinal bacteria, biotin deficiency is rare. However, the heat-labile molecule avidin, found in raw egg whites, binds biotin tightly and blocks its absorption, causing dermatitis, dehydration, and lethargy. Lactic acidosis results as a buildup of lactate due to the lack of functional pyruvate carboxylase when biotin is missing. Vitamin C deficiency leads to scurvy, which causes bleeding gums and bone disease.

Vitamin B_{12} can be deficient due to a lack of intrinsic factor, which is a glycoprotein secreted by gastric parietal cells. A lack of intrinsic factor or a dietary deficiency of cobalamin can cause pernicious anemia and neuropsychiatric symptoms. The only known treatment for intrinsic factor deficiency (vitamin B_{12} deficiency) is intramuscular injection of cyanocobalamin throughout the patient's life.

337. The answer is d. (*Murray, pp 467-481. Scriver, pp 4223-4240.*) People with bowed legs and other bone malformations were quite common in the northeastern United States following the industrial revolution. This was caused by childhood diets lacking foods with vitamin D and by minimal exposure to sunlight due to the dawn-to-dusk working conditions of the textile mills. Vitamin D is essential for the metabolism of calcium and phosphorus. Soft and malformed bones result from its absence. Liver, fish oil, and egg yolks contain vitamin D, and milk is supplemented with vitamin D by law. In adults, lack of sunlight and a diet poor in vitamin D lead to osteomalacia (soft bones). Dark-skinned peoples are more susceptible to vitamin D deficiency (rickets).

Biotin deficiency can be caused by diets with excess egg white, leading to dehydration and acidosis from accumulation of carboxylic and lactic acids. Retinoic acid is a vitamin A derivative that can be helpful in treating acne but not vitamin D deficiency. Leafy vegetables are a source of B vitamins such as niacin and cobalamin.

Hormones and Integrated Metabolism

Questions

338. A 16-year-old teenage female is evaluated because of lack of menstruation (amenorrhea) and is found to have a 46,XY karyotype. DNA testing shows a mutation in the testosterone receptor that is characteristic of testicular feminization or androgen insensitivity syndrome (MIM*300068). Which of the following statements accurately describes sex hormones such as testosterone?

a. They bind specific membrane receptors
b. They interact with DNA directly
c. They cause release of a proteinaceous second messenger from the cell membrane
d. They enhance transcription when bound to receptors
e. They inhibit translation through specific cytoplasmic proteins

339. After a meal and clearance of carbohydrates/chylomicrons from the bloodstream, blood glucose is initially maintained by liver glycogenolysis then sustained by fat mobilization from adipose tissue. Children with glycogen storage disorders have immediate problems with glucose maintenance while those with fatty acid oxidation disorders have later problems after glycogen is depleted. Which of the following mechanisms best explains the coordinate stimulation of glycogenolysis and lipolysis?

a. Cortisol, a glucocorticoid, alters transcription in liver and adipocytes.
b. Cortisol, a glucocorticoid, binds to liver and adipose plasma membrane receptors to increase cAMP.
c. Epinephrine diffuses into the cytosol of liver and adipose cells, activating phosphorylase kinase and triglyceride lipase by allosteric mechanisms.
d. Adenosine 3',5'-cyclic monophosphate (cyclic AMP) is the second messenger in adipocytes, but not in the liver.
e. Epinephrine acts through the second messenger cAMP and protein kinases to stimulate glycogen phosphorylase and triglyceride lipase activities.

340. A 4-year-old Caucasian girl is evaluated for rapid growth and obesity that has developed despite apparently normal food intake. Physical examination shows an unusual fat distribution with a pad over her neck and multiple stretch marks (striae). Based on the probable diagnosis of Cushing syndrome, which of the following would be found by laboratory testing?

a. Decreased production of epinephrine
b. Excessive production of epinephrine
c. Excessive production of vasopressin
d. Excessive production of cortisol
e. Decreased production of cortisol

341. A 3-day-old African American girl is noted to have a narrow distance between the eyes (hypotelorism), malformed nose with a single nostril (proboscis), and a midline cleft lip. These facial changes suggest a brain malformation called holoprosencephaly where the forebrain and related structures fail to develop. The child is noted to have decreased urine output and hypernatremia (high serum sodium concentration). Which of the following hormones is implicated?

a. Cortisol
b. Insulin
c. Vasopressin
d. Glucagon
e. Aldosterone

342. A 22-year-old Caucasian male college student becomes extremely tired after playing golf and seeks evaluation from the student health service. Past medical history reveals normal puberty and genital development. He recalls previous episodes of fatigue that he attributes to dehydration, and his physician obtains a serum glucose of 55 mg/dL (normal 75-105) and serum electrolytes showing Na 142 mEq/L (normal 133-146), K 2.2 mEq/L (normal 3-5.1), Cl 104 mEq/L (normal 98-105), and HCO_3 23 mEq/L (normal 22-28). Which of the following disorders are most likely?

a. Cushing disease with Androstenedione deficiency
b. Cushing disease with 17α-hydroxyprogesterone deficiency
c. Congenital adrenal hyperplasia with estrone deficiency
d. Addison disease with 18-hydroxylase deficiency
e. Addison disease with testosterone excess

343. A 22-year-old African-American female presents with a complaint of muscle weakness following exercise. Neurological examination reveals that the muscles supplied by cranial nerves are most affected. You suspect myasthenia gravis, a diagnosis confirmed by antibodies against which of the following in the patient's blood?

a. Acetylcholinesterase
b. Muscle mitochondrial membranes
c. Cranial nerve synaptic membranes
d. Cranial nerve presynaptic membranes
e. Acetylcholine receptors

344. A 7-month-old Hispanic boy is evaluated for asymmetric skull shape and possible hearing problems. Physical examination reveals a prominent forehead (tower skull) with prominent eyes (exophthalmos) and ridges over his coronal sutures. Premature fusion of the coronal sutures (craniosynostosis) is suspected as part of Crouzon syndrome (MIM*123500), a condition caused by mutations in the fibroblast growth factor receptor-2. Several conditions with disproportionate skeletal growth (dwarfism) or craniosynostosis are caused by mutations in fibroblast growth factors or their receptors. Fibroblast growth factor belongs to which of the following hormone groups?

a. Membrane-soluble hormones interacting with nuclear receptors
b. Membrane-soluble hormones interacting with cytoplasmic receptors
c. Receptor-binding hormones activating calcium/phosphatidyl inositol messengers
d. Receptor-binding hormones activating cAMP/cGMP messengers
e. Receptor-binding hormones activating kinase cascades

345. A 14-year-old African American adolescent has shown weight loss and increased thirst with fatigue and decreased athletic performance. His physician does a urinalysis and the reagent strip is strongly positive for glucose and ketones. A likely diagnosis of diabetes mellitus is made and the patient started on long-acting insulin at night with short-acting insulin at breakfast and lunch. Which of the following statements correctly describes insulin?

a. It is an anabolic signal to cells that glucose is scarce
b. It is converted from proinsulin to insulin primarily following secretion from β-cells
c. It does not have a prohormone form
d. It is a small polypeptide composed of a single chain bridged by disulfide groups
e. Its action is antagonistic to that of glucagon

346. Some individuals with diabetes mellitus are susceptible to rapid drops in blood sugar (hypoglycemia) with lethargy and potential seizures or coma. Such diabetics are called "brittle" and require careful monitoring of glucose levels as proper insulin doses are titrated. Of the many actions of insulin, decrease in which of the following cellular activities best accounts for "brittleness" of certain diabetics?

a. Plasma membrane transfer of glucose
b. Glucose oxidation
c. Gluconeogenesis
d. Lipogenesis
e. Formation of ATP, DNA, and RNA

347. A 50-year-old Caucasian male presents to his physician because of anxiety attacks accompanied by profuse sweating and heart palpitations. His physician documents a high blood pressure of 175/110 (hypertension) and orders ultrasound studies that show an adrenal tumor called pheochromocytoma. The male has also noted weight loss and fatigue over the past month when the attacks began. Knowing that pheochromocytoma releases epinephrine from the adrenal medulla, alteration of which of the following metabolic processes best explains symptoms of decreased energy and weight loss?

a. Glycolysis
b. Lipolysis
c. Gluconeogenesis
d. Glycogenolysis
e. Ketogenesis

348. Which of the following statements about prostaglandins is accurate?

a. They are precursors to arachidonic acid
b. They release arachidonic acid from membranes through the action of phospho-lipase A
c. They were first observed to cause uterine contraction and lowering of blood pressure
d. Although found in many organs, they are synthesized only in the prostate and seminal vesicles
e. They may be converted to leukotrienes by lipoxygenase

349. A 19-year-old African American male college student presents to his physician complaining of fatigue, weight loss, inability to concentrate, and occasional fainting spells. He also has noted a slight brown pigmentation to his skin despite no sun exposure. His physician suspects Addison disease, a multifactorial disorder that causes dysfunction of the adrenal cortex. Which of the following hormones is most likely deficient in Addison disease?

a. ACTH
b. Norepinephrine
c. Aldosterone
d. Testosterone
e. Epinephrine

350. The absorption of glucose from the gut into intestinal mucosal cells is coupled to Na^+, K^+-ATPase. In contrast, the movement of glucose from the intestinal epithelial cells into the submucosal bloodstream occurs through passive transport. Given these facts, which of the following statements is most accurate?

a. Cytosolic levels of glucose in intestinal mucosal cells are regulated by levels of glucose in skeletal muscle cells.
b. Free glucose levels in the lumen of the intestine can never be higher than levels in intestinal cells.
c. Plasma glucose levels are much higher than intestinal cell cytosolic levels of glucose.
d. Levels of glucose in the intestinal lumen are always higher than those in the cytosol of intestinal epithelial cells.
e. Levels of plasma glucose are approximately equal to levels in the cytosol of intestinal epithelial cells.

351. A 35-year-old Caucasian male is evaluated for epilepsy that appeared in his teenage years. He has had reasonable control with antiepileptic medications but recently has had seizures in the late evening. He also has chronic indigestion that requires daily proton pump inhibitors and was noted to have calcium deposits in his lungs when recently evaluated for a respiratory infection. His physician recognizes symptoms of multiple endocrine neoplasia type I (MIM*131100) that involves hypersecretion of multiple pancreatic hormones plus hyperparathyroidism. Which of the following options describes the peptide hormone that regulates stomach acid and the hormone that opposes its secretion?

a. Cholecystokinin, gastrin
b. Gastrin, insulin
c. Insulin, secretin
d. Secretin, insulin
e. Gastrin, secretin

352. A 6-year-old African American boy is evaluated for respiratory distress from refractory asthma and improves after albuterol inhalation therapy. He is discharged with instructions to continue albuterol nebulizer treatments and is given 2 mg/kg oral prednisolone as a 5-day burst. This therapy avoids the side effects of chronic steroid therapy (obesity, hypertension, shock susceptibility) by using short bursts of oral therapy or inhaled steroids that affect nasal/bronchial membranes without systemic absorption. Steroid therapies impact which of the following processes?

a. Conversion of membrane arachidonyl-triglyceride to arachidonic acid
b. Conversion of arachidonic acid to leukotrienes
c. Conversion of arachidonic acid to prostaglandins
d. Peroxidation of prostaglandin precursor
e. Dietary absorption of arachidonic acid

353. A 5-day-old Caucasian boy is kept in the nursery because of persisting neonatal jaundice with atypical elevation of direct-reacting, conjugated bilirubin. Further investigation indicates that the infant has liver disease with simultaneous elevation of liver transaminases. A sibling died with similar symptoms, and an inborn error of bile acid metabolism is suspected (eg, intrahepatic cholestasis with defective conversion of trihydroxyco-prostanic bile acid to cholic acid—MIM*214950). Which of the following compounds is normally used to conjugate bile acids?

a. Acetate
b. Glucuronic acid
c. Glutathione
d. Sulfate
e. Glycine

354. Several weight-loss diets are based on decreased carbohydrate intake to prevent stimulation of insulin secretion; insulin drives the feeling of hunger and also inhibits lipolysis. The suggested way of monitoring the success of low carbohydrate intake during fasting reflects the greatest increase in plasma concentration of which of the following?

a. Palmitate, oleate (free fatty acids)
b. Glucose, galactose
c. Lactate, pyruvate
d. Acetoacetate, β-hydroxybutyrate
e. Triacylglycerols

355. Congestive heart failure can be caused by intrinsic defects of the heart muscle/valves or by pumping against increased pressure as with prolonged hypertension. Which of the following effects of the steroid digitalis is observed after treatment of congestive heart failure?

a. Decrease in cytosolic sodium levels
b. Inhibition of Na^+, K^+-ATPase
c. Decrease in the force of heart muscle contraction
d. Stimulation of the plasma membrane ion pump
e. Decrease in cytosolic calcium

356. Defects in the ability to oxidize fatty acids can be asymptomatic in the presence of frequent feeding; a therapy applied to all but the most severe long chain fatty acid oxidation disorders that are frequently lethal. In asymptomatic children with medium or short chain fatty acid oxidation defects, unintentional fasting due to infections can produce lethargy and even coma after 4 to 6 hours without food. A deficit in which of the following compounds in serum most likely causes these neurologic symptoms?

a. Pyruvate and lactate
b. Free fatty acids
c. Propionate and methylmalonate
d. Glucose and ketone bodies
e. Triacylglycerols

357. A 14-year-old African American girl is evaluated in the emergency room and noted to have increased respiration (tachypnea), vomiting, and confusion. She bleeds from puncture sites during withdrawal of blood for testing, and a urine toxicology screen reveals increased amounts of acetosalicylic acid, ibuprofen, and acetaminophen. Initial blood studies show an elevated pH (alkalosis) with a salicylate level of 75 mg/dL (above 35 considered toxic). She has a past history of depression and suicide attempts. Which of the following enzymes are likely to be inhibited?

a. Lipoprotein lipase
b. Lipoxygenase
c. Cyclooxygenase
d. Phospholipase D
e. Phospholipase A_2

358. A 28-year-old female has had normal progress of her first pregnancy except for some early bleeding that resolved. At 30 weeks gestation, vaginal bleeding recurs and she experiences abdominal cramping suggestive of early labor. Which of the following treatments might be recommended?

a. Linoleic acid dietary supplement
b. Arachidonic acid dietary supplement
c. Prostaglandin therapy
d. Steroid therapy
e. Angiotensin II therapy

359. A 40-year-old Caucasian female is stung by a bee and rushed into the emergency room with a variety of symptoms including increasing difficulty in breathing due to nasal and bronchial constriction. Although your subsequent treatment is to block the effects of histamine and other acute-phase reactants released by most cells, you must also block the slow-reacting substance of anaphylaxis (SRS-A), which is the most potent constrictor of the muscles enveloping the bronchial passages. An SRS-A is composed of which of the following?

a. Thromboxanes
b. Interleukins
c. Complement
d. Leukotrienes
e. Prostaglandins

360. A premature Caucasian male infant of 30 weeks gestation has multiple respiratory complications and remains 2 months in the neonatal intensive care unit. He has received 24 days of total parental alimentation after developing an infection (necrotizing enterocolitis) that necessitates antibiotics and a rested bowel (no feeds) for healing. His nurse reports a plateau in weight gain accompanied by scaly skin on his extremities that is typical of fatty acid deficiency. Which of the following fatty acids would most effectively correct this deficiency?

a. Palmitic acid
b. Linoleic acid
c. Arachidonic acid
d. Oleic acid
e. Eicosatetraenoic acid

361. The 4-ring structure typical of steroids would be found in which of the following hormones?

a. Adrenocorticotropin
b. Aldosterone
c. Epidermal growth factor
d. Insulin
e. Insulin-like growth factor

362. A 25-year-old African American male seeks evaluation for increasing fatigue and muscle aches during exercise. He recalls avoiding athletics when young because he could not keep up with his peers and recently has embarked on an exercise program to help lose weight. Stress testing reveals normal cardiac function but serial blood tests show increased serum lactic acid and ammonia levels when he is at rest. His physician postulates a mitochondrial DNA depletion disorder that affects mitochondrial function due to defects in mitochondrial DNA polymerase or tRNAs. Which of the following options (1) list mitochondrial pathways that would explain the man's blood findings, and (2) name a compound linking these pathways?

a. Glycogenolysis, glycolysis, glucose 1-P
b. Glycogen synthesis, gluconeogenesis, pyruvate
c. Citric acid cycle, electron transport, isocitrate
d. Citric acid and urea cycles, arginine
e. Citric acid and urea cycles, fumarate

363. Which of the following can be converted to an intermediate of either the citric acid cycle or the urea cycle?

a. Tyrosine
b. Lysine
c. Leucine
d. Tryptophan
e. Aspartate

364. An 18-year-old Caucasian female is admitted to the hospital for evaluation of extreme weight loss over the past 6 months. She has decreased subcutaneous tissue, sores on the back of her fingers, severe dental decay, and sparse hair. Her parents report that she jogs each morning despite her weight loss, yet is preoccupied with food. A diagnosis of anorexia nervosa with bulimia is made and the female is started on a counseling program with intravenous feeding. Which of the following pathways would be least affected by this female's catabolic state?

a. Lipolysis
b. Glycolysis
c. β-Oxidation of fatty acids
d. Citric acid cycle
e. Gluconeogenesis

365. A 46-year-old Caucasian female has had spells of irritability, headaches, and trembling when she does not eat for several hours. She is hospitalized overnight for metabolic studies that demonstrate a low blood sugar in the presence of adequate gluconeogenesis. Which of the following would be an indicator of active gluconeogenesis?

a. Increased urea production
b. Increased conversion of alanine to pyruvate
c. Increased conversion of acetyl-CoA to malonyl-CoA
d. Increased conversion of oxaloacetate to citrate
e. Increased conversion of glucose 6-phosphate to glucose 1-phosphate

366. A 60-year-old Egyptian male has a hemoglobin of 12 g/dL (13.5 lower limit of normal) during his annual checkup and was taking Bactrim (antibiotic with trimethoprim folate inhibitor and a sulfonamide) for a skin infection. The medical student who evaluated him had suggested a diagnosis of glucose-6-phosphate dehydrogenase (G6PD) deficiency (MIM*305900), recognizing the patient's Mediterranean origin and exposure to sulfa antibiotics that can precipitate hemolysis in these individuals. The attending suggested G6PD deficiency would give much more severe symptoms of rapid hemolysis, severe anemia, and heart failure. Given that PI II converts glucose 6-phosphate to fructose 6-phosphate and G6PD initiates the reverse conversion (with several subsequent enzymes), which of the following statements do these different clinical presentations support?

a. Chemical conversions in metabolic pathways often use different enzymes and intermediates than reactions proceeding in the reverse direction.
b. The reaction steps for degradative (catabolic) pathways are the exact reverse of those for biosynthetic sequence.
c. Enzymes found in an anabolic pathway are never found in the corresponding catabolic pathway.
d. The first steps in a metabolic pathway are rarely rate limiting or subject to regulation.
e. Steps in both anabolic and catabolic pathways are usually reversible

367. Which of the following statements is true in the well-fed state?

a. NADPH production by the hexose monophosphate shunt is decreased.
b. Acetoacetate is the major fuel for muscle.
c. Glucose transport into adipose tissue is decreased.
d. The major fuel used by the brain is glucose.
e. Amino acids are utilized for glucose production.

368. An 8-year-old Caucasian boy is evaluated for mild short stature and night-time awakening feeling irritable and anxious. His mother's brother is said to have a storage disease that made him short. Physical examination reveals a palpable liver edge about two finger-breadths below the right costal margin and a span of 7 cm by percussion—evidence of hepatomegaly. Fasting values are obtained for glucose (50 mg/dL; 60-100 normal, cholesterol 220 mg/dL; <199 normal for age, uric acid 7.5 mg/dL; 2.5-6 normal) and a diagnosis of X-linked glycogen storage disease is considered (type IXa-MIM*306000-involving liver phosphorylase kinase deficiency). Night-time cornstarch infusion feedings are begun based on knowledge that which of the following is the major source of blood glucose during fasting?

a. Dietary glucose from the intestine
b. Hepatic glycogenolysis
c. Gluconeogenesis
d. Muscle glycogenolysis
e. Glycerol from lipolysis

369. The jinga bean, found in the jungles of Brazil, is unique in that it is composed almost exclusively of protein. Studies have shown that, immediately following a meal composed exclusively of jinga beans, which of the following occurs?

a. A decreased release of epinephrine
b. A complete absence of liver glycogen
c. Hypoglycemia
d. An increased release of insulin
e. Ketosis caused by the metabolism of ketogenic amino acids

370. Approximately 3 hours following a well-balanced meal, blood levels of which of the following are elevated?

a. Fatty acids
b. Glucagon
c. Glycerol
d. Epinephrine
e. Chylomicrons

371. If a homogenate of liver cells is centrifuged to remove all cell membranes and organelles, which of the following enzyme activities will remain in the supernatant?

a. Glucose-6-phosphate dehydrogenase
b. Glycogen synthetase
c. Aconitase
d. Acyl-CoA hydratase
e. Hydroxybutyrate dehydrogenase

372. A 15-month-old African American boy has recently been weaned from breast-feeding to whole milk in addition to a balanced diet of table food. His pediatrician refers him to endocrinology because he is noted to have increasing outward bowing of the legs (genu valgum) and thickened, somewhat tender wrists. Which of the following mechanisms is likely operating in this child?

a. Decreased calcium in the diet
b. Decreased conversion of cholesterol intermediates to previtamin D in the skin
c. Decreased conversion of skin previtamin D to blood cholecalciferol
d. Decreased conversion of cholecalciferol to calcidiol in liver
e. Decreased conversion of calcidiol to calcitriol in kidney

373. Which of the following enzymes is active in adipocytes following a heavy meal?

a. Glycogen phosphorylase
b. Glycerol kinase
c. Hormone-sensitive triacylglyceride lipase
d. Glucose-6-phosphatase
e. Phosphatidate phosphatase

374. A 35-year-old Caucasian female notes a lump in her breast and undergoes biopsy that shows breast cancer. The biopsy tissue is sectioned and shown to react with an antibody to the epidermal growth factor (EGF) receptor-2, also called Her-2. Which of the following describes the most likely treatment strategy for this female?

a. Intravenous infusion of EGF to activate signal transduction in normal breast tissue
b. Intravenous infusion of EGF antibody to block signal transduction in breast cancer tissue
c. Oral dosing of EGF to activate signal transduction in normal and breast cancer tissue
d. Oral dosing of EGFR2 antibody (Herceptin) to block signal transduction in normal breast tissue
e. Intravenous infusion of EGFR2 antibody (Herceptin) to block signal transduction in breast cancer tissue

375. Which of the following statements correctly apply to energy metabolism?

a. Fatty acids can be precursors of glucose.
b. High energy levels turn on glycolysis.
c. Pyruvate is committed to the citric acid cycle by acetylation through pyruvate dehydrogenase.
d. Phosphorylation activates enzymes that store fat and glycogen.
e. Guanosine triphosphate (GTP) is the major donor for enzyme phosphorylation.

376. Which of the following is appropriate for a patient with renal failure?

a. High-carbohydrate diet
b. High-protein diet
c. Low-fat diet
d. High-fiber diet
e. Free water of at least 3 L/d

377. An unfortunate complication of long-term diabetes mellitus is the occurrence of heart attacks and gangrene of the extremities. Which of the following is the most likely cause?

a. Decreased glucose availability to liver cells
b. Decreased glucose availability to extrahepatic tissues
c. Increased catecholamine synthesis
d. Decreased catecholamine synthesis
e. Decreased glucose concentrations in vascular epithelium

378. A 14-year-old African American adolescent presents with abdominal discomfort, abdominal fullness, excess gas, and weight loss. Blood glucose, cholesterol, and alkaline phosphatase levels are normal. There is no jaundice or elevations of liver transaminases. The stool tests positive for reducing substances. Which of the following is the most likely diagnosis?

a. Diabetes mellitus
b. Starvation
c. Nontropical sprue
d. Milk intolerance
e. Gallstones

379. Which of the following diseases reflects the loss of ability to move specific molecules between membrane-separated cellular compartments?

a. McArdle phosphorylase disease
b. Carnitine deficiency
c. Methanol poisoning
d. Ethylene glycol poisoning
e. Diphtheria

380. Which of the following sets of blood values most closely correlates with a patient who has conducted a hunger strike for 1 month? The blood levels listed by option (a) represent the immediate postprandial state—choose option a if blood levels after the hunger strike will remain the same or other options if they will change as specified

	CONCENTRATION OF BLOOD FUELS (mM)			
	Glucose	Free Fatty Acids	Ketone Bodies	Amino Acids
a.	4.5	0.5	0.02	4.5
b.	2.5	3.0	2.0	5.0
c.	14.0	1.5	2.0	5.0
d.	4.5	0.25	0.02	4.5
e.	4.5	3.0	2.0	4.0

Hormones and Integrated Metabolism

Answers

338. The answer is d. (*Murray, pp 429-435. Scriver, pp 4117-4146.*) All steroid hormones, including the sex hormones estrogen, testosterone, and progesterone, can be classified as group I hormones, meaning that they act by binding specific cytoplasmic receptors that enter the nucleus and stimulate transcription by specific DNA binding. Most nonsteroidal hormones, for example epinephrine, are group II hormones that interact with the cell membrane and produce a second-messenger effect. The group II hormones, in contrast to steroids, act in minutes while steroid hormones require hours for a biologic effect. Recent studies have indicated that specific cytoplasmic receptors for steroid hormones have an extraordinarily high affinity for the hormones. In addition, the receptors contain a DNA-binding region that is rich in amino acid residues that form metal binding fingers. Likewise, thyroid hormone receptors contain DNA-binding domains with metal-binding fingers. Like steroid hormones, thyroid hormones are transcriptional enhancers.

339. The answer is e. (*Murray, pp 75-83, 435-438. Scriver, pp 2226-2297.*) Epinephrine (as well as glucagon) in liver stimulates adenylate cyclase and a kinase cascade ending with glycogen phosphorylase to initiate glycogenolysis. In adipose tissue, epinephrine more directly activates cyclic AMP, protein kinase, and triglyceride lipase to initiate lipolysis of stored triacylglycerides. Failure of glycogenolysis in glycogen storage diseases transmits a continuous signal of low glucose and enhanced fatty acid metabolism, causing high cholesterol and triglycerides. Normal glycogenolysis and failure of fat oxidation in fatty acid oxidation disorders causes hypoglycemia after glycogen is depleted, accompanied by deficient energy yield and carnitine depletion (from formation of abnormal acylcarnitines) that leads to lethal liver and heart failure.

Some distinguish between type I hormones like cortisol that diffuse into the cytosol and type II hormones like epinephrine that interact with membrane receptors at the cell surface. The type I hormones form ligand-receptor complexes and mediate action in the cytosol or nucleus while type II hormones often act through second messengers. Epinephrine and glucagon activate G protein complexes, changing cytosolic levels of adenosine 3',5'-cyclic monophosphate (cyclic AMP), and modifying protein kinases. Cyclic AMP functions as a "second messenger" between the cell membrane and cytosolic or nuclear proteins.

340. The answer is d. (*Murray, pp 429-435. Scriver, pp 4029-4240.*) Hypersecretion of cortisol manufactured in the adrenal cortex produces Cushing syndrome with truncal obesity, fat pad below the neck, and striae (incorrect answers a-c, e). Cushing disease is multifactorial with causes including excessive production of adrenocorticotrophic hormone (ACTH) by pituitary tumors, adrenal tumors as would be likely in this female patient, or even specific mutations in G proteins that modulate the cortisol response (see MIM*219080). Epinephrine (adrenalin) is synthesized in the adrenal medulla and does not respond to ACTH.

341. The answer is c. (*Murray, pp 427-429. Scriver, pp 4029-4240.*) Vasopressin, which is also called antidiuretic hormone (ADH), increases the permeability of renal tubules and facilitates reabsorption of water into the bloodstream (incorrect answers a, b and d, e). Vasopressin is secreted by the posterior pituitary (neurohypophysis), which may undergo altered development in concert with brain malformations like holoprosencephaly. Vasopressin is like aldosterone in that its action expands the blood volume. However, aldosterone causes sodium reabsorption rather than water reabsorption and indirectly leads to increased plasma osmolality with water retention. Cortisol is a glucocorticoid that potentiates catabolic metabolism chronically. Epinephrine stimulates catabolic metabolism acutely. Insulin acutely favors anabolic metabolism, in large part by allowing glucose and amino acid transport into cells.

342. The answer is d. (*Murray, pp 429-435. Scriver, pp 4029-4240.*) Patients with Addison disease (MIM*103230) have muscle weakness and fatigue due to overall adrenal dysfunction with insufficiency of several hormones (incorrect answer e) or specific blocks in 21- or 18-hydroxylation of the steroid precursors progesterone or corticosterone. Cushing disease involves excess corticosteroid secretion (incorrect answers a, b) and congenital adrenal hyperplasia would produce changes in the external genitalia and/or pubertal development (incorrect answer c).

Both cortisol and aldosterone contain C-21-hydroxyl groups, the latter an 18-aldehyde group obtained by reduction of 18-hydroxy-corticosterone, another potent mineralocorticoid. Aldosterone secretion is regulated by the renin-angiotensin system through the kidney, acting to increase sodium and thus water resorption in the renal distal tubule. Decreases in renal blood flow prompt renin protease to produce angiotensin I that is converted to angiotensin II in the lungs, a potent pressor agent that acts on the adrenal to produce aldosterone. The sex hormones are synthesized in the ovaries and testicular interstitial cells. In the synthesis of sex hormones, progesterone is converted to 17α-hydrox-yprogesterone and then androstenedione, which may either become estrone or testosterone. Testosterone gives rise to estradiol in the ovaries, while progesterone is produced by the corpus luteum that persists in the ovary after conception.

343. The answer is e. (*Murray, pp 545-565. Scriver, pp 5493-5524.*) The major problem in myasthenia gravis is a marked reduction of acetylcholine receptors on the motor endplate where cranial nerves form a neuromuscular junction with muscles (incorrect answers a-d). In these patients, autoantibodies against the acetylcholine receptors effectively reduce receptor numbers. Normally, acetylcholine molecules released by the nerve terminal bind to receptors on the muscle endplate, resulting in a stimulation of contraction by depolarizing the muscle membrane. The condition is improved with drugs that inhibit acetylcholinesterase.

344. The answer is e. (*Murray, pp 427-429. Scriver, pp 4029-4240.*) Most steroid hormones like gluco- and mineralocorticoids, sex steroids freely enter cells and form receptor complexes that act in the cytosol or nucleus (sometimes called group I hormones, answer e). Water soluble hormones cannot cross cell membranes and act at the plasma membrane by binding to membrane receptors and activating second messengers (sometimes called group II hormones). These include fibroblast growth factors (FGFs—incorrect answers a, b) and epidermal growth factors (EGFs—see Fig. 20 in the High-Yield Facts). Second messengers can include G protein complexes modulating cAMP or cGMP concentrations through adenyl or guanyl cyclases (eg, epinephrine, glucagons, nitric oxide), calcium-phosphatidyl inositols (eg, angiotensin II, vasopressin), or protein kinase cascades as with FGFs (incorrect answers c, d), EGFs, insulin-like growth factors (IGFs), platelet-derived growth factors (PDGFs), as well as growth hormone and insulin. Factors/hormones regulating growth all use kinase cascades as second messengers with the exception that PDGFs also use calcium/ phosphatidyl inositol. In contrast, most steroid hormones (gluco- and mineralocorticoids, sex steroids) freely enter cells and form receptor complexes that act in the cytosol or nucleus (sometimes referred to as group I hormones).

345. The answer is e. (*Murray, pp 438-441. Scriver, pp 1471-1488.*) Early signs of diabetes mellitus reflect the inability of glucose to enter peripheral tissues, accompanied by decreased energy metabolism (fatigue), excess glucagon action, hyperglycemia, increased glucose excretion (polyuria), and dehydration (thirst). The anabolic hormone called insulin is synthesized in pancreatic β-cells in response to signals of glucose availability and is processed to its active form (incorrect answers a, c). The action of insulin is antagonistic to that of glucagon, a catabolic hormone secreted by pancreatic α-cells. Insulin is synthesized as a nascent polypeptide chain called preproinsulin, then cleaved immediately following synthesis to form proinsulin (incorrect answer b). Proinsulin is composed of one continuous polypeptide that contains in sequence an A chain of 21 residues, a connecting peptide (C peptide) of about 30 residues, and a B chain of 30 residues. The molecule is folded so that two disulfide bridges span the A and B chains (incorrect answer d). The proinsulin molecule is transported from the lumen of the endoplasmic reticulum to the Golgi apparatus, where it is packaged into storage granules. In the Golgi apparatus and in the storage granules, proteolysis of the C peptide occurs. Exocytosis of the granules releases insulin as well as C peptides into the bloodstream. Neither proinsulin nor the C peptide is biologically active.

346. The answer is c. (*Murray, pp 131-142, 438-441. Scriver, pp 1471-1488.*) Gluconeogenesis is a catabolic process for the synthesis of glucose, mainly from the amino acids of degraded proteins. Gluconeogenesis is the adaptive response of the organism to low blood levels of glucose and is, therefore, diminished by insulin. Insulin regulates the disposition and utilization of glucose, particularly exogenous glucose. Glucose can enter liver and pancreatic β-cells freely, and high blood glucose signals the latter cells to secrete insulin. This hormone acts through various protein kinase cascades (sometimes called group II hormones) to stimulate entry of glucose and amino acids into certain extra-hepatic tissues that include muscle and fat cells. The presence of glucose stimulates synthesis of glucose oxidation, lipogenesis, and macromolecular precursors such as nucleotides. Chronic insulin therapy as with type I (juvenile onset, insulin-dependent) diabetes may stimulate extrahepatic glucose entry under conditions of inhibited gluconeogenesis, potentiating hypoglycemia while suppressing its correction.

347. The answer is a. (*Murray, pp 435-438. Scriver, pp 4029-4240.*) The actions of epinephrine (adrenaline) and norepinephrine are catabolic; that is, these catecholamines are antagonistic to the anabolic functions of insulin and, like glucagon, are secreted in response to low blood glucose or during "fight or flight" stress. Glycolysis is an anabolic process that is decreased in the presence of elevated catecholamines. The catabolic processes increased by secretion of epinephrine and norepinephrine include glycogenolysis, gluconeogenesis, lipolysis, and ketogenesis (incorrect answers b-e). Products that increase blood sugar or spare it, such as ketone bodies and fatty acids, are increased during catabolism. Adrenergic hormones produce a "hypermetabolic" or catabolic state, favoring energy expenditure/depletion (fatigue) and weight loss; anabolic hormones secreted in the fed state favor inactivity and weight gain.

The β-adrenergic catecholamines like epinephrine act at cell membranes, stimulating second messengers including cAMP and protein kinases (sometimes called group II hormones). These hormones are secreted by the adrenal medulla in keeping with its neural crest derivation and response to neural stimulation (eg, anxiety, fight or flight response). Unlike glucagon, which only acts on the liver, the catecholamines affect most tissues, including liver and muscle.

348. The answer is c. (*Murray, pp 203-207. Scriver, pp 4029-4240.*) Although prostaglandins were originally isolated from prostate glands, seminal vesicles, and semen, their synthesis in other organs has been amply documented; indeed, few organs have failed to demonstrate prostaglandin release. Prostaglandins cause platelet aggregation, smooth-muscle contraction, vasodilation, and uterine contraction. Prostaglandins are synthesized from arachidonic acid, a 20-carbon fatty acid with interspersed carbon double bonds. Signals such as angiotensin II, bradykinin, epinephrine, and thrombin can activate phospholipase A_2 and release arachidonic acid from membrane lipids. The arachidonic acid is cyclized by cyclooxygenase to form prostaglandins. Arachidonic acid can also be oxidized to leukotrienes by the action of lipoxygenases.

349. The answer is c. (*Murray, pp 429-435. Scriver, pp 4029-4240.*) Glucocorticoids (eg, cortisol) and mineralocorticoids (eg, aldosterone) are secreted by zona glomerulosa cells at the outer layer of the adrenal cortex. Aldosterone deficiency will alter sodium/potassium electrolyte balance, contributing to the muscle weakness and fatigue seen with Addison disease. Sex steroids like testosterone are secreted in part by the adrenal cortex but also by the gonads (incorrect answer d), while norepinephrine and epinephrine are secreted by the adrenal medulla (incorrect answers b, e) and have synergy with neural tissues. ACTH-releasing hormone (adreno-corticotropin) is a pituitary hormone that regulates secondary hormone release from target tissues (like thyroid stimulating hormone, growth hormone—incorrect answer a). Lower adrenal hormone action in Addison disease would be associated with higher rather than deficient ACTH secretion. Addison disease has many causes and, like other autoimmune disorders—diabetes mellitus, Hashimoto thyroiditis—shows familial aggregation typical of multifactorial determination. As with these diseases, rare cases show simple Mendelian inheritance, as with a type of Addison disease (MIM*240200) that is probably due to a defect in cortisol synthesis.

350. The answer is e. (*Murray, pp 412-423, 482-488. Scriver, pp 4263-4274.*) Glucose travels from intestinal cells into plasma by passive diffusion, ensuring that plasma glucose levels will be slightly less or equal to those of the intestinal cytosol (incorrect answers b-d). Glucose levels in other tissues of the body (for example, muscle) will not affect those in intestinal cells (incorrect answer a). Absorption of glucose from the intestinal lumen into intestinal epithelial cells uses active transport, coupling glucose import to a sodium gradient glucose. Sodium ions entering the cell in the company of glucose are pumped out again by Na^+, K^+-ATPase. Once in the cytosol of the intestinal cell, the glucose moves across the cell and diffuses out of the cell into the interstitial fluid of the submucosa and then into the plasma of the capillaries underlying the intestinal epithelium.

351. The answer is e. (*Murray, pp 438-441, 459-468. Scriver, pp 4029-4240.*) Gastrin, normally produced in specialized cells of the antral mucosa of the stomach, stimulates parietal cells to produce HCl (approximately 0.16 M) and KCl (0.007 M); it also stimulates secretion of glucagon and insulin (incorrect answers a, c, and d). Production of gastrin is inhibited by secretin (incorrect answer b). Secretin, a circulatory hormone liberated in response to peptides or acid in the duodenum, stimulates the flow of pancreatic juice. Gastrin governs acid production by the stomach, and cholecystokinin causes the gallbladder to contract. Cholecystokinin stimulates this contraction after it is released by the duodenum into the circulation, with subsequent emptying of bile into the intestine. Multiple endocrine neoplasia type I (MIM*131100) has diverse presentations, often having pituitary adenomas that stimulate parathormone production with increased calcium or extragastric adenomas that produce ulcers by hypergastrinemia (either or both states are also known as Zollinger-Ellison syndrome).

352. The answer is a. (*Murray, pp 203-207. Scriver, pp 4029-4240.*) Anti-inflammatory steroids act at many metabolic sites that include inhibition of phospholipase A_2 (incorrect answers b-e). This enzyme is responsible for hydrolyzing arachidonyl-glycerol ester that is found at the second position of some membrane glycerophospholipids. Corticosteroids induce the phospholipase A_2–inhibitory protein lipocortin and inhibit production of all of the derivatives of arachidonic acid (lipoxins, leukotrienes, thromboxanes, and prostaglandins). Steroids also inhibit inflammatory signal transduction pathways as shown in Fig. 20 of the High-Yield facts.

　　Phospholipase liberation of arachidonic acid from membrane phospholipids (stimulated by epinephrine, angiotensin II, etc) or absorbed from the diet is converted to prostaglandin by cyclooxygenase components of prostaglandin synthase. (COX I, II—inhibited by nonsteroidal anti-inflammatory drugs [NSAIDs] such as aspirin, indomethacin, and ibuprofen.) The prostaglandin precursor can be converted to thromboxanes active in platelets or prostacyclins. Alternatively, lipoxygenases act on arachidonic acid to produce lipoxins and leukotrienes.

353. The answer is e. (*Murray, pp 271-284, 609-615. Scriver, pp 2981-2960.*) Bile acids often are conjugated with glycine to form glycocholic acid and with taurine to form taurocholic acid. In human bile, glycocholic acid is by far the more common. The presence of the charged carboxyl group of glycine or the charged sulfate of taurine adds to the hydrophilic nature of the bile acids, thereby increasing their ability to emulsify lipids during the digestive process. Glucuronic acid is used to conjugate bilirubin and many xenobiotics (foreign chemicals), such as polychlorinated biphenyls (PCBs) and insecticides. A hydroxyl group is added to the xenobiotic by the cytochrome P450 system and then conjugated with glucuronide, sulfate, acetate, or glutathione to make it water-soluble for excretion in urine. A group of rare inborn errors affect the enzymes of bile acid synthesis, resulting in accumulation of toxic acids in liver. Patients with these disorders may have lethal accumulation of abnormal bile acids and conjugated bilirubin in liver due to cholestasis (abnormal concentration of bile acids in gall bladder), illustrated by infants with defective cholic acid synthesis (MIM*214950) that live 4 to 6 months on average.

354. The answer is d. (*Murray, pp 131-142.*) Urine ketone measurements by dipstick were recommended for monitoring of success in limiting carbohydrate intake (incorrect answers a-c, e). Under fed conditions, glucose is the preferred fuel for most tissues. However, under starvation conditions, glucose must be reserved for use by the central nervous system. There is a small initial decrease in plasma glucose upon starvation but the concentration levels off after a time because of conversion of glycogen in the liver. Under starvation conditions, ketone bodies are made in the liver and provide a major metabolic fuel source for skeletal and heart muscle and can serve to meet some of the brain's energy needs. Another effect of starvation and carbohydrate limitation is accelerated lipogenesis and elevated serum cholesterol/triglycerides, which was exaggerated by substituting fat (meat, eggs) in one famous low-carbohydrate diet. These effects may have contributed to the sudden collapse and death of the diet's founder; low-fat, heart-friendly low carbohydrate diets have since been promoted.

355. The answer is b. (*Murray, pp 412-123, 444-458. Scriver, pp 5433-5452.*) Treatment of patients with congestive heart failure is often based on the use of cardiotonic steroids such as digitalis. Digitalis is derived from the foxglove plant and has been used as an herbal treatment for heart problems since ancient times. Digitalis and ouabain are cardiotonic steroids that inhibit the Na^+, K^+-ATPase pump located in the plasma membrane of cardiac muscle cells. They specifically inhibit the dephosphorylation reaction of the ATPase when the cardiotonic steroid is bound to the extracellular face of the membrane. Because of inhibition of the pump, higher levels of sodium are left inside the cell, leading to a diminished sodium gradient. This results in a slower exchange of calcium by the sodium-calcium exchanger. Subsequently, intracellular levels of calcium are maintained at a higher level and greatly enhance the force of contraction of cardiac muscle.

356. The answer is d. (*Murray, pp 184-192. Scriver, pp 2297-2326.*) The brain uses glucose as its major energy source but can also use ketone bodies to provide up to 20% of its energy needs. Other metabolites are not efficient energy sources (incorrect answers a-c, e). Glucose is the preferred metabolic fuel for most tissues. However, extrahepatic tissues such as heart prefer ketone bodies and fatty acids as energy sources over glucose. Children with medium or short chain fatty acid oxidation defects can breakdown glycogen over the first 1 to 3 hours of fasting to maintain glucose, but have deficient fat breakdown when glycogen is depleted. They have normal lipases and can mobilize triacylglycerols but cannot metabolize the fatty acid side chains. Some abnormal ketones are produced as expected from sequential breakdown of fatty acyl-CoAs in 2-carbon steps—dehydrogenase to make β-double bond, enolase to make β-hydroxyl, dehydrogenase to make β-ketone, thiolase to cleave off acetyl-CoA and an acyl-CoA 2 carbons shorter. A block like that in medium chain-CoA dehydrogenase (MCAD) deficiency (MIM*201450) will cause accumulation of 8 to 12 carbon β-hydroxyl and ketone β-compounds, but these will have much less serum concentrations and metabolic efficiency than the normal 4-carbon acetoacetate, β-hydroxybutyrate, and 2-carbon acetone. Even greater deficiency of ketone bodies with long chain oxidation defects may explain their early and lethal cardiac failure. Lactate but not pyruvate will be deficient in mitochondrial pyruvate dehydrogenase deficiency (eg, MIM*300502), while propionate and methylmalonate will accumulate in disorders like methylmalonic aciduria (MIM*251000).

357. The answer is c. (*Murray, pp 203-207, 609-615. Scriver, pp 4029-4240.*) Aspirin (acetosalicylic acid) inhibits the cyclooxygenase (COX) that converts arachidonic acid to prostaglandins while nonsteroidal anti-inflammatory drugs (NSAIDs) like ibuprofen and indomethacin compete for arachidonate and influence both cyclooxygenase and the lipoxygenase that produces leukotrienes (incorrect answers a, b, d, and e). Additional effects of aspirin in toxic doses include uncoupling of oxidative phosphorylation and inhibition of the tricarboxylic acid cycle. Stimulation of the respiratory center causes tachypnea which blows off carbon dioxide and produces respiratory alkalosis as in this teen. Although aspirin and ibuprofen overdoses can be treated effectively, acetaminophen (Tylenol) causes irreversible liver damage and failure above certain levels and requires liver transplant.

Eicosanoids consist of C20 unsaturated fatty acids that include prostaglandins, thromboxanes, leukotrienes, and lipoxins. They can be synthesized from essential linoleic and linolenic (C18) fatty acids in the diet or from (C20) arachidonic acid. Arachidonate can also come from diet or from elongation of linolenic acid released from the 2' position of membrane acyltriglyceride phospholipids by the action of phospholipase A_2. The lipoxygenase pathway that produces leukotrienes/lipoxins competes with the cyclooxygenase (prostaglandin synthetase) pathway for available arachidonate.

358. The answer is d. (*Murray, pp 203-207. Scriver, pp 4029-4240.*) Steroids inhibit synthesis of prostaglandins, metabolites that stimulate uterine contraction, increase bronchoconstriction, relax gastrointestinal smooth muscle, and decrease gastric acid secretion (prostaglandins may be used to induce abortion–incorrect answer c). Dietary linoleic and arachidonic acids are precursors to prostaglandins (incorrect answers a, b) although their major pathway of synthesis is from arachidonic acid liberated from membrane phospholipids by phospholipase A_2 hydrolysis. The latter process is stimulated by angiotensin II (incorrect answer e) and inhibited by steroids. Progesterone is often used to prevent premature abortion/delivery and administration of glucocorticoids enhances fetal lung maturation.

In mammals, arachidonic (5,8,11,15-eicosatetraenoic) acid can be synthesized from dietary essential fatty acids (linoleic—9,12-octadecadienoic or C18 with 2 double bonds, linolenic—9,12,15-octadecatrienoic or C18 with 3 double bonds). These fatty acids are essential because the fatty acid synthase system in mammals lacks desaturases to produce the requisite fatty acyl double bonds. Arachidonic acid occurs in vegetable oils and animal fats with linoleic and linolenic acids, and can also be synthesized from linoleic acid following liberation from membrane phospholipids by phospholipase A_2 cleavage at the 2'-carbon of glycerol. Oleic, palmitic, and stearic acids are all nonessential fatty acids that can be manufactured by the fatty acid synthase system but cannot be desaturated or elongated to produce arachidonate.

359. The answer is d. (*Murray, pp 203-207. Scriver, pp 4029-4240.*) Leukotrienes C_4, D_4, and E_4 together compose the slow-reacting substance of anaphylaxis (SRS-A), which is thought to be the cause of asphyxiation in individuals not treated rapidly enough following an anaphylactic shock. SRS-A is up to 1000 times more effective than histamines in causing bronchial muscle constriction. Anti-inflammatory steroids are usually given intravenously to end chronic bronchoconstriction and hypotension following a shock. The steroids block phospholipase A_2 action, preventing the synthesis of leukotrienes from arachidonic acid. Acute treatment involves epinephrine injected subcutaneously initially and then intravenously. Antihistamines such as diphenhydramine are administered intravenously or intramuscularly.

360. The answer is b. (*Murray, pp 203-207. Scriver, pp 2297-2326.*) The essential fatty acid linoleic acid with 18 carbons and two double bonds at carbons 9 and 18 is absorbed and converted to eicosatrienoic acid, the precursor of eicosanoids (20-carbon compounds) that include prostaglandins, thromboxanes, and leukotrienes (incorrect answers a, c-e). The scientific name of arachidonic acid is eicosatetraenoic acid. Arachidonic acid can only be synthesized from essential fatty acids obtained from the diet. Palmitic acid (C16) and oleic acid (C18) can be synthesized by the tissues.

361. The answer is b. (*Murray, pp 429-435. Scriver, pp 4029-4240.*) Steroid hormones such as aldosterone are ultimate derivatives of cholesterol, a four-ring compound synthesized from the 5-carbon isoprene unit mevalonic acid or derived from the diet. Cholesterol is the precursor of all steroids involved in mammalian metabolism, including the bile acids, and steroid hormones like cortisol, aldosterone, progesterone, testosterone, and vitamin D (incorrect answers a, c-e). Cholesterol cannot be metabolized to carbon dioxide and water in humans. It must be excreted as a component of bile. Adrenocorticotropin (ACTH) is a peptide hormone from the adenohypophysis that stimulates secretion of corticosteroids while insulin, insulin-like growth factor, and epidermal growth factor are proteins that interact with specific membrane receptors to trigger anabolic cell responses.

362. The answer is e. (*Murray, pp 131-142, 165-173, 234-238. Scriver, pp 1909-1964.*) The citric acid and urea cycle are located primarily in the mitochondria while pathways for glycogen and glucose metabolism are primarily in the cytosol (incorrect answers a, b). Isocitrate and fumarate are intermediates of the citric acid cycle but only fumarate is an intermediate of both the citric acid and urea cycles (incorrect answer c). Fumarate and arginine are produced from argininosuccinate in the urea cycle, after which arginine is converted to ornithine to yield urea and fumarate is converted to malate and then oxaloacetate in the citric acid cycle. Depending upon the organism's needs, oxaloacetate can either enter gluconeogenesis or react with acetyl-CoA to form citrate and traverse the citric acid cycle with generation of NADH and then energy through oxidative phosphorylation. Starvation will simultaneously increase urea cycle activity to remove ammonia from protein degradation and increase fumarate for oxaloacetate production; the oxaloacetate is then available for gluconeogenesis to maintain glucose levels that are essential for brain metabolism. Depletion of mitochondrial pathway functions will mainly impact electron transport and cause more dependence on glycolysis and lactate production as exercise depletes blood oxygen saturation. A vicious cycle of exercise intolerance leading to muscle inactivity with fewer mitochondria exacerbates myopathy (muscle weakness and incoordination) in mitochondrial disorders.

363. The answer is e. (*Murray, pp 239-247. Scriver, pp 1909-1964.*) Aspartate is a glucogenic amino acid that is also used to carry NH_4^+ into the urea cycle. Aspartate aminotransferase catalyzes the direct transamination of aspartate to oxaloacetate:

$$aspartate + \alpha\text{-ketoglutarate} \rightarrow oxaloacetate + glutamate$$

Oxaloacetate may either be utilized in the citric acid cycle or undergo gluconeogenesis. Argininosuccinate synthetase catalyzes the condensation of citrulline and aspartate to form argininosuccinate:

$$citrulline + aspartate + ATP \rightarrow argininosuccinate + AMP + PP_i$$

In this manner, one of the two nitrogens of urea is introduced into the urea cycle.

364. The answer is d (*Murray, pp 131-142. Scriver, pp 1327-1406.*) The citric acid cycle generates energy (through production of NADH/FADH2) and precursors of anabolic pathways (like succinic acid); it also catabolizes compounds like acetyl-CoA to carbon dioxide and water. For these reasons, the citric acid cycle is often called an amphibolic pathway. Catabolic pathways degrade protein, lipid, and carbohydrate to acetyl-CoA to produce energy and conserve essential molecules like glucose when there are caloric deficits as in starvation or eating disorders (incorrect answers a-c, e). Anabolic pathways store energy through conversion of foodstuffs to glycogen or fat during caloric excess (fed states). In general, the catabolic and anabolic pathways may share metabolites but involve different enzyme steps and cofactors that yield or consume energy (glycolysis versus gluconeogenesis, lipolysis and β-oxidation of fatty acids versus fatty acid synthesis, glycogenolysis versus glycogenesis).

365. The answer is b. (*Murray, pp 131-142, 239-247. Scriver, pp 1327-1406.*) Transamination of alanine to pyruvate, like that of other amino acids provides citric acid cycle intermediates leading to oxaloacetate and gluconeogenesis. Urea is excreted (incorrect answer a) although fumarate from the urea cycle is a precursor to oxaloacetate, conversion of acetyl-CoA to malonyl-CoA initiates fatty acid synthesis (incorrect answer c), and diversion of oxaloacetate to citrate rather than pyruvate or glucose 6-P to glucose 1-P rather than glucose would decrease gluconeogenesis (incorrect answers d, e). Many amino acids are degraded and transaminated to yield citric acid cycle intermediates, including arginine, histidine, proline, glutamine to glutamate and then α-ketoglutarate, tyrosine and phenylalanine to fumarate, asparagine to aspartate, and then to oxaloacetate. Others, like cysteine, glycine, serine, and threonine can be converted to alanine and transaminated to pyruvate that directly contributes to gluconeogenesis (through pyruvate carboxylase and phosphoenolpyruvate carboxykinase).

During the early phases of starvation, the catabolism of proteins is at its highest level. Anabolic enzymes, which are not utilized during starvation, are targeted for degradation (with ubiquitin) and their synthesis repressed. The transamination of amino acids is a first step in amino acid degradation and also yields ketoacids for gluconeogenesis. The protein and amino acid degradation with ketogenesis results in a negative nitrogen balance, increasing ammonia and urea levels in the urine (from the urea cycle). The glucose formed from gluconeogenic amino acids becomes the major source of blood glucose following depletion of liver glycogen stores. Complete oxidation of this glucose, as well as the ketone bodies formed from ketogenic amino acids, leads to a relative increase in the CO_2 and H_2O formed from amino acid carbon skeletons.

366. The answer is a. (*Murray, pp 131-142. Scriver, pp 1327-1406.*) Chemical conversions in metabolic pathways usually employ different enzymes and intermediates than those occurring in the reverse direction (eg, phosphohexose isomerase—PHI enzyme) (MIM*172400) converting glucose 6-phosphate to fructose 6-phosphate but several enzymes including G6PD (MIM*305900) to accomplish the reverse conversion (incorrect answers b, e). The first steps of metabolic pathways are often rate limiting and subject to regulation, allowing shifts to the appropriate pathway during times of energy excess/depletion or synthetic product excess/deficiency (incorrect answer d). Thus, oxaloacetate or pyruvate can be diverted toward the citric acid cycle to generate energy or toward gluconeogenesis to generate glucose, using different enzymes and intermediates in each case. Some enzymes like PHI occur in different pathways but are not rate limiting (incorrect answer d).

367. The answer is d. (*Murray, pp 131-142. Scriver, pp 1327-1406.*) Glucose is the major fuel for the brain in the well-fed state. The brain requires a continuous supply of glucose at all times. In fact, if glucose drops to a low level, convulsions may follow. However, during starvation or fasting, the brain is capable of obtaining approximately 75% of its energy from circulating ketone bodies. During the absorptive phase, ketone bodies such as acetoacetate and 3-hydroxybutyrate are low (with glucose rather than these ketones used by muscle—incorrect answer b). Circulating amino acids are utilized for protein synthesis, not glucose production (incorrect answer e). Liver production of NADPH is at a high level because it is needed for fatty acid synthesis (incorrect answer a). Glucose is actively transported into all cells, including adipocytes, which require it to form glycerol-3-phosphate for esterifying fatty acids into triacylglyceride (incorrect answer c).

368. The answer is b. (*Murray, pp 131-142. Scriver, pp 1471-1488.*) During overnight or other fasting, the major source of blood glucose is hepatic glycogen (incorrect answers a, c-e). Through the effects of glycogenolysis, which are mediated by glucagon, hepatic glycogen is slowly parceled out as glucose to the bloodstream, keeping blood glucose levels normal. After a meal, glucose is absorbed from the intestine into the blood system. Much of this glucose is absorbed into cells and, in particular, into the liver via the action of insulin, where it is stored as glycogen. Once the effects of daytime eating have subsided and all the glucose from absorption has been stored, the normal overnight fast begins. During this period, the major source of blood glucose is hepatic glycogen. In contrast, muscle glycogenolysis has no effect on blood glucose levels because no glucose-6-phosphatase exists in muscle and hence phosphorylated glucose cannot be released from muscle into the bloodstream. Following a more prolonged fast or in the early stages of starvation, gluconeogenesis is needed to produce glucose from glucogenic amino acids and the glycerol released by lipolysis of triacylglycerides in adipocytes. This is because the liver glycogen is depleted and the liver is forced to turn to gluconeogenesis to produce the amounts of glucose necessary to maintain blood levels.

369. The answer is d. (*Murray, pp 131-142. Scriver, pp 1471-1488.*) High blood levels of amino acids, in addition to glucose, promote the release of insulin through their action on receptors at the surface of the β-cells of the pancreas. Although insulin alone could lead to a hypoglycemic effect, hypoglycemia should not be observed because glucagon is also released in response to the elevated levels of circulating amino acids (incorrect answer c). The balance of glucagon and glucose tends to keep blood levels of glucose within normal ranges while amino acid transport into cells is promoted. Because of the normal insulin levels in the fed state, ketosis and depletion of liver glycogen are not observed (incorrect answers b, e). Both of these events occur during fasting and starvation due to the abundance of glucagon and epinephrine (incorrect answer a) in the blood as opposed to the low levels of insulin.

370. The answer is e. (*Murray, pp 131-142. Scriver, pp 1471-1488.*) Following digestion, the products of digestion enter the bloodstream. These include glucose, amino acids, triacylglycerides packaged into chylomicrons from the intestine, and very low density lipoproteins from the liver. The hormone of anabolism, insulin, is also elevated because of the signaling of the glucose and amino acids in the blood, which allows release of insulin from the β-cells of the pancreas. Insulin aids the movement of glucose and amino acids into cells. In contrast, all the hormones and energy sources associated with catabolism are decreased in the blood during this time. Long chain fatty acids and glycerol released by lipolysis from adipocytes are not elevated. Glucagon and epinephrine are not released. The only time glucose levels rise significantly above approximately 80 mM is following a well-balanced meal when glucose is obtained from the diet. The concentration of glucose reaches a peak 30 to 45 min after a meal and returns to normal within 2 hours after eating. This response of blood glucose after eating (mimicked by giving 50 g of oral glucose) is the basis for the glucose tolerance test. In the event of insulin deficiency (diabetes mellitus), the peak glucose concentration is abnormally high and its return to normal is delayed.

371. **The answer is a.** (*Murray, pp 131-142. Scriver, pp 1327-1406.*) Centrifugation of a cellular homogenate at a force of 100,000 X g will pellet all cellular organelles and membranes. Only soluble cellular molecules found in the cytosol will remain in the supernatant. Thus, the enzymes of glycolysis and most of those of gluconeogenesis, fatty acid synthesis, and the pentose phosphate pathway will be in the supernatant. Glucose-6-phosphate dehydrogenase, which results in the formation of 6 phosphoglucono-δ-lactone from glucose 6-phosphate, is the committed step in the pentose phosphate pathway. In the pellet will be the enzymes within mitochondria, including those of the citric acid cycle (aconitase), fatty acid β-oxidation (acyl-CoA hydratase), and ketogenesis (hydroxybutyrate dehydrogenase). Enzymes of glycogen degradation and synthesis (glycogen synthetase) will also be in the pellet associated with glycogen particles.

372. The answer is b. (*Murray, pp 467-481. Scriver, pp 4029-4240.*) The most common cause of vitamin D deficiency is dietary deficiency compounded by decreased UV-dependent manufacture of previtamin in the skin. The latter process is most likely in African Americans with their darker skin that protects them from UV light (incorrect answers a, c-e). Calcium is plentiful in milk but its intestinal absorption is stimulated and its renal excretion inhibited by active vitamin D (1,25-hydroxycholecalciferol or calcitriol). Answer options a to e summarize the steps of calcium uptake by the intestine, conversion of vitamin D to previtamin D in skin then absorbed as cholecalciferol in blood, conversion of cholecalciferol to 25-hydroxycholecalciferol (calcidiol) in liver, conversion of calcidiol to calcitriol in kidney. Mutations in the enzymes can cause autosomal recessive rickets that is very rare, and mutations in proteins that form membrane channels for chloride or phosphate transport can produce X-linked rickets (eg, MIM*307800). Calcium is present as a divalent cation when soluble and as hydroxyapatite (calcium phosphate) when insoluble in bone formation. A major function for soluble calcium is muscle contraction; it is sequestered into the sarcoplasmic reticulum during relaxation and actively transported by a calcium-ATPase across the sarcoplasmic reticulum.

373. The answer is e. (*Murray, pp 193-199. Scriver, pp 1471-1488.*) The enzyme phosphatidate phosphatase converts phosphatidic acid to diacylglycerol during synthesis of triacylglycerides. The function of adipose tissue is the storage of fatty acids as triacylglycerols in times of plenty and the release of fatty acids during times of fasting or starvation. Fatty acids taken in by adipocytes are stored by esterification to glycerol-3-phosphate. Glycerol-3-phosphate is derived almost entirely from the glycolytic intermediate dihydroxyacetone phosphate through the action of glycerol-3-phosphate dehydrogenase. Glycolytic enzymes are active in adipocytes during triglyceride synthesis, but those of glycogen degradation (low levels in adipocytes) and gluconeogenesis (ie, glucose-6-phosphatase) are not. Glycerol kinase is not present to any great extent in adipocytes, so that glycerol freed during lipolysis is not used to reesterify the fatty acids being released. The enzyme triacylglyceride lipase is turned on by phosphorylation by a cyclic AMP-dependent protein kinase following epinephrine stimulation.

374. The answer is d. (*Murray, pp 446-454. Scriver, pp 1471-1488.*) Epidermal growth factor (EGF) can interact with four receptors including EGF receptor-2 (Her-2) as shown in Fig. 20 of the High-Yield Facts. The resulting signal transduction cascade promotes cell survival and growth, so provision of EGF (intravenously since oral proteins will be degraded in the intestine) would promote growth of normal and cancer cells (incorrect answers a-d). Cancer cells are now tested for protein or microRNA markers that can forecast prognosis and responses to therapy. Some marker proteins like the Her-2 receptor in breast cancer become targets for antibody therapy, illustrated by Herceptin in breast cancer and Gleevec antibody to the fusion oncogenic protein in chronic myelogenous leukemia (MIM*608232).

375. The answer is c. (*Murray, pp 131-142. Scriver, pp 1471-1488.*) The acetylation of pyruvate to citric acid by pyruvate dehydrogenase rather than its reduction by lactate dehydrogenase is a key regulatory step between high energy yields of citric acid cycle/oxidative phosphorylation or lower energy yields of glycolysis (incorrect answers a, b, d). GTP can be a phosphate donor (eg, in the phosphoenolpyruvate carboxykinase reaction of gluconeogenesis) but ATP is much more common (incorrect answer e).

There are certain properties of metabolism that are considered truisms:

(1) Futile cycles involving useless synthesis and degradation of a fuel do not occur simultaneously.

(2) Acetyl-CoA or substances that produce it, such as fatty acids or ketogenic amino acids, cannot be precursors of glucose.

(3) ATP is a major phosphate donor and energy source; it must be present in cells at all times in order for them to function.

(4) Protein phosphorylation inactivates enzymes that store glycogen and fat and activates enzymes that increase blood glucose and fatty acids.

(5) Low blood glucose stimulates gluconeogenesis and glycogenolysis.

(6) Low energy levels stimulate glycolysis and lipolysis.

(7) High energy levels inhibit glycolysis and β-oxidation of fatty acids.

376. The answer is a. *(Murray, pp 131-142. Scriver, pp 5467-5492.)* A diet high in carbohydrate and fats spares glucose use and inhibits gluconeogenesis, thereby preventing protein catabolism and nitrogen production. A major function of the kidneys is to excrete nitrogen catabolized from proteins in the form of urea. Indeed, the major clinical measures of renal function are products of protein catabolism (blood urea nitrogen [BUN] and blood creatinine). A diet for a patient with renal failure should therefore minimize protein and nitrogen load. Although 3 L/d of fluid is a normal intake for adults with healthy kidneys, glomerular filtration and water excretion are decreased in renal failure. Water and salt intake (particularly potassium) must therefore be limited in renal failure. Excess water or salt intake in patients with renal disease is manifest clinically by edema (swollen eyelids, swollen lower limbs).

377. The answer is b. *(Murray, pp 131-142, 438-441. Scriver, pp 1471-1488.)* Decreased insulin synthesis (juvenile onset, insulin-dependent type I diabetes) or increased resistance to insulin action (adult onset, type II diabetes) results in decreased glucose entry into extrahepatic tissues and increased serum glucose levels. Glucose can enter hepatic or pancreatic β-cells directly, regulating insulin release in the latter cells. Decreased glucose entry into extrahepatic tissues forces increased lipid catabolism with associated increases in serum cholesterol. The combination of increased cholesterol and perhaps hyperglycemia leads to the process of blood vessel damage called atherosclerosis. The blood vessel lining (intima) becomes damaged with buildup of plaques, deposit of cholesterol, and increased aggregation of platelets and other blood constituents. The atheroma then blocks blood flow in the affected vessels, potentially causing coronary artery obstruction (coronary thrombosis) and myocardial infarction, carotid artery obstruction and strokes, or extremity artery obstructions with leg pains (claudication) and tissue hypoxia (nonhealing sores, gangrene).

378. The answer is d. (*Murray, pp 438-441, 459-468. Scriver, pp 1623-1650.*) Milk intolerance may be due to milk protein allergies during infancy, but it is commonly caused by lactase deficiency in older individuals. Intestinal lactase hydrolyzes the milk sugar lactose into galactose and glucose, both reducing sugars that can be detected as reducing substances in the stool. The symptoms of lactose intolerance (lactase deficiency) and other conditions involving intestinal malabsorption include diarrhea, cramps, and flatulence due to water retention and bacterial action in the gut. In nontropical sprue, symptoms seem to result from the production of antibodies in the blood against fragments of wheat gluten. It seems likely that a defect in intestinal epithelial cells allows tryptic peptides from the digestion of gluten to be absorbed into the blood, as well as to exert a harmful effect on intestinal epithelia. Gallbladder inflammation (cholecystitis) usually presents with acute abdominal pain (colic) with radiation to the right shoulder. The normal composition of bile is about 5% cholesterol, 15% phosphatidylcholine, and 80% bile salt in a micellar liquid form. Increased cholesterol from high-fat diets or genetic conditions can upset the delicate micellar balance, leading to supersaturated cholesterol or cholesterol precipitates that cause gallstone formation. Removal of the gallbladder is a common treatment for this painful condition. Mobilization of fats with the production of ketone bodies occurs during fasting and starvation, but ketone production is well controlled. During uncontrolled diabetes mellitus, ketogenesis proceeds at a rate that exceeds the buffering capacity of the blood to produce ketoacidosis.

379. The answer is b. (*Murray, pp 184-192. Scriver, pp 2297-2326.*) A deficiency in carnitine, carnitine acyltransferase I, carnitine acyltransferase II, or acylcarnitine translocase can lead to an inability to oxidize long chain fatty acids. This occurs because all of these components are needed to translocate activated long chain (>10 carbons long) fatty acyl-CoA across mitochondrial inner membrane into the matrix where β-oxidation takes place. Once long chain fatty acids are coupled to the sulfur atom of CoA on the outer mitochondrial membrane, they can be transferred to carnitine by the enzyme carnitine acyltransferase I, which is located on the cytosolic side of the inner mitochondrial membrane. Acylcarnitines are transferred across the inner membrane to the matrix surface by translocase. At this point, the acyl group is reattached to a CoA sulfhydryl by the carnitine acyltransferase II located on the matrix face of the inner mitochondrial membrane.

McArdle disease (deficiency of muscle glycogen phosphorylase) is one of several glycogen storage diseases. Muscle cramping and fatigue after exercise are characteristics of muscle glycogen storage diseases (types V and VII), whereas hypoglycemia, hyperuricemia, and liver disease are characteristics of liver glycogen storage diseases (types I, III, IV, VI, and VIII)—see Table 6 of the High-Yield Facts.

Wood alcohol (methanol) is a cause of death or serious illness (including blindness) among patients who ignorantly substitute it for ethanol or mistakenly ingest it. Ingestion of automotive antifreeze (ethylene glycol) can also result in death if not treated. In both cases, death or serious injury can be averted by quickly administering an intoxicating dose of ethanol. The success of this treatment is based on the fact that methanol and ethylene glycol are not poisons as such. First, they must be converted by the action of the enzyme alcohol dehydrogenase to precursors of potentially toxic substances. Administration of large doses of ethanol inhibits oxidation of both methanol and ethylene glycol by effectively competing as a preferred substrate for the active sites of alcohol dehydrogenase. Over time, methanol and ethylene glycol are excreted.

One of the primary killers of children prior to immunization was upper respiratory tract infections by *Corynebacterium diphtheriae*. Toxin produced by a lysogenic phage that is carried by some strains of this bacteria causes the lethal effects. It is lethal in small amounts because it blocks protein synthesis. The viral toxin is composed of two parts. The B portion binds a cell's surface and injects the A portion into the cytosol of cells. The A portion ADP ribosylates a unique histidine-derived amino acid of the elongation factor 2 (EF-2) known as diphthamide. This action completely blocks the ability of EF-2 to translocate the growing polypeptide chain.

380. The answer is e. (*Murray, pp 131-142. Scriver, pp 1171-1488.*) In a normal postabsorptive patient, blood fuel values are 4.5 mM glucose, 0.5 mM free fatty acids, 0.02 mM ketone bodies, and 4.5 mM amino acids as shown beside answer a; fasting will elevate levels of ketone bodies, making answer a incorrect. Following several days of starvation, a catabolic home-ostasis has set in, such that free fatty acids ketone bodies have increased concentrations with glucose remaining the same (incorrect answers b-d). At this point, glycogen stores have been depleted. Blood glucose is maintained at about 4.5 mM during starvation by gluconeogenesis of amino acids from protein breakdown. Most of the brain's fuel supply still derives from glucose at this time—a considerable demand because the brain accounts for at least 20% of the body's total consumption of fuel. Following prolonged starvation, utilization of glucose and hence catabolism of protein is spared by the induction of brain enzymes that utilize ketone bodies. In prolonged starvation, the blood concentration of amino acids decreases, whereas that of free fatty acids and ketone bodies increases with preservation of blood glucose (correct answer e). A diabetic could have blood values of free fatty acids, ketone bodies, and amino acids but not high levels of blood glucose shown in answer c (answer c incorrect). The lack of insulin does not allow glucose to enter cells (aside from liver), stimulating lipolysis, glycogenolysis, gluconeogenesis, and ketogenesis.

Inheritance Mechanisms/Risk Calculations

Questions

381. A 35-year-old Caucasian female develops aching and numbness in her legs at night which she at first ascribes to fatigue from exercise. She then experiences the same symptoms in her arms. Her physician suspects amyotrophic lateral sclerosis (ALS, Lou Gehrig disease) and the female, who was adopted, seeks information on her biological parents. She locates her biological mother, who tells her that her father died from a neurologic disease in his thirties, leaving her destitute and forcing her to place the new baby for adoption. ALS usually occurs as an isolated case with onset at older ages but occasionally presents in younger people, following an auto-somal dominant inheritance pattern. There is a slight predominance of males. Which of the following best summarizes this information?

a. ALS is a genetic disease.
b. ALS is an autosomal dominant disease with occasional new mutations.
c. ALS is a sporadic disease.
d. ALS is a congenital disease.
e. ALS exhibits multifactorial determination with occasional dominant inheritance.

382. Diabetes mellitus is caused by insulin deficiency or resistance with decreased import of glucose into extrahepatic tissues. Type I diabetes with earlier onset often follows a viral infection with inflammation of the pancreatic β-cells while later onset type II diabetes is strongly associated with obesity. Each type exhibits genetic predisposition with a 40% to 50% concordance rate in monozygous twins and clustering in families. Diabetes mellitus is best described as which of the following types of disorders?

a. Congenital disorder
b. Multifactorial disorder
c. Mendelian disorder
d. Sporadic disorder
e. Sex-limited disorder

383. Which of the following characteristics is most typical of multifactorial inheritance?

a. Sex predilection
b. Mitochondrial inheritance
c. Recurrence risks reflect the number of affected relatives
d. Major cause of miscarriages
e. Maternally derived

384. Assume that D and d alleles derive from a single locus and that the presence of one D allele causes deafness. Match the mating of a genotype Dd father with a genotype dd mother and their probabilities for genotypes in offspring.

a. 1 DD
b. $\frac{1}{2}$ Dd, $\frac{1}{2}$ dd
c. $\frac{1}{4}$ DD, $\frac{1}{2}$ Dd, $\frac{1}{4}$ dd
d. $\frac{1}{2}$ DD, $\frac{1}{2}$ Dd
e. 1 dd

385. A couple has three girls, the last of whom is affected with cystic fibrosis. The first-born daughter marries her first cousin—that is, the son of her mother's sister—and they have a son with cystic fibrosis. The father has a female cousin with cystic fibrosis on his mother's side. Which of the following pedigrees represents this family history?

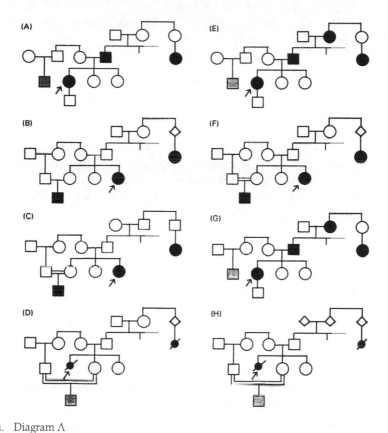

a. Diagram A
b. Diagram B
c. Diagram C
d. Diagram D
e. Diagram E
f. Diagram F
g. Diagram G
h. Diagram H

386. Huntington disease (MIM*143100) is an autosomal dominant, progressive neurodegenerative disease that causes uncontrolled physical movements and mental deterioration with usual onset in middle age. A husband and wife have three children, two boys and one girl. The husband was diagnosed with Huntington disease in his mid-fifties, as was his father. The wife has no symptoms and no family history of Huntington disease Assuming 100% penetrance, what is the probability that all three of his children will eventually develop Huntington disease?

a. $\frac{1}{8}$
b. $\frac{1}{4}$
c. $\frac{1}{2}$
d. $\frac{3}{4}$
e. Virtually 0

387. A couple is referred to the physician because their first three pregnancies have ended in spontaneous abortion. Chromosomal analysis reveals that the wife has two cell lines in her blood, one with a missing X chromosome (45,X) and the other normal (46,XX). Her chromosomal constitution is best described as which of the following?

a. Chimeric
b. Polyploid
c. Trisomic
d. Mosaic
e. Euploid

388. A 3-day-old Caucasian girl has a cleft palate, heart defect, extra fifth fingers, scalp defect (absent skin exposing underlying flesh), and unusual face with narrow distance between the eyes. Her physician orders a routine karyotype which shows 46 chromosomes with extra material on one homologue of the chromosome 5 pair. This chromosomal abnormality is best described by which of the following terms?

a. Polyploidy
b. Balanced rearrangement
c. Ring formation
d. Mosaicism
e. Unbalanced rearrangement

389. A 10-year-old African American boy is referred to the physician because of learning problems and some behavior changes. His family history is unremarkable. Physical examination reveals tall stature with few anomalies except for single palmar creases of the hands and curved fifth fingers (clinodactyly). The physician decides to order a karyotype. Which of the following indications for obtaining a karyotype best explains the physician's decision in this case?

a. A couple with multiple miscarriages or a person who is at risk for an inherited chromosome rearrangement
b. A child with ambiguous genitalia who needs genetic sex assignment
c. A child with an appearance suggestive of Down syndrome or other chromosomal disorder
d. A child with mental retardation and/or multiple congenital anomalies
e. A child who is at risk for cancer

390. A 10-year-old Caucasian girl with early developmental and speech delay is able to progress to third grade but is failing fourth grade. Evaluation shows an elongated body habitus like her mother with somewhat lax joints. Genetic evaluation is suggested, and a chromosomal analysis reveals a 47,XXX karyotype with normal fragile X DNA studies. Which of the following descriptions best fits this abnormality?

a. A female with mosaicism
b. A female with polyploidy
c. Sex chromosome aneuploidy
d. A female with Turner syndrome
e. A female with X monosomy

391. The parents of a 13-year-old Caucasian adolescent are asked to have their child evaluated because of poor grades and aggressive, defiant behaviors at school. A neuropsychology evaluation reveals poor fine motor coordination with dysgraphia (poor handwriting) and borderline IQ of 91. A parental questionnaire suggests characteristics of oppositional-defiant disorder, prompting pediatric genetic evaluation that reveals a 47,XYY karyotype. Which of the following options correctly describe the origin of the 47,XYY karyotype in this child?

a. Meiosis division I of paternal spermatogenesis
b. Meiosis division I of maternal oogenesis
c. Meiosis division II of paternal spermatogenesis
d. Meiosis division II of maternal oogenesis
e. Meiosis division II in either parent

392. A physician evaluates a 16-year-old Caucasian adolescent with a slightly unusual facial appearance and poor school performance. A peripheral blood chromosome study reveals a karyotype of 46,XY/47,XY,+8 mosaicism, with 10% of 100 examined cells showing the extra chromosome 8. Which of the following options is most appropriate for the physician during the counseling session that follows the chromosome result?

a. Recommend karyotyping of the parents.
b. Explain that the recurrence risk for such chromosomal aberrations is about 1%.
c. Urge that the school receive a copy of the karyotype since these boys often have behavior problems.
d. Recommend special education.
e. Inform the parents that their child will be sterile.

393. A 4-year-old Caucasian girl presents with short stature, web neck, and other features suggestive of Turner syndrome, but also has mild mental disability. Her chromosome studies reveal 90,XX/92,XXXX with about 10% abnormal cells in blood and 20% in skin. These results can be described as which of the following?

a. Aneuploidy
b. Haploidy
c. Triploidy mosaicism
d. Tetraploidy without mosaicism
e. Trisomy with mosaicism

394. Which of the following is the proper cytogenetic notation for a female with Down syndrome mosaicism?

a. 46,XX,+21/46,XY
b. 47,XY,+21
c. 47,XXX/46,XX
d. 47,XX,+21/46,XX
e. 47,XX,+21(46,XX)

395. A female with Turner syndrome is denoted by which of the following cytogenetic notations?

a. 47,XX,+21
b. 45,X
c. 47,XXX
d. 46,XX,t(14;21)
e. 45,XX, −21

Questions 396 and 397

Refer to the figure below for the next two questions.

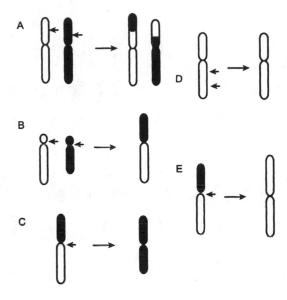

396. Which of the diagrams above depicts a reciprocal translocation?

a. Diagram A
b. Diagram B
c. Diagram C
d. Diagram D
e. Diagram E

397. A 15-year-old Hispanic adolescent with manifestations of Turner syndrome is found to have a karyotype described as 46,XX,i(Xq). This best fits with which of the lettered diagrams above?

a. Diagram A
b. Diagram B
c. Diagram C
d. Diagram D
e. Diagram E

Questions 398 to 400

Refer to the figure below to answer the next three questions.

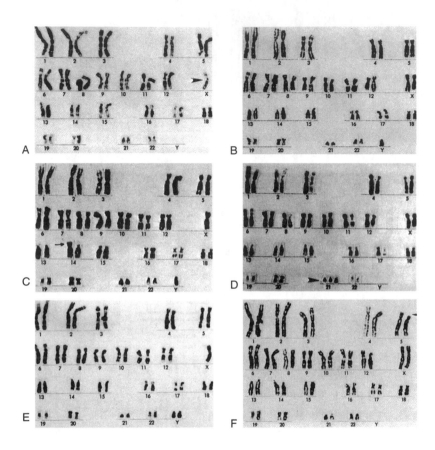

398. A 1-day-old newborn Caucasian girl has swelling of the dorsal areas of her feet in the nursery; later follow-up showed the swelling resolved and she did well during childhood. She also has delayed menstruation, broad neck and chest, mild short stature, and decreased peripheral pulses that suggest the possibility of coarctation of the aorta. Ovaries could not be seen on pelvic ultrasound, and the uterus was thin. Her physician suspects a chromosomal disorder and orders a karyotype. Which of the results pictured is most likely?

a. Result A
b. Result B
c. Result C
d. Result D
e. Result F

399. A 1-day-old Caucasian boy feeds poorly, turning blue and choking after breast-feeding. He is also very floppy (hypotonic), has a loud heart murmur, and has some unusual physical findings. These include a flat occiput (brachycephaly), folds over the inner corners of the eyes (epicanthal folds), single creases on the palms (single palmar creases), and a broad space between the first and second toes. Significant in the family history is that one of the parents' three prior children had Down syndrome. After obtaining a chromosome analysis, which of the results pictured is most likely?

a. Result A
b. Result B
c. Result C
d. Result D
e. Result F

400. A 2-week-old African American girl is hospitalized for inadequate feeding and poor growth. The parents are concerned by the child's weak cry. An experienced grandmother accompanies them, saying she thought the cry sounded like a cat's meow. The grandmother also states that the baby doesn't look much like either parent. The physician orders a karyotype after noting a small head size (microcephaly) and subtle abnormalities of the face. Which of the results pictured is most likely?

a. Result A
b. Result B
c. Result C
d. Result D
e. Result F

401. Children with type IV glycogen storage disease (MIM*232500) accumulate abnormal glycogen, causing them to have progressive liver damage in addition to the low blood glucose (hypoglycemia), increased triglycerides and cholesterol (hyperlipidemia), and high uric acid (hyperuricemic) due to deficient glycogenolysis (see High-Yield Facts Table 6). Type IV glycogen storage is autosomal recessive. Autosomal recessive conditions are correctly characterized by which of the following statements?

a. They are often associated with deficient enzyme activity.
b. Both alleles contain the same mutation.
c. They are more variable than autosomal dominant conditions.
d. Most persons do not carry any abnormal recessive genes.
e. Affected individuals are likely to have affected offspring.

402. Gardner syndrome or adenomatous polyposis of the colon (MIM*175100) is an autosomal dominant condition characterized by retinal changes, extra teeth, skin cysts, and multiple colonic polyps with high rates of malignant transformation. A family is encountered in which a great-grandfather, grandmother, and father are affected with Gardner syndrome and develop intestinal cancer in their thirties. The father brags that none of his four children have inherited Gardner syndrome because they lack skin cysts and have not had cancer. The chance that at least one child has inherited the Gardner syndrome allele and the reason the children have not manifested cancer are which of the following?

a. $1/4$, ascertainment bias
b. $1/2$, variable cancer predisposition
c. $3/4$, early-onset disease manifestation
d. $1/16$, incomplete medical evaluation
e. $15/16$, later-onset disease manifestation

403. Ectrodactyly causes missing middle fingers (lobster claw malformation) and exhibits genetic heterogeneity with autosomal dominant and recessive forms. One type of ectrodactyly (split hand-foot malformation) is an autosomal dominant trait (MIM*183600). A grandfather and grandson have this form of ectrodactyly, but the intervening father has normal hands by x-ray. Which of the following terms applies to this family?

a. Incomplete penetrance
b. New mutation
c. Variable expressivity
d. Germinal mosaicism
e. Anticipation

404. A 4-year-old Caucasian boy presents to the physician's office with coarse facies, short stature, stiffening of the joints, and mental retardation. The physician performs a urine screen that shows elevated mucopolysaccharides and makes a tentative diagnosis of mucopolysaccharidosis. The boy's parents, a 10-year-old sister, and an 8-year-old brother all appear unaffected but the mother had a brother who died at 15 years of age with similar findings that seemed to worsen with age. Mother also has a nephew (her sister's son) who exhibits similar clinical findings. During the evaluation of her son, mother reveals she is 5 months pregnant. Based on the probable mode of inheritance, which of the following is the risk that her fetus is affected?

a. 100%
b. 67%
c. 50%
d. 25%
e. Virtually 0

405. A couple comes to the physician's office after having had two sons affected with a similar disease. The first-born son is tall and thin and has dislocated lenses and an IQ of 70. He has also experienced several episodes of deep vein thromboses. The chart mentions deficiency of the enzyme cystathionine-β-synthase, but a diagnosis is not given. The second son was treated from an early age with pyridoxine (vitamin B_6) and is less severely affected. No other family members are affected. While taking a family history, the physician discovers that the parents are first cousins. The 38-year-old mother is pregnant, and amniocentesis has demonstrated that the fetus has a 46,XY karyotype. What is the risk that the fetus will be affected with the same disease?

a. 100%
b. 67%
c. 50%
d. 25%
e. Virtually 0

406. A 35-year-old African American male affected with Crouzon syndrome (MIM*123500) has craniosynostosis (ie, premature closure of the skull sutures) along with unusual facies that includes proptosis secondary to shallow orbits, hypoplasia of the maxilla, and a prominent nose. His son and brother are also affected, although two daughters and his wife are not. The patient and his wife are considering having another child. Their physician counsels them that their child might inherit Crouzon syndrome from his father. Which of the following risk percentages are most likely?

a. 100%
b. 67%
c. 50%
d. 25%
e. Virtually 0

407. A 51-year-old Hispanic male presents to the physician's office to ask questions about color blindness. The patient is color-blind, as is one of his brothers. His maternal grandfather was color-blind, but his mother, father, daughter, and another brother are not. His daughter is now pregnant. What is the risk that her child will be color-blind?

a. 100%
b. 50%
c. 25%
d. 12.5%
e. Virtually 0

408. Little People of America (LPA) is a support group for individuals with short stature that conducts many workshops and social activities. Two individuals with achondroplasia (MIM*100800), a common form of dwarfism, meet at an LPA convention and decide to marry and have children. What is their risk of having a child with dwarfism?

a. 100%
b. 75%
c. 50%
d. 25%
e. Virtually 0

409. A 23-year-old Caucasian female with cystic fibrosis (MIM*219700) marries her first cousin. What is the risk that their first child will have cystic fibrosis?

a. $\frac{1}{2}$
b. $\frac{1}{4}$
c. $\frac{1}{8}$
d. $\frac{1}{16}$
e. $\frac{1}{32}$

410. A 22-year-old Caucasian female with no family history of color blindness (MIM*304000) marries a color-blind male. What is the risk for this couple of having a son or daughter who is color-blind?

a. 100%
b. 75%
c. 50%
d. 25%
e. Virtually 0

411. A family presents with an unusual type of foot-drop and lower leg atrophy that is unfamiliar to their physician. The pedigree below is obtained. Based on the pedigree, what is the risk of individual III-3 having an affected child?

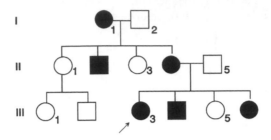

a. 100%
b. 75%
c. 50%
d. 25%
e. Virtually 0

412. A 3-year-old Caucasian boy is evaluated by an ophthalmologist and is found to have retinitis pigmentosa, a disorder characterized by pigmentary granules in the retina and progressive vision loss. The pedigree below is obtained and the family comes in for counseling. What is the risk for individual II-2 of having an affected child if he impregnates an unrelated female?

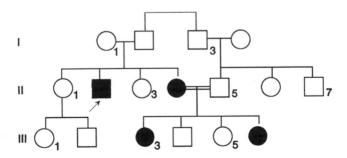

a. 100%
b. 75%
c. 50%
d. 25%
e. Virtually 0

413. A different family with retinitis pigmentosa is encountered, and the pedigree shown below is documented. What is the risk that a son born to individual III-3 would be affected?

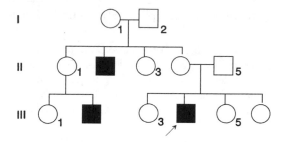

a. 100%
b. 75%
c. 50%
d. 25%
e. Virtually 0

414. Osteogenesis imperfecta (MIM*166200) is an autosomal dominant disorder that causes thin, bluish sclerae (whites of the eyes), deafness, and multiple bone fractures. Parents have two children with osteogenesis imperfecta, but themselves exhibit no signs of the disease. Which of the following genetic mechanisms is the most likely explanation for two off-spring of normal parents to have an autosomal dominant disease?

a. Variable expressivity
b. Uniparental disomy
c. New mutations
d. Germinal mosaicism in one parent
e. Incomplete penetrance

415. Females occasionally have symptoms of X linked recessive diseases such as Duchenne muscular dystrophy, hemophilia, or color blindness. Which of the following is the most common explanation?

a. Nonrandom lyonization
b. X-chromosome trisomy (47,XXX)
c. X autosome–balanced translocation that disrupts the particular X-chromosome locus
d. Turner syndrome (45,X)
e. 46,XY karyotype in a female

416. Incontinentia pigmenti (MIM*308300) is an X-linked disorder that is lethal in utero for affected males. The findings vary in females and include pigmented skin lesions, dental abnormalities, patchy areas of alopecia, and mental retardation. Approximately 45% of cases are the result of new mutations. Which of the following descriptions of incontinentia pigmenti is most accurate?

a. X-linked recessive inheritance with spontaneous abortions and few isolated cases
b. X-linked dominant inheritance; 3:1 ratio of females to males in affected sibships
c. X-linked recessive inheritance with spontaneous abortions and many isolated cases
d. X-linked dominant inheritance, 1.5:1 ratio of females to males in affected sibships
e. X-linked dominant inheritance with spontaneous abortions and many isolated cases

417. A couple present for genetic counseling because three of their first four children have had pyloric stenosis, a narrowing of the valve between stomach and duodenum that presents with severe vomiting and loss of gastric hydrochloric acid (hypochloremic alkalosis). When parents with three affected children have a higher recurrence risk than parents with one affected child, the disease in question is likely to exhibit which of the following modes of inheritance?

a. Autosomal dominant inheritance
b. Autosomal recessive inheritance
c. X-linked recessive inheritance
d. X-linked dominant inheritance
e. Multifactorial determination

418. Two parents are both affected with albinism (MIM*203100 and MIM*203200), but have a normal child. Which of the following terms best describes to this situation?

a. Allelic heterogeneity
b. Locus heterogeneity
c. Variable expressivity
d. Incomplete penetrance
e. New mutation

419. Waardenburg syndrome (MIM*193500) is an autosomal dominant condition that accounts for 1.4% of cases of congenital deafness. In addition to deafness, patients with this condition have an atypical facial appearance, including lateral displacement of the inner canthi (eye corners), hypertelorism (widely spaced eyes), poliosis (white forelock), and white patches of skin on the ventral midline (partial albinism or piebaldism). A mother has Waardenburg syndrome, her husband is unaffected, and they plan to have a family with three children. What is the probability that only one of the three children will be affected?

a. $\frac{1}{8}$
b. $\frac{1}{4}$
c. $\frac{3}{8}$
d. $\frac{1}{3}$
e. $\frac{1}{2}$

420. The major blood group locus in humans produces types A (genotypes AA or AO), B (genotypes BB or BO), AB (genotype AB), or O (genotype OO). For parents who are type AB and type O, what are the possible blood types of their offspring?

a. Type AB child
b. Type B child
c. Type O child
d. Type A or B child
e. Type B or AB child

421. Phenylketonuria (PKU—MIM*261600) is an autosomal recessive disease that causes severe mental retardation if it is undetected. Two normal parents are told by their state neonatal screening program that their third child has PKU. Assuming that the initial screening is accurate, what is the risk that their first child is a carrier for PKU?

a. 100%
b. 67%
c. 50%
d. 25%
e. Virtually 0

422. A Caucasian couple presents for genetic counseling after their first child, a son, is born with short limb dwarfism and diagnosed with autosomal dominant achondroplasia (MIM*100800). The physician obtains the following family history: the husband is the firstborn of four male children, and his next oldest brother has cystic fibrosis (MIM*219700). The wife is an only child, but she had DNA screening because a second cousin had cystic fibrosis and she knows that she is a carrier. There are no other medical problems in the couple or their families. The physician should now draw the pedigree with the female member of any couple on the left. The generations are numbered with Roman numerals and individuals with Arabic numerals; individuals affected with achondroplasia or cystic fibrosis are indicated. Which of the following risk figures applies to the next child born to this husband and wife?

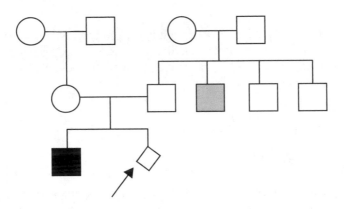

a. Achondroplasia $\frac{1}{2}$, cystic fibrosis $\frac{1}{4}$
b. Achondroplasia $\frac{1}{2}$, cystic fibrosis $\frac{1}{8}$
c. Achondroplasia virtually 0, cystic fibrosis $\frac{1}{4}$
d. Achondroplasia virtually 0, cystic fibrosis $\frac{1}{6}$
e. Achondroplasia virtually 0, cystic fibrosis $\frac{1}{8}$

423. A 6-month-old Caucasian boy of Ashkenazi Jewish origin plateaus in his development, exhibits a "startle" response to hand-claps, and is noted to have a central red area in his retina surrounded by white (cherry red spot). His physician suspects autosomal recessive Tay-Sachs disease (MIM*272800) and initiates evaluation that demonstrates deficiency of the lysosomal enzyme hexaminidase A. This deficiency leads to accumulation of complex glycolipids in brain and produces a ring of white, lipid-infiltrated cells around normal central retina (the macula). What is the risk that the grandmother of an affected child is a carrier (heterozygote) for Tay-Sachs disease?

a. 100%
b. 67%
c. 50%
d. 25%
e. Virtually 0

424. Isolated cleft lip and palate (meaning no other congenital anomalies are present) is a multifactorial trait. The recurrence risk of isolated cleft lip and palate is which of the following?

a. The same in all families
b. Not dependent on the number of affected family members
c. The same in all ethnic groups
d. The same in males and females
e. Affected by the severity of the cleft

425. Individuals with achondroplastic dwarfism have about 80% fewer viable offspring than do normal persons, but the incidence of achondroplasia seems to have remained constant for generations. Achondroplasia is an autosomal dominant disorder caused by mutations in the fibroblast growth factor receptor-2. What do these observations imply about the population genetics of achondroplasia?

a. Decreased fitness, negative selection, and relatively high mutation rates
b. Increased fitness, negative selection, and relatively high mutation rates
c. Decreased fitness, positive selection, and relatively low mutation rates
d. Increased fitness, positive selection, and relatively low mutation rates
e. Decreased fitness, positive selection, and relatively high mutation rates

426. A family is seen for routine prenatal counseling because the mother of two normal children is of age 35, the arbitrary "advanced maternal age" when the approximate 1 in 100 risk for fetal chromosome disorders is deemed significant. Family history reveals that the mother's parents and her husband all have had onset of high blood pressure (hypertension) at early ages, and two of mother's grandparents died of strokes that may be hypertension related. The mother also had some hypertension in the third trimester of her last pregnancy. Recognizing that hypertension is a multi-factorial trait, which of the following is the most appropriate explanation and counseling for the couple?

a. Multifactorial determination indicates an interaction between the environment and a single gene, implying a 50% risk for eventual hypertension in mother and offspring.

b. Multifactorial determination indicates an interaction between the environment and multiple genes, implying a 5% to 10% risk for eventual hypertension in mother and offspring.

c. Multifactorial determination results from multiple postnatal environmental factors, implying a 75% to 100% risk for eventual hypertension in mother and a 5% to 10% risk to offspring.

d. Multifactorial determination results from multiple pre- and postnatal environmental factors, implying a 75% to 100% risk for eventual hypertension in mother and a 5% to 10% risk to offspring.

e. Multifactorial determination implies action of multiple genes independent of environmental factors, implying low risks for hypertension in mother's next pregnancy but a 5% to 10% risk for eventual hypertension in offspring.

427. Availability of DNA testing for many single disease traits has allowed routine prenatal screening of couples for disorders prevalent in their ethnic group. Which of the following genetic disorders has a similar incidence in different ethnic groups and would not be subject to different criteria for screening?

a. Cystic fibrosis
b. Thalassemias
c. Tay-Sachs disease
d. Down syndrome
e. Sickle cell anemia

428. The incidence of a genetic form of diabetes insipidus (MIM*304800) in North Americans was hypothesized to be related to immigration of affected individuals on the ship Hopewell that arrived in Halifax, Nova Scotia several hundred years ago. If the disease allele were known as A, and residents near Halifax had 10 times the frequency of this allele as did those on mainland Canada, which of the following terms best describes this phenomenon?

a. Selection for allele A
b. Linkage disequilibrium with allele A
c. Linkage to allele A
d. Founder effect for allele A
e. Assortative mating for allele A

429. Increased resistance to malaria is seen in persons with hemoglobin AS, where A is the normal allele and S is the allele for sickle hemoglobin. Which of the following terms applies to this situation?

a. Founder effect
b. Heterozygote advantage
c. Genetic lethal
d. Fitness
e. Natural selection

430. Assume that frequencies for the different blood group alleles are as follows: A = 0.3; B = 0.1; O = 0.6. What is the expected percentage of individuals with blood type B?

a. 7%
b. 13%
c. 27%
d. 36%
e. 45%

431. A 1-month-old Caucasian male infant is being considered for adoption, and his older half sister is known to have developed hydrocephalus, an accumulation of cerebrospinal fluid in the brain ventricles. Hydrocephalus is a multifactorial disorder, and the prospective parents wish to know the chance the boy will develop hydrocephalus. In order to estimate this risk, the physician must determine what proportion of genes the brother and half sister have in common. What is this proportion?

a. 1
b. $\frac{1}{2}$
c. $\frac{1}{4}$
d. $\frac{1}{8}$
e. $\frac{1}{16}$

432. A 23-year-old Caucasian male whose brother has cystic fibrosis (MIM*219700) wants to know his risk of having an affected child. The prevalence of cystic fibrosis is 1 in 1600 individuals. Which of the following is the risk in this case?

a. $\frac{1}{8}$
b. $\frac{1}{16}$
c. $\frac{1}{60}$
d. $\frac{1}{120}$
e. $\frac{1}{256}$

433. An African American couple with a normal family history wants to know their chance of having a child with sickle cell anemia (MIM*603903). The incidence of sickle cell trait is 1 in 8 for African Americans. Which of the following is the risk in this case?

a. $\frac{1}{8}$
b. $\frac{1}{16}$
c. $\frac{1}{60}$
d. $\frac{1}{120}$
e. $\frac{1}{256}$

434. A 22-year-old Caucasian female who married her first cousin wants to know the risk of having a child with cystic fibrosis (MIM*219700) because her grandmother, who is also her husband's grandmother, died of cystic fibrosis. Which of the following is her risk?

a. $\frac{1}{8}$

b. $\frac{1}{16}$

c. $\frac{1}{60}$

d. $\frac{1}{120}$

e. $\frac{1}{256}$

Inheritance Mechanisms/Risk Calculations

Answers

381. The answer is e. (*Lewis, pp 132-151. Scriver, pp 193-202.*) Amyotrophic lateral sclerosis (ALS) is not always sporadic (isolated cases—incorrect answer c), not always genetic (incorrect answers a, b), and not present at birth (congenital—incorrect answer d). When counseling families, the physician should realize that lay people often assume that a normal family history excludes the possibility of genetic disease despite the frequent occurrence of autosomal or X-linked recessive mutations.

Many common disorders including both forms of diabetes mellitus, schizophrenia, and most isolated birth defects like cleft palate exhibit multifactorial determination: multiple genes (polygenic inheritance) plus environmental factors interact to determine susceptibility to disease. Often one or more of these determining genes can sustain mutations that have a major effect on susceptibility as when LDL receptor mutations overwhelm dietary and coagulation factors to cause heart attacks at a young age (familial hypercholesterolemia-MIM*14010). Disorders that exhibit multifactorial determination have a recurrence risk that depends on the number of affected relatives—a first child with birth defect like cleft palate confers a 3% to 5% recurrence risk, a risk that is doubled if a parent and first child are affected. Current research is defining molecular markers that associate with susceptibility to common multifactorial diseases, allowing risk modification in the way that HLA type B27 indicates higher risk for ankylosing spondylitis (MIM*106300—many multifactorial disorders are listed in Online Mendelian Inheritance in Man). The superoxide dismutase gene may be mutated in rare cases of familial (autosomal dominant), early-onset ALS (MIM*105400).

382. The answer is b. (*Lewis, pp 132-151. Scriver, pp 1471-1488.*) Diabetes mellitus clusters in families (incorrect answer d), is not be purely

Mendelian (less than 100% concordance in genetically identical twins (incorrect answer c), affects both sexes (incorrect answer e), and is usually not present at birth (incorrect answer a). Diabetes mellitus is associated with various risk factors, from autoimmune mechanisms with specific HLA haplotype associations to obesity. The multifactorial causation and hereditary tendency reflects multiple genes (polygenic inheritance) and environmental factors, termed multifactorial determination. Many common diseases are caused by a combination of environmental and genetic factors, and are described as multifactorial diseases. Examples include diabetes mellitus, schizophrenia, alcoholism, and many common birth defects such as cleft palate or congenital dislocation of the hip. The proportion of genetically identical monozygous twins who share (are concordant for) a trait such as diabetes mellitus provides a measure of the genetic contribution to etiology (heritability)—often 40% to 60% twin concordance in multifactorial disorders. Mendelian disorders are more completely determined by the genotype of an individual and often exhibit 100% concordance in identical twins.

383. The answer is c. *(Lewis, pp 132-151. Scriver, pp 193-202.)* Disorders exhibiting multifactorial determination (polygenic inheritance plus environmental factors) frequently show sex predilection, an ill-defined pattern in pedigrees, higher but not 100% identical twin concordance, and empiric recurrence risks that increase as more affected family members are ascertained. Mitochondrial disorders can exhibit autosomal recessive or X-linked inheritance if they affect nuclear gene products imported into mitochondria; they can exhibit maternal inheritance if they derive from alterations of the mitochondrial DNA (transmitted only from the mother). Over 60% of first trimester abortuses (miscarriages) are due to chromosome aberrations, although some will derive from multifactorial maternal conditions (lupus, toxemia) and some from single gene causes (mostly undefined).

Recurrence risks for multifactorial diseases are empiric, that is, determined by population studies. An approximate risk of 3% applies to offspring of individuals affected with the majority of multifactorial diseases—a figure that is similar to the 2% to 3% risk for birth defects in the average pregnancy. This approximate risk can be tailored to the disease (ie, 5% for a parent with juvenile diabetes) using appropriate tables, and increased if there are other relatives affected besides the parent (ie, 10% risk to offspring of two parents with juvenile diabetes). It can also be tailored to the degree of relationship, falling off rapidly (as would befit the requirement for cotransmission of multiple causative alleles) with the affected being a twin (40%-60% chance of concordance), parent or sibling (first-degree relative, 3%-5% risk), grandparent/aunt/uncle (second-degree relative, 0.5%-0.7% risk), or cousin (third-degree relative, close to background 0.1% incidence of many multifactorial diseases).

384. The answer is b. *(Lewis, pp 70-82, 70-94. Scriver, pp 3-45.)* The phenotype refers to individual traits or characteristics and the genotypes to gene combinations that determine them. Genetic loci are positions on chromosomes that contain genes; since all chromosomes are paired in humans except the XY of males, most genes are paired and have structures (now defined as DNA sequences) called alleles. During meiotic segregation, each parental gamete receives one paired gene (one allele) from every genetic locus (except males who receive paired alleles from the small homologous XY short arm regions and single alleles from the nonpaired X or Y. The probability of a parental allele being transmitted to offspring is thus one-half, and the probability of a given genotype appearing in offspring is the joint probability of maternal and paternal allele transmission.

For a paternal Dd versus maternal dd mating, the probability of maternal alleles D or d being transmitted is one-half and the probability of transmission of the paternal allele d is 1. The joint probability for a Dd genotype in offspring is thus one-half for D from mother multiplied by 1 for d from father equals one-half. A similar calculation would apply to the joint probability for the dd genotype, giving probabilities of one-half for Dd and one-half for dd, expected ratios of 1 Dd:1 dd in offspring, or a recurrence risk for father's deaf phenotype of one-half or 50%. More than 30 genes causing deafness have been characterized in humans, with over 75% exhibiting autosomal recessive inheritance rather than the dominant inheritance implied here.

385. The answer is f. *(Lewis, pp 70-82. Scriver, pp 3-45.)* It is important that the pedigree be an accurate reflection of the family history and that information not be recorded unless specifically mentioned. Pedigree B in the figure below Question 385 omits the double line needed to indicate consanguinity, and pedigree C assumes that the father's affected cousin is the offspring of his uncle rather than being unspecified. Pedigree F correctly illustrates the birth order (third) of the affected female (indicated by arrow) and the consanguinity (double line) represented by the first-cousin marriage. Cystic fibrosis is an autosomal recessive disease that causes progressive lung disease and intestinal malabsorption due to deficiencies of multiple pancreatic enzymes (MIM*219700). Autosomal recessive diseases are much more common with consanguinity because the related couple has a greater chance to inherit the same rare allele.

386. The answer is a. (*Scriver, pp 5677-5702. Lewis, pp 63-65, 70-86.*) The individual probability for each child developing Huntington disease is $\frac{1}{2}$ and the probability that all three children will develop the disease is $\frac{1}{2} \times \frac{1}{2} \times \frac{1}{2} = \frac{1}{8}$ (incorrect answers b-e). Huntington disease exhibits autosomal dominant inheritance, meaning that heterozygotes with one normal and one Huntington allele will develop the disease. The husband most likely inherited a normal allele from his mother and a Huntington allele from his father, making him a heterozygote (homozygous affected individuals with Huntington disease are extremely rare because both parents must be affected). The wife most likely has two normal alleles since she has no family history and no symptoms of disease (she could theoretically have a Huntington allele that has not yet caused disease but this is unlikely given the incidence of 1 in 15-25,000). Note that the presence of an abnormal allele in the wife could not be discounted if this were an autosomal or X-linked recessive disorder.

387. The answer is d. (*Lewis, pp 248-261. Scriver, pp 3-45.*) The case described represents one of the more common chromosomal causes of reproductive failure, Turner syndrome mosaicism. Turner syndrome involves short stature, anomalies including webbed neck (pterygium colli), heart defects such as coarctation of the aorta, short fourth and fifth knuckles (metacarpals), and streak ovary with infertility. Turner syndrome is produced by monosomy for all or a portion of the X chromosome, causing several genes to be present in a single rather than double dose (haploinsufficiency). Mosaicism (ie, two or more cell lines with different karyotypes in the same individual) is common, including 46,XX/45,X or 46,XX/45,X/46,XY that poses risk for gonadal cancer due to the presence of a Y chromosome. Chimerism is extremely rare and occurs when two cell lines in an individual arise from different zygotes; some cases may reflect fraternal twins who do not separate. Trisomy refers to three copies of a chromosome rather than the normal two (eg, 47,XXX), and monosomy to a missing chromosome as in the most common cause of Turner syndrome (45,X). Polyploidy refers to entire extra sets of haploid (23) chromosomes as in 69,XXX triploidy or 92,XXYY polyploidy; polyploidy occurs naturally in some tissues like liver. Euploidy refers to a normal chromosome number and composition.

388. The answer is e. (*Lewis, pp 243-248. Scriver, pp 3-45.*) Chromosomal abnormalities may involve changes in number (ie, polyploidy and aneuploidy) or changes in structure (ie, rearrangements such as translocations, rings, and inversions). Extra material (ie, extra chromatin) seen on chromosome 5 implies recombination of chromosome 5 DNA with that of another chromosome to produce a rearranged chromosome. Since this rearranged chromosome 5 takes the place of a normal chromosome 5, there is no change in number of the autosomes (nonsex chromosomes) or sex chromosomes (X and Y chromosomes). The question implies that all cells examined from the patient (usually 11-25 cells) have the same chromosomal constitution, ruling out mosaicism. The patient's clinical findings are similar to those occurring in trisomy 13 or Patau syndrome, suggesting that the extra material on chromosome 5 is derived from the long arm of chromosome 13 (the acrocentric chromosomes 13-15 and 21-22 have small short arms that contain repetitive DNA). With this interpretation, or by comparing banding patterns of the extra and 13 material, the aberration would be more specifically described as duplication 13q [dup(13q)] or as partial trisomy for 13q.

389. The answer is d. (*Lewis, pp 248-261. Scriver, pp 3-45.*) The hallmarks of children with chromosomal anomalies are mental disability (developmental delay in children) with multiple congenital anomalies. The described individual has learning problems that are not yet described as mental disability, and many such children are mistakenly assumed to have poor motivation rather than cognitive problems that could be defined by IQ testing. Parents also may resist the classification as mental disability, particularly when the harsher term retardation is used. The hand changes can be classified as minor anomalies rather than major birth defects that cause cosmetic or surgical problems, but minor anomalies are significant in that several indicate abnormal development and an increased possibility of a birth defect pattern or syndrome. The physician was astute to suspect a chromosomal anomaly with subtle cognitive and physical changes, and this boy would be typical of 47,XYY individuals with tall stature, variable anomalies, and aggressive or antisocial behaviors. Other indications for peripheral blood chromosome studies include couples with three or more pregnancy losses, relatives of individuals with chromosome rearrangements, and children with ambiguous external genitalia. Fetal chromosomes will be considered with triple/quad screen and/or ultrasound abnormalities, while bone marrow/solid tumor chromosomes are now examined in most cancers as a guide to tumor type, chemotherapy, and prognosis.

390. The answer is c. (*Lewis, pp 248-261. Scriver, pp 3-45.*) The 47,XXX karyotype is an example of sex chromosome aneuploidy, which as a trisomy (47,XXX; 47, XXY; 47XYY) produces fewer anomalies and milder mental disability than autosomal trisomies like Down syndrome, for example, 47,XX,+21 or trisomy 21; Patau syndrome, for example, 47,XX,+13 or trisomy 13; and Edward syndrome, for example, 47,XY,+18 or trisomy 18. Triploidy with a 69,XXX karyotype would be an example of a female with polyploidy, presenting as an spontaneous abortus or severely malformed, short-lived infant. Turner syndrome, most commonly 45,X, would be an example of a female with X monosomy and 45,X/46,XX an example of mosaicism—producing in this case a milder form of Turner syndrome that may have no abnormal signs or symptoms except for infertility.

391. The answer is c. (*Lewis, pp 152-167, 248-261. Scriver, pp 3-45.*) The sex chromosomes with differently named homologues allow easy visualization of chromosome sorting during meiosis. Female meiosis only involves X chromosomes; thus, Y chromosomal abnormalities must arise during paternal meiosis or occur spontaneously in offspring. During meiosis I, the newly replicated homologous chromosomes line up at the metaphase plate and then migrate to opposite poles of the cell. Nondisjunction at paternal meiosis I produces XY secondary spermatocytes and a 24,XY gamete. Fertilization with a 23,X ovum yields a 47,XXY individual (Klinefelter syndrome). In meiosis II, the replicated chromosomes line up at the equator of the cell and the sister chromatids separate. Thus, only nondisjunction at paternal meiosis II can produce a 24,YY gamete that yields a 47,XYY individual after fertilization.

392. The answer is b. (*Lewis, pp 248-261. Scriver, pp 3-45.*) The recurrence risk for simple extra or missing chromosomes (whole chromosome aneuploidies) is about 1% in addition to the maternal age-related risk. It is not known why the risk for aneuploidy increases slightly after an affected child is born, but parental karyotypes are almost always normal. Parental chromosome studies are thus not indicated in this case, especially with the low degree of mosaicism that might have arisen after conception. The empiric risk of 1% is comparable to that of females over 35 (ironically called advanced maternal age!) for fetal chromosome aberrations, so pre-natal diagnosis should be discussed as an option for the parents. The school should not be given a copy of the karyotype unless the parents request it and sign a release of medical records. Some parents prefer to keep diagnoses of genetic disease or attention deficit-hyperactivity disorders confidential so their child will not be labeled as different by school person-nel. Trisomy 8 mosaicism can have a very mild phenotype, so special edu-cation should not be recommended unless cognitive testing demonstrates a lower IQ (below 75 is often required for special education).

393. The answer is a. (*Lewis, pp 248-261. Scriver, pp 3-45.*) Aneuploidy involves extra or missing chromosomes that do not arise as increments of the haploid chromosome number n and thus would fit the 90,XX cell line since tetraploidy without aneuploidy would imply a 92,XXXX or 92,XXYY karyotype. Polyploidy involves multiples of n, such as triploidy (3n = 69,XXX) or tetraploidy (4n = 92,XXXX). Diploidy (46,XX) and haploidy (23,X) are normal karyotypes in gametes and somatic cells, respectively. A 92,XXXX/90,XX karyotype represents mosaicism with a tetraploid cell line and an aneuploid line with tetraploidy minus two X chromosomes, which was observed in a patient with features of Turner syndrome. The mental disability, unusual in Turner syndrome, may reflect the usual trend toward greater severity when sex chromosome aneuploidy involves more extra chromosomes (eg, 47,XXY Klinefelter to 48,XXXY and 49,XXXXY Kline-felter variants).

394. The answer is d. (*Lewis, pp 248-261. Scriver, pp 3-45.*) Mosaicism occurs when a chromosomal anomaly affects one of several precursor cells of an embryo or tissue. The two or more karyotypes that characterize the mosaic cells are separated by a slash in cytogenetic notation. The notation 47,XX,+21 denotes a cell line typical of a female with trisomy 21 (Down syndrome), whereas 46,XX is the karyotype expected for a normal female. XY sex chromosomes refer to a male (incorrect answers a, b) and incorrect answer e employs parenthesis for the second cell line. Incorrect answer b does not have two cell lines characteristic of mosaicism, and incorrect answer c refers to 47,XXX (triple X) mosaicism.

395. The answer is b. (*Lewis, pp 248-261. Scriver, pp 3-45.*) Cytogenetic notation provides the chromosome number (eg, 46), the sex chromosomes, and a shorthand description of anomalies. Examples include the following:

45,X indicates a female with monosomy X or Turner syndrome; 47,XX+21 indicates a female with trisomy 21 or Down syndrome; 46,XX,t(14;21) indicates a female with translocation Down syndrome; 45,XX–21 indicates a female with monosomy 21. Note the absence of spaces between symbols, and the use of 47,XXX for sex chromosomal aneuploidy ("triple X" syndrome) rather than the more awkward 47,XX+X. (Note also that 45,X is sufficient for X-chromosome monosomy, since absence of an X is indicated by the convention of listing sex chromosomes). Translocations that join two chromosomes with minuscule short arms (acrocentric chromosomes—13, 14, 15, 21, and 22) are called Robertsonian translocations. The joined acrocentric chromosomes in a Robertsonian translocation have a single centromere between them and are counted as one chromosome. A normal person who "carries" a Robertsonian translocation therefore has a chromosome number of 45, as in 45,XX,t(14;21).

396. The answer is a. (*Lewis, pp 248-261. Scriver, pp 3-45.*) Reciprocal translocations (diagram A in figure below Questions 396 and 397) involve the exchange of segments between two chromosomes. Robertsonian translocations (diagram B) involve the joining of two acrocentric chromosomes by breakage and reunion of their short arms. Translocations that produce no duplication or deficiency are called balanced. Individuals who have balanced translocations are called "carriers"; they have normal phenotypes unless the translocation alters the expression of an important gene at the breakpoint region. Isochromosomes involve duplication of short (diagram C) or long (diagram E) arms, which produces perfectly metacentric chromosomes deficient in long- or short-arm material, respectively. Paracentric inversions (diagram D) alter the banding pattern but not the shape of the chromosome because they do not involve the centromere.

397. The answer is e. (*Lewis, pp 248-261. Scriver, pp 3-45.*) The abbreviations i and t describe isochromosomes and translocation chromosomes, respectively. Isochromosomes create chromosomes with mirror-image duplications of the long arm (diagram E below Questions 396 and 397) or short arm (diagram C). The child with 46,XX,i(Xq) would have an isochromosome composed of two X long arms fused together, thus having Xp material only on her normal chromosome and being haploinsufficient for those genetic loci. Individuals with isochromosome Xq and especially those with isochromosome Xp will have milder manifestations of Turner syndrome than those with full monosomy X. Reciprocal translocations (diagram A) involve exchange of segments between two chromosomes. A semicolon (;) indicates this exchange and is placed between the breakpoints, as in 46,XX,t (2;6)(q23;p14). Robertsonian translocations join together two acrocentric chromosomes to form a metacentric chromosome (diagram B). Carriers of balanced reciprocal translocations have a normal chromosome number, whereas carriers of balanced Robertsonian translocations have only 45 chromosomes.

398. The answer is a. (*Lewis, pp 248-261. Scriver, pp 3-45.*) In most cases of Turner syndrome there is a lack of one X chromosome, as in panel A of the figure below Questions 398 to 400, which shows one X (arrow) and no Y chromosome. A chromosome study or karyotype delineates the number and kinds of chromosomes in one cell karyon (nucleus). Blood is conveniently sampled, so most chromosomal studies or karyotypes are performed on peripheral leukocytes in blood. The buffy coat of leukocytes is removed after centrifugation, stimulated to grow in tissue culture media with lectins, arrested in metaphase with colchicine, swollen in hypotonic solution, dropped onto glass slides to rupture nuclei and spread metphase chromosomes, and stained with various dyes (usually Giemsa) to bring out bands (G-bands). Well-spread chromosomes are selected for karyotyping by eye (10-25, depending on the laboratory), representative photographs taken, and chromosome images arranged by computer in order of size from the #1 pair to the #22 pair; this ordered array is also called a karyotype. Except in cases of mosaicism (different karyotypes in different tissues), the peripheral blood karyotype is indicative of the germ-line karyotype that is characteristic for an individual.

399. The answer is c. (*Lewis, pp 248-261. Scriver, pp 3-45.*) Panel C in the figure below Questions 398 to 400 demonstrates normal X and Y sex chromosomes, but one pair of autosomes is not homologous (arrow). Given the family history of Down syndrome, the appearance of extra material on the short arm of chromosome 14 (arrow) can be interpreted as material from chromosome 21. Together with the two normal chromosomes 21, this extra 21 material would give three doses of chromosome 21 and result in Down syndrome. The abnormal chromosome 14 can thus be interpreted as a Robertsonian 14;21 translocation that was inherited by this child and by the previous child with Down syndrome (ie, karyotypes of 46,XY,t[14;21] causing Down syndrome). Karyotyping the parents would then be important to determine which was the carrier of the 14;21 translocation—

45,XX,t(14;21) or 45,XY,t(14;21). Genetic counseling using the appropriate recurrence risk (5%-10% for male carriers, 10%-20% for female carriers) could include the option of prenatal diagnosis (fetal karyotyping) for future pregnancies.

400. The answer is e. *(Lewis, pp 248-261. Scriver, pp 3-45.)* Cri-du-chat syndrome is caused by deletion of the terminal short arm of chromosome 5(46,XX,del[5p]), also abbreviated as 5p⁻ as depicted in panel F of the figure below Questions 398 to 400. Children with chromosome abnormalities often exhibit poor growth (failure to thrive) and developmental delay with an abnormal facial appearance. This baby is too young for developmental assessment, but the cat-like cry should provoke suspicion of cri-du-chat syndrome. When a partial deletion or duplication like this one is found, the parents must be karyotyped to determine if one carries a balanced reciprocal translocation. Most disorders involving excess or deficient chromosome material produce a characteristic and recognizable phenotype as in Down, cri-du-chat, or Turner syndromes. The mechanism(s) by which imbalanced chromosome material produces a distinctive phenotype are not well defined.

401. The answer is a. *(Lewis, pp 70-82. Scriver, pp 1521-1552. Murray, pp 157-164.)* Autosomal recessive conditions tend to have a horizontal pattern in the pedigree. Males and females are affected with equal frequency and severity. Autosomal and X-linked recessive inheritance is seen in almost all metabolic diseases as illustrated by type IV glycogen storage disease (MIM*232500). Traits like deafness that can follow any of the three major Mendelian inheritance mechanisms (genetic heterogeneity) tend to be more severe in recessive rather than dominant forms, and recessive conditions are less variable than dominant phenotypes. Both alleles are defective but do not necessarily contain the exact same mutation. All individuals carry 6 to 12 mutant recessive alleles. Fortunately, most matings involve persons who have mutations at different loci. Since related persons are more likely to inherit the same mutant gene, consanguinity increases the possibility of homozygous affected offspring.

402. The answer is e. *(Lewis, pp 82-86, 355-377. Scriver, pp 1063-1076, Murray, pp 621-624.)* The father is affected with Gardner syndrome (MIM*175100), an autosomal dominant disease. Therefore, each of his four children has a half chance of receiving the allele that causes Gardner syndrome and a half chance of receiving the normal allele. The probability that none of his four children received the allele for Gardner syndrome is thus the joint probability of four independent events, computed by the product $\frac{1}{2} \times \frac{1}{2} \times \frac{1}{2} \times \frac{1}{2} = \frac{1}{16}$. The probability that at least one child has received the abnormal Gardner syndrome allele is thus $1 - \frac{1}{16} = \frac{15}{16}$. Gardner syndrome is one of many genetic disorders that may not be obvious in early childhood. Intestinal cancer in particular has a later onset, with 50% of patients being affected by age 30 to 35. More extensive evaluation of the children for internal signs of disease (eg, the bony tumors) is required before the father can conclude that he has not transmitted the gene. The evaluations would be important; many patients choose colonectomy to avoid lethal colonic cancers. A recent option for the family would be DNA diagnosis for mutations in the adenomatous polyposis coli (APC) gene. Presymptomatic DNA diagnosis offers a new approach to genetic diseases of later onset, but is ethically controversial when minors are involved.

403. The answer is a. *(Lewis, pp 91-98. Scriver, pp 3-45.)* Incomplete penetrance applies to a normal individual who is known from the pedigree to have an allele responsible for an autosomal dominant trait. Variable expressivity refers to family members who exhibit signs of the autosomal dominant disorder that vary in severity. When this severity seems to worsen with progressive generations, it is called anticipation. A new mutation in the grandson would be extremely unlikely given the affected grandfather. The father could be an example of somatic mosaicism if a back mutation occurred to allow normal limb development, but there is no reason to suspect mosaicism of his germ cells (germinal mosaicism). Split hand-foot malformation (MIM*183600) is one of many human birth defects that have been traced to mutations in developmental genes homologous to those in simpler organisms like the fruit fly—for example, Sonic hedgehog (SHH—MIM*600725).

404. The answer is d. *(Lewis, pp 110-126. Scriver, pp 3421-3452. Murray, pp 533-537.)* The fact that the mother of the affected child has an affected brother and an affected nephew through her sister suggests X-linked recessive inheritance. Given X-linked recessive inheritance, the mother must have the abnormal allele on one of her X chromosomes (she is an obligate carrier) in order for her son and brother to be affected. The fetus thus has a one-half chance of being a boy and a one-half chance of being affected if male, resulting in a one-fourth (25%) overall risk of being affected.

An X-linked recessive form of mucopolysaccharidosis is Hunter syndrome (MPS type II-MIM*309900). When evaluating the possibility of an X-linked disorder, it is important to remember the pattern of inheritance of the X chromosome. Females have two X chromosomes, which are passed along in a random fashion. They pass any given X chromosome to 50% of their sons and 50% of their daughters. For an X-linked recessive condition, those daughters who inherit the affected allele are heterozygous carriers of the disorder but are not affected (in practice, some female carriers show mild expression). Since males have only one X chromosome, those who inherit the affected allele are affected with the disorder.

405. The answer is d. *(Lewis, pp 70-82. Scriver, pp 2007-2056. Murray, pp 239-247.)* The family history and the likelihood that the boys have a metabolic disease suggest autosomal recessive inheritance. Autosomal recessive conditions tend to have a horizontal pattern in the pedigree. Although there may be multiple affected individuals within a sibship, parents, offspring, and other relatives are generally not affected. Most autosomal recessive conditions are rare; however, consanguinity greatly increases the likelihood that two individuals will inherit the same mutant allele and pass it along to their offspring. The recurrence risk for the fetus will be that for an autosomal recessive condition with carrier parents—one-fourth or 25%. This risk is not affected by the sex of the fetus. The disease caused by cystathionine-β-synthase (CS) deficiency is homocystinuria (MIM*236300). S-adenosylmethionine accepts methyl groups and is converted to S-adenosylhomocysteine, which yields homocysteine; homocysteine is converted to cystathionine by CS. Methionine and homocysteine (dimerized to homocystine) accumulate, and homocystine is excreted in urine. Pyridoxine is a cofactor for CS and is beneficial in some forms of homocystinuria. Other causes of homocystinuria include deficient methionine synthase, which can be ameliorated with its cofactors tetrahydrofolate and cobalamin (vitamin B_{12}).

406. The answer is c. *(Lewis, pp 70-82. Scriver, pp 6117-6146.)* In an autosomal dominant pedigree, there is a vertical pattern of inheritance. Assuming the disorder is not the result of a new mutation, every affected person has an affected parent. The same is true of X-linked dominant pedigrees. However, male-to-male transmission, as seen in this family, excludes the possibility of an X-linked disorder. A person with an autosomal dominant phenotype has one mutant allele and one normal allele. These people randomly pass one or the other of these alleles to their offspring, giving a child a 50% chance of inheriting the mutant allele and therefore being affected with the disorder. This risk is unaffected by the genotypes of the previous offspring.

407. The answer is c. (*Lewis, pp 110-126. Scriver, pp 3-45.*) Males always transmit their single X chromosome to their daughters. Therefore, a daughter of a male affected with an X-linked disorder is an obligate carrier for that disorder. When the condition is X-linked recessive, as with most forms of color blindness, the daughter is unlikely to show any phenotypic evidence that she is carrying this abnormal gene. Offspring of female carriers are of four types: (1) female carrier with one normal and one mutant allele, (2) normal female with two normal alleles, (3) affected male with a single mutant allele, and (4) normal male with a single normal allele. The chance of having an affected child is thus one-fourth or 25%. If the obligate carrier female gives birth to a son, the chance of the son being color-blind is 50%.

408. The answer is b. (*Lewis, pp 70-82. Scriver, pp 5379-5398.*) The genotype of each individual with achondroplasia can be represented as Aa, with the uppercase A representing the achondroplasia allele. The Punnett square below demonstrates that $^3/_4$ of the possible gamete combinations yield individuals with at least one A allele. Homozygous AA achondroplasia is a severe disease that is usually lethal in the newborn period. The increased likelihood of individuals with achondroplasia marrying each other because of their similar phenotypes is an example of assortative mating.

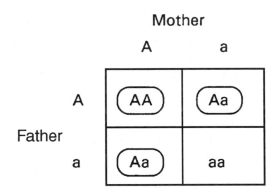

409. The answer is c. *(Lewis, pp 82-86. Scriver, pp 5121-5188. Murray, pp 624-626.)* The McKusick number for cystic fibrosis (MIM*219700) begins with 2, indicating an autosomal recessive disorder. The genotype of the affected female with cystic fibrosis is therefore best represented as the two lowercase letters cc. Her parents are obligate carriers for the disorder (genotypes Cc), and one of her grandparents must also be a carrier (barring new mutations). Her first cousin then has a one-fourth chance of being a carrier, since one of their common grandparents is a carrier, one of his parents has a one-half chance of being a carrier, and he has a one-half chance of inheriting the c allele from his parent. The affected female can only transmit c alleles to her fetus, while her cousin has one-half chance of transmitting his c allele if it is present. Thus, the probability that the first child will have cystic fibrosis is one-fourth (cousin is carrier) × one-half (cousin transmits c allele) = one-eighth (fetus has cc genotype).

410. The answer is e. *(Lewis, pp 110-126. Scriver, pp 5955-5976.)* The common forms of color blindness are X-linked recessive, as indicated by the initial 3 of the McKusick number (MIM*304000). The couple's daughters will be obligate carriers—that is, carriers implied by the pedigree. Using a lowercase c to represent the recessive color blindness allele, the female is most likely X^CX^c, while her husband is X^cY. The Punnett square below indicates that all daughters will be carriers (X^cX^c), while sons will be normal (X^CY). Note again that loci on the X chromosome cannot be transmitted from father to son, since the son receives the father's Y chromosome.

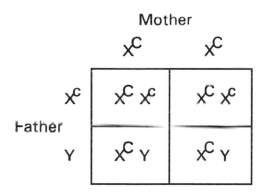

411. The answer is c. (*Lewis, pp 82-86. Scriver, pp 5759-5788.*) Autosomal dominant inheritance is suggested by the pedigree because of the vertical pattern of affected individuals and the affliction of both sexes. Autosomal recessive inheritance is ruled out by transmission through three generations, and X-linked recessive inheritance is made unlikely by the presence of affected females. Maternal inheritance should demonstrate transmission to all or most offspring of affected mothers. Polygenic or multifactorial inheritance is not associated with such a high frequency of transmission. Note that X-linked dominant inheritance would also be an explanation for the pedigree. Because the most likely mechanism responsible for the pedigree is autosomal or X-linked dominant inheritance, individual III-3 in the figure accompanying the question is affected with the disorder, and she has a 50% risk of transmitting the disease. Discrimination between autosomal and X-linked dominant inheritance could be made by noting the offspring of affected males, such as individual III-4. If X-linked dominant inheritance were operative, affected males would have normal sons and affected daughters. The likely diagnosis is an autosomal dominant form of Charcot-Marie-Tooth disease (MIM*118200). Charcot-Marie-Tooth disease exhibits genetic heterogeneity and can exhibit autosomal dominant, autosomal recessive (MIM*214380), and X-linked inheritance (MIM*302800). Note that the physician could provide counseling based on knowledge of genetics even though the disease is unfamiliar.

412. The answer is e. (*Lewis, pp 82-86. Scriver, pp 5903-5934.*) The presence of consanguinity (double line in the figure) is a red flag for autosomal recessive inheritance because, although disease-causing alleles are rare, the probability of a homozygous individual escalates dramatically when the same rare allele descends through two branches of a family. Using a lowercase r to denote the retinitis pigmentosa allele, the affected male (individual II-2 in the figure accompanying the question) has a genotype of rr. His prospective mate has a very low risk to be a carrier for this rare disease, making her genotype RR. Their children will all have genotypes Rr, making them carriers but not affected. Retinitis pigmentosa is another disease manifesting genetic heterogeneity, with autosomal dominant (MIM*180100), autosomal recessive (MIM*268000), and X-linked recessive (MIM*312650) forms. Carriers of autosomal recessive diseases are heterozygotes with one normal and one abnormal allele. Many autosomal recessive diseases involve enzyme deficiencies, indicating that 50% levels of enzymes found in heterozygotes are sufficient for normal function. The probability that an affected individual will encounter a mate who is a carrier is approximately twice the square root of the disease incidence. This figure derives from the Hardy-Weinberg law. Since most recessive diseases have incidences lower than 1 in 10,000, the risk for unrelated mates to be carriers is less than 1 in 50, and the chance of having an affected child is less than $^1/_{50} \times ^1/_4$ = less than 1 in 200. Disorders that are fairly common in certain ethnic groups, such as cystic fibrosis, are exceptions to this very low risk.

413. The answer is d. (*Lewis, pp 110-126. Scriver, pp 5903-5934.*) X-linked recessive inheritance is characterized by a predominance of affected males and an oblique pattern. Transmission must be through females with no evidence of male-to-male transmission. The lack of affected females would make autosomal dominant inheritance less likely, and the sex ratio plus transmission through three generations would eliminate autosomal recessive inheritance. Polygenic inheritance usually exhibits less frequent transmission, although it is certainly not ruled out in this pedigree. The many normal offspring of affected females rule out maternal inheritance. Individual II-4 in the figure accompanying the question is an obligate carrier because she has an affected brother and affected son. This means that her daughter (III-3) has a one-half chance of inheriting the X chromosome with an abnormal allele and one-half chance of inheriting the X chromosome with the normal allele. If individual III-3 is a carrier, she has a one-half chance of transmitting her abnormal allele to her son. The risk that her son will be affected is thus one-half × one-half = one-fourth or 25%. Because the daughters of individual III-3 might be carriers (one-half chance) but will not be affected, individual III-3 has a one-half chance of having an affected child.

414. The answer is d. (*Lewis, pp 82-86. Scriver, pp 5241-5287.*) If a mutation occurs in the primordial germ cells, then these cells may have abnormal alleles despite the lack of these alleles in the rest of the body tissues (germinal mosaicism). A parent with germ-line mosaicism for an autosomal dominant disorder may thus present more than one gamete with the disease allele for fertilization and have several children with the disease. Incomplete penetrance refers to the lack of a disease phenotype after all relevant medical evaluations in a person who must have the disease allele (eg, parent whose father and daughter has the disease—incorrect answer e). Variable expressivity denotes variable severity among individuals with disease alleles in the same family, and would apply if one of the parents had very mild disease compared to their children (incorrect answer a). Uniparental disomy reflects transmission of one parental chromosome to comprise both homologues in a child (first occurring as a trisomy in the embryo with subsequent correction). Uniparental disomy may rarely produce a child with autosomal recessive disease when only one parent is a carrier. However, uniparental disomy and new mutations would be very unlikely to occur twice (incorrect answers b, c).

Germinal mosaicism was thought to be very rare until testing for type I collagen gene mutations in osteogenesis imperfecta allowed verification of germinal mosaicism in this condition. Germinal mosaicism explained why autosomal recessive inheritance had been incorrectly postulated for families with normal parents and multiple affected children with type II or lethal osteogenesis imperfecta. The characterization of mutations in the $\alpha 1$ or $\alpha 2$ chains of type I collagen in osteogenesis imperfecta allowed proof of germ-line mosaicism through paternal sperm studies.

415. The answer is a. *(Lewis, pp 110-126. Scriver, pp 3-45, Murray, pp 545-565, 628-629.)* The Lyon hypothesis predicts that X inactivation is early, irreversible, and random, but some females exhibit nonrandom X inactivation and inactivate only the X chromosome carrying the normal allele (incorrect answers b-e). Females have two alleles for each locus on the X chromosome because of their 46,XX karyotype. One normal allele is by definition sufficient for normal function in X-linked recessive disorders, so that females with one abnormal allele are heterozygous and usually unaffected—they are said to "carry" the disease. Only when the companion normal allele is disrupted or missing does the abnormal allele cause disease. X autosome translocations may disrupt an X chromosome locus and cause disease because the translocated autosome must remain active to avert embryonic death—this and the possibility of Turner syndrome with a single X is less likely than nonrandom inactivation of the normal X chromosome. Conversely, females with triple X or trisomy X syndrome have three alleles at each X chromosome locus and are not affected with X-linked recessive disorders.

416. The answer is e. *(Lewis, pp 110-126. Scriver, pp 3-45.)* Females who are heterozygous at an X-chromosome locus will have a one-half chance to transmit their abnormal allele to sons or daughters with each pregnancy. When heterozygous females show disease symptoms, they are considered affected and the disorder is considered to be X-linked dominant. When an abnormal X-chromosome allele is sufficiently severe to affect heterozygous females, the hemizygous males often do not survive the embryonic period and present as unrecognized early losses or later miscarriages. If the disorder does not affect the in utero viability of females, twice as many females as males are born. The decreased survival of affected males and reduced reproductive fitness of affected females also implies a high rate of new mutations and means that many isolated cases will occur. In disorders such as incontinentia pigmenti (MIM*308300), where affected individuals have variable manifestations, careful examination of the mother is required before assuming that an affected daughter is a new mutation. A pregnancy history will also be helpful, in that a history of early pregnancy losses would suggest the mother was a mildly affected heterozygote. The distinction between X-linked dominant and X-linked recessive diseases is somewhat arbitrary, since heterozygous females may show mild symptoms in disorders such as Duchenne muscular dystrophy (MIM*310200) or hemophilia A (MIM*306700). Severe symptoms in some female heterozygotes, together with male lethality, are good criteria for classification as X-linked dominant (as for Goltz syndrome—MIM*305600, Aicardi syndrome—MIM*304050, and incontinentia pigmenti).

417. The answer is e. (*Lewis, pp 132-151. Scriver, pp 193-202.*) An increasing recurrence risk according to the number of relatives affected is characteristic of polygenic inheritance. The more affected relatives there are, the more evidence there is that an individual's genetic background is shifted toward the threshold for a particular trait; for example, the expectation for tall parents with tall grandparents is to have tall children. Inheritance risks for Mendelian disorders are unaffected by outcomes in prior offspring because they reflect segregation ratios for a known (or deduced) pair of alleles (chance has no memory). Pyloric stenosis was once a lethal disease but now is easily repaired by surgery (recently, by less invasive laparoscopic surgery). The diagnosis can be difficult, often requiring palpation of the abdomen for 20 to 30 minutes when the baby has vomited and is relaxed. The characteristic "olive" mass can be felt in the mid-abdomen and can now be confirmed by ultrasound study.

418. The answer is b. (*Lewis, pp 70-82. Scriver, pp 5587-5628.*) Albinism is one of many genetic diseases that exhibit locus heterogeneity, which means that mutations at several different loci can produce identical phenotypes. The two McKusick numbers provide a clue that there is more than one locus for albinism, both causing autosomal recessive disease. Each parent must be homozygous for a mutant allele from one albinism locus but heterozygous or homozygous normal at the other locus. Their child would then be an obligate carrier for each type of albinism. A new mutation in the child is also possible, converting one of the parental mutant alleles to normal, but this would be very rare. Autosomal dominant disorders often vary in severity within families (variable expressivity) but occasionally are clinically silent in a person known to carry the abnormal allele (incomplete penetrance).

419. The answer is c. (*Lewis, pp 70-82. Scriver, pp 6097-6116.*) For each pregnancy, the probability that the child will be affected is one-half. Therefore, the probability that all three children will be affected is the product of the three independent events—that is, $\frac{1}{2} \times \frac{1}{2} \times \frac{1}{2} = \frac{1}{8}$. The probability that all three children will be unaffected is the same. When evaluating the probability that one of the three children will be affected, it must be noted that there are three of eight possible birth orders that have one affected child (Www, wWw, wwW). For two of three children to be affected, there are also three of eight possible birth orders (WWw, WwW, wWW). The ventral midline hair and skin patches relate to the fact that neural crest cells provide melanin, and that migration of these cells from the dorsal midline (neural tube) of the embryo is slowed in disorders like Waardenburg syndrome (MIM*193500) and piebald trait (MIM*172800).

420. The answer is d. (*Lewis, pp 70-82. Scriver, pp 3-45.*) Diploid persons have two alleles per autosomal locus, with one being transmitted to each gamete (Mendel's law of segregation). The key to blood group problems is to recognize that a blood type is ambiguous regarding possible alleles— type A persons may have AA or AO genotypes. Once the possible genotypes are deduced from the blood types, potential offspring will represent all combinations of parental alleles. Parents with AB and OO genotypes can only have offspring with genotypes AO (type A) or BO (type B).

421. The answer is b. (*Lewis, pp 70-82, 287-299. Scriver, pp 1667-1724.*) If the abnormal allele is represented as p and the normal as P, an infant affected with phenylketonuria (PKU) has the genotype pp. Parents must be heterozygotes or carriers (Pp) for the child to inherit the p allele from both the mother and father (assuming correct paternity and the absence of unusual chromosomal segregation). Subsequent children have a one-half chance of inheriting allele p from the mother and a one-half chance of inheriting allele p from the father; the chance that both events will occur to give genotype pp is thus $\frac{1}{2} \times \frac{1}{2} = \frac{1}{4}$ or 25%. A normal sibling may be genotype PP (one-fourth probability) or Pp (one-half probability since two different combinations of parental alleles give this genotype). The ratio of these probabilities results in a two-thirds chance (67%) of genotype Pp. Note that genotype pp is excluded because a normal sibling (the first child) is specified. Neonatal screening is mandated for disorders like phenylketonuria (MIM*261600) because they are difficult to recognize clinically and early dietary treatment prevents severe mental disability.

422. The answer is d. (*Lewis, pp 82-86. Scriver, pp 5379-5398.*) The figure beneath Question 422 shows the correctly drawn pedigree with generations indicated by Roman numerals and individuals by Arabic numbers. As the McKusick numbers indicate, achondroplasia (MIM*100800) is autosomal dominant, cystic fibrosis (MIM*219700) autosomal recessive. Since neither parent is affected with achondroplasia, the risk for their next child to be affected is virtually zero (rare chances for germ-line mosaicism or incomplete penetrance are ignored). The person who prompted genetic concern is the proband (III-1). The husband has a brother with cystic fibrosis, making his parents (I-3, I-4) obligate carriers. He has a one-fourth chance of being normal, a two-fourths chance of being a carrier, and a one-fourth chance of being affected with cystic fibrosis. Since the possibility of him being affected is eliminated by circumstance (he is normal), his odds of being a carrier are two-thirds. The wife is definitely a carrier, giving their next child a one-sixth chance to have cystic fibrosis (two-thirds chance husband is a carrier X; one-fourth chance the child is affected if both are carriers). Although the ΔF_{508} (three–base pair deletion of phenylalanine codon at position #508 in the cystic fibrosis transmembrane regulator gene) accounts for 70% of cystic fibrosis mutations in Caucasians, husband's family may have a different mutation than was detected by DNA analysis in his wife. Their child may therefore have a risk of being a compound heterozygote (two different abnormal cystic fibrosis alleles) but will still be affected. Current DNA analysis for cystic fibrosis would likely clarify this issue, since over 30 mutations can be screened in Caucasians.

423. The answer is c. (*Lewis, pp 82-86. Scriver, pp 3827-3876.*) Inborn errors of metabolism often reflect enzyme deficiencies with resulting autosomal recessive inheritance. Parents of children with autosomal recessive disorders are obligate carriers if nonpaternity and rare examples of uniparental disomy (inheritance of both chromosomal homologues from the same parent) are excluded. Normal siblings have a two-thirds chance of being carriers because they cannot be homozygous for the abnormal allele. Grandparents have a one-half chance of being carriers because one or the other must have transmitted the abnormal allele to the obligate carrier parent. First cousins share a set of grandparents of whom one must be a carrier. There is a one-half chance for the aunt or uncle to be a carrier and a one-fourth chance for the first cousin. Half-siblings share an obligate carrier parent and have a one-half chance of being carriers. These calculations assume a lack of new mutations and a lack of coincidental alleles (lessened if the parents are not related but of concern in certain Jewish communities where carrier rates for Tay-Sachs can be high).

424. The answer is e. (*Lewis, pp 132-151. Scriver, pp 193-202.*) Cleft lip with or without cleft palate is one of the most common congenital malformations. Because of the genetic component of this trait, it tends to be more common in certain families. The more family members affected and the more severe the cleft, the higher the recurrence risk. In addition, cleft lip with/without cleft palate is more common in males and in certain ethnic groups (ie, Asians > Caucasians > African Americans).

425. The answer is a. (*Lewis, pp 287-299. Scriver, pp 3-45.*) If an abnormal allele is as likely to be transmitted to the next generation as its corresponding normal allele, it is said to have a fitness of 1. Loss of fitness (decrease in allele frequency after one generation) is also referred to as negative selection. The decreased fitness of achondroplast alleles that are eliminated by negative selection must be balanced by new mutations if the disorder has not disappeared or declined in incidence. Thus, the mutation rate of achondroplasia would be expected to be high relative to those of more benign dominant diseases.

426. The answer is b. (*Lewis, pp 132-151. Scriver, pp 193-202.*) Many common disorders tend to run in families but are not single-gene or chromosomal disorders. These disorders exhibit multifactorial determination, a theoretical mechanism envisioned as the interaction of multiple genes (polygenic inheritance) and environmental factors. For quantitative traits like height, it is easy to visualize how the alleles at multiple loci plus environmental factors (eg, nutrition) might make additive contributions toward a given stature. For qualitative traits such as cleft lip/palate and other congenital anomalies, a threshold is envisioned that divides normal from abnormal phenotypes. Individuals with more clefting alleles, in combination with an unfavorable intrauterine environment, can cross the threshold and manifest the anomaly. Environmental factors in multifactorial determination are thus prenatal as well as postnatal. For adult diseases like coronary artery disease, strokes, or hypertension, the quantitative trait can be viewed as degree of artery occlusion or blood pressure and the threshold as events like myocardial or cerebral infarction. The likelihood of inheriting hypertension-promoting alleles is increased if there are several affected relatives as in the family under discussion, translating the usual 3% to 5% risk for a multifactorial disorder in a first-degree relative to the 5% to 10% risk estimated in answer b. Recurrence risks for multifactorial disorders are modified by family history because the multiple predisposing alleles cannot be determined by testing. Current research is attempting to find single nucleotide polymorphisms (SNPs) that travel with these multiple predisposing alleles, allowing more definitive susceptibility testing and risk prediction for the occurrence and transmission of multifactorial traits.

427. The answer is d. (*Lewis, pp 248-261. Scriver, pp 3-45.*) Down syndrome, a chromosomal disorder, has virtually the same frequency of 1 in 600 births in all ethnic groups. Screening for Down syndrome is carried out during pregnancy with triple test/quad screens offered to all individuals (with less sensitivity or specificity) and chorionic villus sampling/amniocentesis (with high accuracy but some miscarriage risk) to females above age 35. Allele frequencies may differ among populations when there has been geographic isolation, founder effect, or selection for certain alleles based on different environments. Although African Americans have intermixed with Caucasians in the United States for over 400 years, they retain a higher frequency of sickle cell alleles (MIM*603903), which are thought to protect individuals from malarial infection. Each ethnic group has frequencies of polymorphic alleles that reflect its origin; for example, Ashkenazi Jews have a higher frequency of Tay-Sachs alleles (MIM*272800); Greeks and other Mediterranean peoples of β-thalassemia alleles (MIM*603902);

Asian peoples of α-thalassemia alleles (MIM*141800); and Caucasians of cystic fibrosis alleles (MIM*219700). Specific genetic differences (polymorphisms) in the mitochondrial and Y chromosomes have allowed reconstruction of migrations that show correlations between genetic homogeneity and language.

428. The answer is d. *(Lewis, pp 287-299. Scriver, pp 3-45.)* Founder effects represent a special case of genetic drift in which rare alleles are introduced into a small population by the migration of ancestors. These founder mutant alleles can overcome selective disadvantage because they begin with high frequency in a small gene pool. Linkage disequilibrium describes an association between a particular polymorphic allele and a trait. Many autoimmune diseases exhibit association with particular human leukocyte antigen (HLA) alleles (ie, HLA-B27 and ankylosing spondylitis). The association is not necessarily cause and effect (eg, when viral infections that trigger a disease preferentially infect certain HLA genotypes). Genetic linkage implies physical proximity of the allele locus to the gene causing the disease. Linkage differs from allele association in that either allele A or a may be linked in a given family, depending on which allele is present together with the offending gene. Neither assortative mating (preferential mating by genotype) nor selection (advantageous alleles) applies to the situation under discussion. Later research using DNA polymorphisms has refuted the Hopewell hypothesis, showing that families with this form of diabetes insipidus (MIM*304800) are not related to ancestors from Halifax.

429. The answer is b. *(Lewis, pp 287-299. Scriver, pp 3-45.)* Sickle cell anemia (MIM*603903) is the classic example of a disorder with a high frequency in a specific population because of heterozygote advantage. Persons who are heterozygous for this mutant allele (hemoglobin AS) have increased resistance to malaria and are therefore at an advantage in areas where malaria is endemic. Founder effect is a special type of genetic drift. In these cases, the founder or original ancestor of a population has a certain mutant allele. Because of genetic isolation and inbreeding in populations such as the Pennsylvania Amish, certain disorders such as maple syrup urine disease (MIM*248600) are maintained at a relatively high frequency. Fitness is a measure of the ability to reproduce. A genetic lethal implies that affected individuals cannot reproduce and, therefore, cannot pass on their mutant alleles. Natural selection is a theory introduced by Charles Darwin, which postulates that the fittest individuals have a selective advantage for survival.

430. The answer is b. (*Lewis, pp 333-354. Scriver, pp 3-45. Murray, pp 593-608.*) It is important to remember that individuals with blood type A can have either genotype AA or AO, and individuals with blood type B can have either genotype BB or BO. Therefore, the frequency of blood type A is the frequency of homozygotes—that is, 0.3×0.3—plus the frequency of heterozygotes—that is, $2(0.3) \times 0.6$—for a total of 0.45. The frequency of blood type B is 0.1×0.1 (homozygotes) plus that for heterozygotes ($2[0.1]) \times 0.6$), yielding a total of 0.13. The frequency of individuals with blood type O is simply the frequency of homozygotes—that is, $0.6 \times 0.6 = 0.36$.

431. The answer is c. (*Lewis, pp 132-151. Scriver, pp 3-45.*) Although all individuals, other than identical twins, are genetically unique, each individual will have some genes in common with their relatives. The more closely related, the more genes individuals have in common. First-degree relatives, such as siblings, parents, and children, share one-half of their genes. Second-degree relatives share one-fourth, and third-degree relatives share one-eighth. Full siblings will have half their genes in common, half siblings (with only one common parent) one-fourth. Risks for multifactorial disorders like hydrocephalus falloff rapidly with decreasing degrees of relationship, with average figures of 3% to 5% for first-degree relatives (sharing one-half their genes), 0.5% to 0.7% for second-degree relatives (sharing one-fourth their genes as for this child and his sister), dropping to near baseline incidence (1-3 per thousand for congenital anomalies) for third-degree relatives like first cousins.

432. The answer is d. (*Lewis, pp 267-270. Scriver, pp 3-45.*) According to the Hardy-Weinberg equilibrium, the frequency of heterozygotes ($2pq$) is twice the square root of the rare homozygote frequency (q^2). The male in the question has a two-thirds chance of being a carrier. His wife has a one-twentieth chance of being a carrier. The rare homozygote frequency is $1/600$, so the square root is $1/40$ and the frequency of heterozygotes is thus $2 \times 1/40 = 1/20$. His risk for an affected child is $2/3 \times 1/20 \times 1/4 = 1/20$.

433. The answer is e. (*Lewis, pp 81-87. Scriver, pp 4571-4636.*) The African American male and female each have a one-eighth chance of having sickle trait. They have a $\frac{1}{64} \times \frac{1}{4} = \frac{1}{256}$ chance of having a child with sickle cell anemia. There is also a $\frac{1}{64} \times \frac{1}{2} = \frac{1}{128}$ chance that their child will have sickle trait.

434. The answer is b. (*Lewis, pp 82-86. Scriver, pp 3-45.*) The grand-mother has cystic fibrosis, so her children are obligate carriers. Each cousin therefore has a one-half chance of being a carrier. The female's risk is $\frac{1}{2} \times \frac{1}{2} \times \frac{1}{4} = \frac{1}{16}$ chance of having an affected child. This illustrates the effects of consanguinity.

Genetic and Biochemical Diagnosis

Questions

435. A 66-year-old African American female is diagnosed with Parkinson disease (PD-MIM*168601) and there are no other cases in her family. She requests genetic counseling and/or testing to assess risks that her middle-aged children will develop Parkinsonism. Her physician explains that 1% of people over 50 may contract the disease, that rare families exhibit autosomal dominant inheritance, and that usual risks are increased three- to fourfold for first-degree relatives of affected individuals. Based on this information, which of the following options provide appropriate genetic counseling for this patient?

a. Likely multifactorial determination in your family with a 3% to 4% risk for your middle-aged children to develop PD.
b. Likely multifactorial determination in your family with a 1% risk for your middle-aged children to develop PD.
c. Likely autosomal dominant inheritance in your family with a 50% risk for your middle-aged children to develop PD.
d. Likely autosomal dominant inheritance in your family with a 25% risk for your middle-aged children to develop PD.
e. Likely multifactorial determination in your family with a 10% risk for your middle-aged children to develop PD.

436. Individuals with Parkinson disease (PD-MIM*168601) have dopamine deficiency in the substantia nigra of the central nervous system. Which of the following would comprise the best strategy for therapy?

a. Feedback inhibition of dopamine oxidation
b. Competitive inhibition of biosynthesis from histidine
c. Provision of metabolites in the tyrosine pathway
d. Stimulation of monoamine oxidase
e. Provision of metabolites in the alanine pathway

437. A 3-year-old Caucasian girl is scheduled for a tonsillectomy. As she is prepared for the operating room, her father becomes agitated and insists on accompanying her. He says that he lost a son several years ago when the child did not wake up after an operation. Which of the following options is the best response to the father's anxiety?

a. Postpone the operation until the psychiatric state of the father can be evaluated.
b. Proceed after explaining that problems in a previous child are unlikely to be present in his daughter.
c. Proceed after reassuring the father that drug reactions are environmental and unlikely to have a genetic basis.
d. Postpone the operation until a more detailed family history is obtained.
e. Proceed after explaining that modern anesthetic procedures are much safer than in the past.

438. In the operating room, a 5-year-old Hispanic boy receives succinyl-choline as a muscle relaxant to facilitate intubation and anesthesia. The operation proceeds until it is time for recovery, when the child does not begin breathing. A hurried discussion with the father discloses no additional problems in the family, but he does say that he and his wife are first cousins. Which of the following is the most likely possibility?

a. An autosomal dominant disorder that interferes with succinylcholine metabolism
b. An autosomal recessive disorder that interferes with succinylcholine metabolism
c. An X-linked disorder that interferes with succinylcholine metabolism
d. A lethal gene transmitted through consanguinity that affects the respiratory system
e. Mismanagement of halothane anesthesia during the operation

439. Pharmacogenetics, or the study of drug-induced disease due to genetic variation, is receiving increased attention particularly with regard to population or at least preoperative screening. The frequency of heterozygotes for variant butyrylcholinesterase (BChE) alleles in Caucasians is about 4 per 100, implying an incidence of individuals with potential for severe apnea of which of the following?

a. 1 in 5000
b. 1 in 2500
c. 1 in 1250
d. 1 in 500
e. 1 in 50

440. A 32-year-old Caucasian male of Scandinavian origin exhibits increased fatigue with shortness of breath during his usual jogging routine. His physician suspects early-onset emphysema and performs protein electrophoresis for analysis of α_1-antitrypsin (AAT) deficiency (MIM*107400). The result shows two electrophoretic bands that react with AAT, one at the normal position and one at an abnormal position. Which of the following best describes this result?

a. The male is homozygous and has normal AAT activity
b. The male is heterozygous and has normal AAT activity
c. The male is homozygous and has deficient AAT activity
d. The male is homozygous and has an altered AAT protein
e. The male is heterozygous and has an altered AAT protein

441. A 6-month-old Caucasian girl of Ashkenazi Jewish background seems to plateau in development after a normal gestation, delivery, and early infancy. She rolled over well with smiling and good interaction but became less active and does not maintain a sit. Her pediatrician notes low muscle tone and claps her hands to elicit an exaggerated extension of her arms (Moro reflex—enhanced startle response). Ophthalmologic examination reveals a central red area of the retina surrounded by white tissue (cherry red spot). A diagnosis of lipid storage disease (neurolipidosis) is suspected. If the diagnosis is correct, what is the risk that the next child of these parents will be affected with the same disease?

a. $1/2$
b. $1/4$
c. $3/4$
d. $1/12$
e. $1/24$

442. The cause of Tay-Sachs disease (MIM*272800) is best described by which of the following?

a. Excess of a lysosomal enzyme in blood due to defective uptake
b. Deficiency of a lysosomal enzyme that digests proteoglycans
c. Deficiency of a membrane receptor that takes up proteoglycans
d. Deficiency of a mitochondrial enzyme that degrades glycogen
e. Deficiency of a mitochondrial triglyceride lipase

443. The frequency of carriers of Tay-Sachs disease (MIM*272800) in Ashkenazi Jewish populations is 1 in 30. Some Jewish communities offer carrier testing for young adults so they will know their status before marriage. A known carrier female becomes involved with an exchange student from Russia who also is Ashkenazi Jewish but who has not had carrier testing. What is the chance that a child of this union will have Tay-Sachs disease?

a. 1 in 2 $1/_{120}$
b. 1 in 15 $1/_{240}$
c. 1 in 30 $1/_{3600}$
d. 1 in 60 $1/_{9000}$
e. 1 in 120 $1/_{36,000}$

444. The parents of a girl with Tay-Sachs disease (MIM*272800) decide to pursue bone marrow transplantation in an attempt to provide a source for the missing lysosomal enzyme. Preliminary testing of the girl's normal siblings is performed to assess their carrier status and their human leukocyte antigen (HLA) locus compatibility with their affected sister. What is the chance that one of the three siblings is homozygous normal (ie, has a good supply of enzyme) and HLA-compatible?

a. $1/_2$
b. $1/_3$
c. $1/_4$
d. $1/_6$
e. $1/_{12}$

445. A sibling donor is found for a patient with Tay-Sachs disease (MIM*272800), and the physician writes to the patient's insurance company explaining the diagnosis of Tay-Sachs disease and the reasons for the bone marrow transplant. Not only does the insurance company refuse payment for transplantation, it also discontinues coverage for the family based on anticipated medical expenses. From the ethical perspective, these events fall under which of the following categories?

a. Patient confidentiality
b. Nondisclosure
c. Informed consent
d. Failure to provide ongoing care
e. Discrimination

446. A couple decide to have prenatal diagnosis because their previous child has Tay-Sachs disease (MIM*272800). Which of the following prenatal diagnostic techniques is optimal for fetal diagnosis?

a. Chorionic villus sampling (CVS)
b. Percutaneous umbilical blood sampling
c. Amniotic fluid α-fetoprotein levels
d. Maternal serum α-fetoprotein (MSAFP)
e. Fetal x-rays

447. A 14-year-old Caucasian adolescent presents to his physician for a sports physical examination that will approve his participation in football. He is noted to have a tall, thin body habitus, loose joints, and arachnodactyly (spider fingers). Ophthalmologic examination reveals lens dislocation. Echocardiogram reveals dilation of the aortic root. A family history reveals that the patient's parents are medically normal, but that his paternal grandfather and great-grandfather died in their forties with lens dislocation and dissecting aortic aneurysms. A sister is found to have a similar body habitus, dilation of the aortic root, and normal lenses. The physician suspects Marfan syndrome (MIM*154700) and declines to approve his athletic participation until he has cardiology evaluation. Different findings in the boy's relatives who likely have the same disease are best described by which of the following terms?

a. Pleiotropy
b. Founder effect
c. Variable expressivity
d. Incomplete penetrance
e. Genetic heterogeneity

448. Marfan syndrome is caused by which of the following mechanisms?

a. Mutation that prevents addition of carbohydrate residues to the fibrillin glyco-protein
b. Mutation in a carbohydrate portion of fibrillin that interferes with targeting
c. Mutation that disrupts the secondary structure of fibrillin and blocks its assembly into microfibrils
d. Mutation in a lysosomal enzyme that degrades fibrillin
e. Mutation in a membrane receptor that targets fibrillin to lysosomes

449. The diagnosis of osteogenesis imperfecta (MIM*166200) is most accurately performed by which of the following?

a. PCR amplification and DNA sequencing of type I collagen gene segments to look for point mutations
b. Gel electrophoresis of labeled type I collagen chains synthesized in fibroblasts
c. PCR amplification and ASO hybridization to detect particular mutant alleles
d. Northern blotting to evaluate type I collagen mRNAs
e. Purification and trypsin digestion of type I collagen chains to visualize altered peptides after two-dimensional gel electrophoresis

450. Studies of the eye tumor retinoblastoma have revealed an Rb locus on the long arm of chromosome 13 that influences retinoblastoma occurrence. Patients with retinoblastoma 13q–deletions often develop bilateral tumors (both sides), in contrast to more common forms of retinoblastoma that occur at one site. Which of the following phrases best explains this phenomenon?

a. *Rb* is an oncogene.
b. *Rb* is a tumor suppressor gene.
c. Rb mutations ablate a promoter sequence.
d. Rb mutations ablate an enhancer sequence.
e. Rb mutations must always involve chromosome abnormalities.

451. In Burkitt lymphoma, there is increased expression of a hybrid protein with an amino-terminus similar to immunoglobulin (Ig) heavy chain and an unknown carboxy-terminus. Which of the following best explains this phenomenon?

a. Chromosome translocation that brings together an Ig heavy chain with an oncogene
b. Chromosome duplication involving a segment with an oncogene
c. Chromosome translocation involving a segment with Ig heavy chains
d. Chromosome deletion removing an oncogene
e. Chromosome deletion removing a tumor suppressor gene

452. A couple request genetic counseling because the wife has contracted early-onset breast cancer at age 23. The husband has a benign family history, but the wife has several relatives who developed cancers at relatively early ages. Affected relatives include a sister (colon cancer, age 42), a brother (colon cancer, age 46), mother (breast cancer, age 56), maternal aunt (leukemia, age 45), maternal uncle (muscle sarcoma, age 49), and a nephew through the brother with colon cancer (leukemia, age 8). Which of the following is an accurate conclusion from the family history?

a. No genetic predisposition to cancer since most individuals have different types of cancer
b. Possible autosomal dominant inheritance or multifactorial inheritance of cancer predisposition
c. Germ-line mutations in an oncogene, with somatic mutations that suppress the oncogene
d. Germ-line mutations in a tumor suppressor gene, with neoplasia from chemical exposure
e. Mitochondrial inheritance of tumor predisposition evidenced by the affected maternal relatives

453. A normal 6-year-old girl has a strong family history of cancer, including several relatives with Li-Fraumeni syndrome, an autosomal dominant condition that predisposes to breast and colon cancer. Her parents request that she have genetic testing for a possible cancer gene. Which of the following is the major ethical concern about such testing?

a. Nonmaleficence
b. Beneficence
c. Autonomy
d. Informed consent
e. Confidentiality

454. A 45-year-old male is hospitalized for treatment of myocardial infarction. His father and a paternal uncle also had heart attacks at an early age. His cholesterol is elevated, and lipoprotein electrophoresis demonstrates an abnormally high ratio of low- to high density lipoproteins (LDL to HDL). Which of the following is the most likely explanation for this problem?

a. Mutant HDL is not responding to high cholesterol levels.
b. Mutant LDL is not responding to high cholesterol levels.
c. Mutant caveolae proteins are not responding to high cholesterol levels.
d. Mutant LDL receptors are deficient in cholesterol uptake.
e. Intracellular cholesterol is increasing the number of LDL receptors.

455. A patient with myocardial infarction is treated with nitroglycerin to dilate his coronary arteries. Which of the following best describes the action of nitroglycerin?

a. Methylation occurs to produce S-adenosylmethionine.
b. GTP hydrolysis accomplishes oxidation of LDL proteins.
c. Arginine is converted to a neurotransmitter that activates guanyl cyclase.
d. Acetyl-CoA and choline are condensed to form a neurotransmitter.
e. Tyrosine is converted to serotonin.

456. A female presents with fatigue, pallor, and pale conjunctival blood vessels. She gives a recent history of metrorrhagia (heavy menstrual periods). Which of the following laboratory findings is most likely?

a. High serum haptoglobin
b. High serum iron
c. High numbers of transferrin receptors
d. High saturation of transferrin
e. High serum ferritin

457. A male is evaluated for mild liver disease, arthritis, fatigue, and grayish skin pigmentation. A liver biopsy shows marked increase in iron. Which of the following laboratory values is most likely?

a. Low serum iron
b. High serum copper
c. Low saturation of transferrin
d. High serum ferritin
e. Low serum haptoglobin

458. The regulation of transferrin receptors is studied in tissue culture. There is increased synthesis of transferrin receptor protein with no changes in transferrin mRNA transcription. Which of the following is the most plausible explanation?

a. Change in amounts or types of transcription factors
b. Allosteric regulation of transferrin receptor function
c. Activation of transferrin receptor function by a protein kinase
d. Stabilization of transferrin mRNA
e. Increased GTP levels to accelerate protein elongation

459. A 2-year-old child is hospitalized for evaluation of poor growth and low muscle tone. The most striking physical finding is unruly, "kinky" hair, but the child also has increased joint laxity and thin skin. Which of the following laboratory findings is most likely?

a. High ceruloplasmin
b. High tissue copper
c. Low serum iron
d. Low saturation of transferrin
e. Low serum haptoglobin

460. Deletions of 11p13 may result in Wilm tumor, aniridia, genitourinary malformations, and mental retardation (WAGR syndrome). In some patients, however, not all features are seen. Additionally, individual features of this syndrome may be inherited separately in a Mendelian fashion. Limited features may also be seen in patients without visible chromosomal deletions. Which of the following is the most likely mechanism for this finding?

a. Mitochondrial inheritance
b. Imprinting
c. Germ-line mosaicism
d. Uniparental disomy
e. Contiguous gene syndrome

461. Polycystic kidney disease (MIM*173900) is a significant cause of renal failure that presents from early infancy to adulthood. Early-onset cases tend to affect one family member or siblings, whereas adult-onset cases often show a vertical pattern in the pedigree. Which of the following offers the best explanation of these facts?

a. Pleiotropy
b. Allelic heterogeneity
c. Locus heterogeneity
d. Multifactorial determination
e. Variable expressivity

462. A male child presents with delayed development and scarring of his lips and hands. His parents have restrained him because he obsessively chews on his lips and fingers. Which of the following is likely to occur in this child?

a. Increased levels of 5-phosphoribosyl-1-pyrophosphate (PRPP)
b. Decreased purine synthesis
c. Decreased levels of uric acid
d. Increased levels of hypoxanthine-guanosine phosphoribosyl transferase (HGPRT)
e. Glycogen storage

463. A couple request prenatal diagnosis because a maternal uncle and a male cousin on the wife's side were diagnosed with Lesch-Nyhan syndrome (MIM*308000). DNA analysis of the family is performed using Southern blotting with VNTR probes near the *HGPRT* gene, shown below. What is the chance that the fetus will have Lesch-Nyhan syndrome?

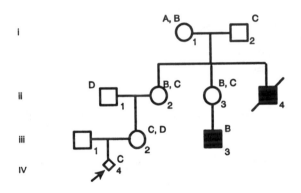

a. 100%
b. 50%
c. 33%
d. 25%
e. Virtually 0%

464. A 6-year-old girl is referred to a physician for evaluation. She is known to have mild mental retardation and a ventricular septal defect (VSD). On physical examination, the patient is noted to have some facial dysmorphism, including a long face, a prominent nose, and flattening in the malar region. In addition, the patient's speech has an unusual quality. Which of the following descriptions best explains the patient's condition?

a. Sequence
b. Syndrome
c. Disruption
d. Deformation
e. Single birth defect

465. A standard karyotypic analysis is ordered for a girl with heart defects, developmental delay, and an unusual appearance. The results are normal, but a colleague recommends performing fluorescent in situ hybridization (FISH) analysis on the patient's chromosomes, using probes for chromosome 22. Only one signal is seen for each chromosomal spread. Which of the following statements best summarizes these analyses?

a. The initial karyotype results are inconsistent with the FISH results.
b. This is a normal result.
c. A small deletion is present on one of the patient's number 22 chromosomes.
d. FISH is only helpful when the initial karyotype results are abnormal.
e. The chromosome with the positive signal is paternal in origin.

466. As exemplified by HLA-DQβ haplotypes in type I diabetes mellitus, an individual's HLA status may be relevant to genetic counseling for certain multifactorial diseases. The relation of HLA haplotypes to disease and the use of this information in genetic counseling are referred to as which of the following?

a. Genetic linkage and the frequency of recombination
b. Allele association and risk modification
c. Positional cloning and gene isolation
d. Gene mapping and gene segregation
e. Genotyping and phenotypic correlation

467. Screening of an African American population in Minnesota yields allele frequencies of $^7/_8$ for the A globin allele and $^1/_8$ for the sickle globin allele. A companion survey of 6400 of these people's ancestors in central Africa reveals 4600 individuals with genotype AA, 1600 with genotype AS (sickle trait), and 200 with genotype SS (sickle cell disease—MIM*603903). Compared to their descendants in Minnesota, the African population has which of the following?

a. A lower frequency of AS genotypes consistent with inbreeding
b. A lower frequency of AS genotypes consistent with malarial exposure
c. A higher frequency of AS genotypes consistent with heterozygote advantage
d. A higher frequency of AS genotypes consistent with selection against the S allele
e. Identical A and S allele frequencies as predicted by the Hardy-Weinberg law

468. A prominent chemist once suggested that individuals who carry or are affected with sickle cell anemia (MIM*603903) have tattoos on their foreheads so they will avoid mating, thus eliminating the disease from the population. If all SS individuals in a population were counseled to avoid reproducing naturally, the SS genotype frequency in the next generation would be which of the following?

a. Reduced by $^2/_3$
b. Reduced by $^1/_2$
c. Reduced by $^1/_3$
d. Reduced to 0
e. Approximately the same

469. A newborn Caucasian girl presents with poor feeding, vomiting, jaundice, and an enlarged liver. The urine tests positive for reducing substances, indicating the presence of sugars with aldehyde groups. Which of the following processes is most likely to be abnormal?

a. Conversion of glucose to galactose
b. Conversion of lactose to galactose
c. Conversion of activated galactose to activated glucose
d. Excretion of glucose by the kidney
e. Excretion of galactose by the kidney

470. The frequency of galactosemia is approximately 1 in 40,000 live births. The frequency of the carrier state can be calculated as which of the following?
a. 1 in 50 live births
b. 1 in 100 live births
c. 1 in 200 live births
d. 1 in 500 live births
e. 1 in 1000 live births

471. A female who has two brothers with hemophilia A (MIM*306700) and two normal sons is again pregnant. She requests counseling for the risk of her fetus to have hemophilia. What is the risk that her next child will have hemophilia?
a. 1
b. $\frac{1}{2}$
c. $\frac{1}{4}$
d. $\frac{1}{8}$
e. $\frac{1}{16}$

472. Which of the following statements best describes hemophilia A (MIM*306700)?
a. The extrinsic clotting pathway is impaired
b. The cleavage of fibrinogen is impaired
c. Tissue factor activation is impaired
d. Activation of factor XII is impaired
e. Activation of factor X is impaired

473. A female who is at risk to be a carrier of hemophilia A desires prenatal diagnosis. She does not want her extended family to know about her pregnancy if the fetus is affected. Which of the following prenatal diagnostic techniques should be advised?
a. Amniocentesis with western blot analysis of factor VIII
b. Chorionic villus sampling with DNA analysis for factor VIII mutations
c. Percutaneous umbilical blood sampling with testing of factor VIII levels
d. Amniocentesis with DNA analysis for factor VIII mutations
e. Chorionic villus sampling with assay of factor VIII activity

474. The figure below shows a pedigree that includes individuals with Charcot-Marie-Tooth disease (CMT), a neurologic disorder that produces dysfunction of the distal extremities with characteristic footdrop. If individual III-4 becomes pregnant, what is her risk of having a child with CMT?

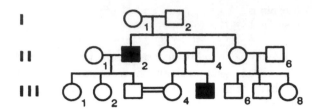

a. $\frac{1}{2}$
b. $\frac{1}{4}$
c. $\frac{1}{8}$
d. $\frac{1}{16}$
e. Virtually 0

475. In another family with Charcot-Marie-Tooth disease (CMT), restriction analysis using sites flanking the *CMT* gene on chromosome 17 yields one large abnormal fragment and one smaller fragment that is seen in controls. What is the probable inheritance mechanism in this family?

a. X-linked recessive
b. Autosomal dominant
c. Autosomal recessive
d. Multifactorial
e. X-linked dominant

476. A 4-year-old African American girl presents with Prader-Willi syndrome obesity, short stature, hypogonadism, and mental disability. Despite a normal gestation and delivery, she had extremely low tone (hypotonia) in the newborn nursery and had to be tube-fed until age 6 months. At age 3 years, she began eating too much, taking food from her parents' plates and even foraging in the garbage for food. Her physician suspects the diagnosis of Prader-Willi syndrome, and recalls that about 60% of Prader-Willi patients have a small deletion on the proximal long arm of chromosome 15. Which of the following techniques would be most accurate in testing for this deletion?

a. Standard karyotyping of peripheral blood leukocytes
b. Northern blotting of mRNAs transcribed from the deletion region
c. Restriction analysis to detect DNA fragments from the deletion region
d. Rapid karyotyping of bone marrow
e. Fluorescent in situ hybridization (FISH) analysis of peripheral blood lymphocytes using fluorescent DNA probes from the deleted region

477. A child is referred for evaluation because of low muscle tone and developmental delay. Shortly after delivery the child was a poor feeder and had to be fed by tube. In the second year, the child began to eat voraciously and became obese. He has a slightly unusual face with almond-shaped eyes and downturned corners of the mouth. The hands, feet, and penis are small, and the scrotum is poorly formed. The diagnostic category and laboratory test to be considered for this child are which of the following?

a. Sequence, serum testosterone
b. Single birth defect, serum testosterone
c. Deformation, karyotype
d. Syndrome, karyotype
e. Disruption, karyotype

478. A 14-year-old Caucasian adolescent has mild disability requiring resource classes and is obese because the parents have had great difficulty controlling her food intake at school and in her grandmother's house where she goes after school. Her physician decides to test for Prader-Willi syndrome and knows that the paternal imprint on chromosome 15 is absent in this condition as opposed to the maternal imprint in Angelman syndrome. A fluorescent in situ hybridization (FISH) test for chromosome 15 deletion had been normal when developmental delay was first suspected, but the physician decides that the girl's increased appetite may reflect uniparental disomy (two chromosome 15 from one parent) that has caused a milder form of Prader-Willi syndrome. Southern blotting is performed to determine the origin of the patient's number 15 chromosomes. In the figure below, a hypothetical Southern blot with DNA probe D15S8 defines which of four restriction fragment length polymorphisms (RFLPs) are present in DNA from mother (M), child (C), and father (F). Which of the following accurately conveys the result of this test?

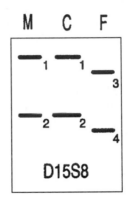

a. Biparental origin of chromosomes 15 confirming a diagnosis of Prader-Willi syndrome
b. Origin of both chromosomes 15 from father suggesting a diagnosis of Angelman syndrome
c. Origin of both chromosomes from the mother suggesting a diagnosis of Prader-Willi syndrome
d. Absence of a paternal chromosome 15, diagnosing nonpaternity and excluding a diagnosis of Prader-Willi syndrome
e. Indeterminate result because the D15S8 locus is deleted in the child

479. The figure in Question 478 demonstrates that the child is missing both paternal chromosome 15 alleles; nonpaternity is a more plausible explanation than uniparental disomy. The hypothetical Southern blot shown below illustrates a DNA "fingerprinting" analysis to examine paternity, where maternal (M), child (C), and paternal (F) DNA samples have been restricted, blotted, and hybridized simultaneously to the probes D7Z5 and D20Z1. The distributions of restriction fragment alleles suggest which of the following?

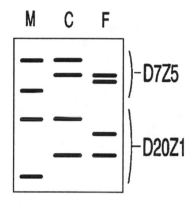

a. The child is adopted
b. False maternity (ie, baby switched in the nursery)
c. False paternity
d. Correct maternity and paternity
e. None of the above

480. Many family studies employing DNA have the potential to demonstrate nonpaternity. If the physician ordering these analyses does not discuss this possibility with the couples involved, he or she is in violation of which of the following?

a. Patient confidentiality
b. Patient rights
c. Informed consent
d. Standards of care
e. Malpractice guidelines

481. The genesis of Prader-Willi syndrome by inheritance of two normal chromosomes from a single parent is a consequence of which of the following?

a. Germinal mosaicism due to paternal mutation
b. Genomic imprinting due to uniparental disomy
c. Chromosome deletion
d. Chromosome rearrangement
e. Anticipation

482. A child with severe epilepsy, autistic behavior, and developmental delay has characteristics of a condition known as Angelman syndrome (MIM*105830). Because of the syndromic nature of the disorder and the developmental delay, a karyotype is performed that shows a missing band on one chromosome 15. Which of the following best describes this abnormality?

a. Interstitial deletion of 15
b. Terminal deletion of 15
c. Pericentric inversion of 15
d. Paracentric inversion of 15
e. 15q⁻

483. An infant with severe muscle weakness is born to a mother with mild muscle weakness and myotonia (sustained muscle contractions manifested clinically by the inability to release a handshake). The mother's father is even less affected, with some frontal baldness and cataracts. Worsening symptoms in affected individuals of successive generations suggest which of the following inheritance mechanisms?

a. Genomic imprinting
b. Heteroplasmy
c. Unstable trinucleotide repeats
d. Multifactorial inheritance
e. Mitochondrial inheritance

484. A child is born with spina bifida, a defect in the lower spinal cord and meninges that may cause bladder and lower limb dysfunction. The family history reveals that the father had a small spina bifida that was repaired by surgery. Which of the following is the most critical aspect of the medical evaluation as it pertains to genetic counseling?

a. A search for additional anomalies to determine if the child has a syndrome
b. A karyotype on the child
c. A serum folic acid level on the child
d. A spinal x-ray on the mother
e. A spinal x-ray on the father

485. Most isolated congenital anomalies exhibit which of the following?

a. Mendelian inheritance
b. Chromosomal inheritance
c. Multifactorial inheritance
d. Maternal inheritance
e. Atypical inheritance

486. A newborn Caucasian girl has bilateral club feet (feet deviated inward and malformed) with minimal movement of her lower extremities. She has a midline bulge over her lower spine that by MRI shows absent vertebrae with extrusion of spinal cord tissue and surrounding dura as a subcutaneous cyst. The lesion is diagnosed as spina bifida occulta and is known to follow the usual multifactorial determination of spina bifida and other common birth defects. Spina bifida exhibits female predilection with an incidence of 1 in 1000 Caucasian individuals and recurrence risks of 3% for first-degree relatives and 0.5% for second-degree relatives. The risk can be decreased by two-thirds if mother takes folic acid before conception. What is the risk that the parent's second child will have spina bifida if mother takes folic acid before becoming pregnant?

a. 1 in 1000
b. 3 in 1000
c. 1 in 100
d. 3 in 100
e. Less than 0.1%

487. Neural tube defects, such as spina bifida and anencephaly, are best diagnosed by which of the following laboratory tests?

a. Chorionic villus biopsy and karyotype at 10 weeks after the last menstrual period (LMP)
b. Maternal serum α-fetoprotein (MSAFP) levels and ultrasound at 16 weeks after conception
c. Amniotic fluid α-fetoprotein (AFP) levels and ultrasound at 16 weeks after the LMP
d. Amniotic fluid acetylcholinesterase levels at 16 weeks after conception
e. Amniotic fluid karyotype and ultrasound at 16 weeks after the LMP

488. Every prenatal evaluation should include which of the following diagnostic procedures?

a. Level I ultrasound
b. Chorionic villus sampling (CVS)
c. Doppler analysis
d. Amniocentesis
e. Genetic counseling

489. A couple has a child who has been diagnosed with medium chain acyl-coenzyme A (CoA) dehydrogenase deficiency (MCAD-MIM*201450), a condition that affects the body's ability to metabolize medium chain fatty acids. This couple is now expecting another child. What is the risk that this child will have MCAD?

a. $^2/_3$
b. $^1/_2$
c. $^1/_3$
d. $^1/_4$
e. $^1/_5$

490. A 1-year-old child develops fever and vomiting and is unable to keep food down for 2 days. The physical examination discloses no congenital anomalies, and the baby resembles his parents. Which of the following laboratory findings are most likely if the child has a disorder of fatty acid oxidation?

a. Hypoglycemia, acidosis, and elevated urine dicarboxylic acids
b. Alkalosis and elevated serum ammonia
c. Acidosis and elevated urine reducing substances
d. Hypoglycemia, acidosis, and elevated serum leucine, isoleucine, and valine
e. Hepatomegaly, elevated serum liver enzymes, and elevated tyrosine

491. Laboratory tests on a sick child reveal a low white blood cell count, metabolic acidosis, increased anion gap, and mild hyperammonemia. Measurement of plasma amino acids reveals elevated levels of glycine, and measurement of urinary organic acids reveals increased amounts of propionic acid and methyl citrate. Which of the following processes is most likely?

a. Diabetes mellitus
b. A fatty acid oxidation disorder
c. Vitamin B_{12} deficiency
d. Propionic acidemia
e. A disorder in glycine catabolism

492. In the treatment of propionic acidemia, which of the following is contraindicated?

a. Antibiotics
b. A diet high in fatty acids
c. Caloric supplementation
d. Aggressive fluid and electrolyte management
e. Hemodialysis

493. DNA analysis is performed on a family because the first child has propionic acidemia. The parents desire prenatal diagnosis, and the fetal DNA is also analyzed for polymorphic alleles A and B that are linked to the causative mutation (see the figure below). The results are shown below. Which of the following risk figures reflect the risk of the fetus being affected before and after testing?

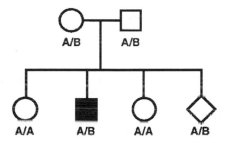

a. $^{1}/_{2}$, virtually 0
b. $^{1}/_{4}$, $^{2}/_{3}$
c. $^{1}/_{4}$, $^{1}/_{2}$
d. $^{1}/_{4}$, $^{2}/_{3}$
e. $^{1}/_{4}$, virtually 0

494. Neonatal screening is mandated in all states, but examines different numbers of diseases. Most commonly tested are phenylketonuria (PKU-MIM*261600), galactosemia (MIM*230400), congenital hypothyroidism, and sickle cell anemia (MIM*603903). Recently, a supplemental newborn screen using tandem mass spectrometry is being adopted by many states, allowing recognition of the more common organic acidemias and fatty acid oxidation disorders. Which of the following is the most important characteristic to qualify a disorder for newborn screening?

a. A highly accurate diagnostic test
b. A high frequency of disease
c. An advantage for treatment from early diagnosis
d. Use of microbial technology like the Guthrie method
e. A minimal incidence of false positive tests

495. The development of DNase therapy has dramatically improved survival and frequency/severity of lung infections in children with cystic fibrosis (MIM*219700). Early diagnosis also allows supplementation of missing pancreatic enzymes with better lipid absorption and improved IQ measures. Over 97 common mutant alleles for Caucasians with cystic fibrosis have now been characterized at the DNA level, allowing screening of pregnant couples with high sensitivity. Which of the following techniques is used to screen couples and newborns for cystic fibrosis?

a. Fluorescent in situ hybridization (FISH) for deletions surrounding the disease locus
b. Subtelomeric FISH analysis
c. Multiplex PCR with high sensitivity
d. Southern analysis to display mutant alleles
e. Comparative genomic hybridization (CGH)-microarray analysis

496. Which of the following is most likely in an untreated child with PKU?

a. Elevated tyrosine
b. Increased skin pigmentation
c. Decreased skin pigmentation
d. Normal phenylalanine hydroxylase levels
e. Elevated alanine

497. A newborn presents with ambiguous genitalia, having an enlarged clitoris or small phallus and labial fusion or hypoplastic scrotum. The newborn's sex can most reliably be established by which of the following?

a. Buccal smear to determine if there are one or two Barr bodies
b. Buccal smear to determine if there is one Barr body or none
c. Peripheral blood karyotype
d. Bone marrow karyotype
e. Polymerase chain reaction (PCR) using primers specific for the long arm of the Y chromosome

498. The dot-blot shown below examines DNA from a child with ambiguous genitalia after polymerase chain reaction (PCR) amplification and hybridization with DNA probes from the X and Y chromosome. In this case, the Y chromosome probe (DXS14) is from the SRY region of Yp that contains the male-determining region. DNA from control male and female patients is also applied to the dot-blot. Based on the dot-blot results, which is the most likely conclusion?

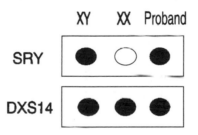

a. The proband is a genetic male.
b. The proband is a genetic female.
c. The proband is male.
d. The proband is female.
e. The proband is mosaic 46,XX/46,XY.

499. A child has ambiguous genitalia including an apparent small phallus and scrotum. The child's DNA hybridizes to probes from the sex-determining region of the Y (SRY). Based on the clinical findings and dot-blot analysis, which of the following terms applies?

a. Female pseudohermaphroditism
b. Male pseudohermaphroditism
c. True hermaphroditism
d. XY female
e. XX male

500. A newborn with ambiguous genitalia and a 46,XY karyotype develops vomiting, low serum sodium concentration, and high serum potassium. Which of the following proteins is most likely to be abnormal?

a. 21-Hydroxylase
b. An ovarian enzyme
c. 5β-Reductase
d. An androgen receptor
e. A testicular enzyme

Genetic and Biochemical Diagnosis

Answers

435. The answer is a. (*Lewis, pp 132-151. Scriver, pp 1366-1368.*) The data indicate that Parkinson disease (PD-MIM*168601) exhibits multifactorial determination with rare families showing autosomal dominant inheritance; the patient could represent a new mutation for the rare dominant form but most likely has multifactorial disease (incorrect answers c-e). First-degree relatives (parent-child, siblings) share 50% of their genes, giving the female's children a 3% to 4% risk to develop PD (3-4 times the baseline 1% risk, incorrect answer b). Were the female a rare example of mutation for autosomal dominant PD, each child would have a 50% risk to inherit her abnormal PD allele (not 25 as in incorrect answer d) and be affected (and a 50% risk to inherit her normal allele, with a background 1% risk to be affected).

Genetic counseling is fundamentally an educational process in which the physician discusses likely inheritance risks, potential testing, and reproductive options. Because humans have small family sizes, genetic information is often incomplete and requires judgment about likelihood. Genetic counseling always depends upon a correct medical diagnosis. In the case of common multifactorial diseases like PD, DNA testing for rare mutations like that in the α-synuclein gene (MIM*168601) might be performed to exclude autosomal dominant inheritance. Another approach is to search for DNA markers (eg, single nucleotide polymorphisms = SNPs that occur every 2-300 bp in human DNA) that allows modification of risk for multifactorial PD. The connection of PD with low CNS dopamine levels prompted a successful search for SNPs near loci encoding enzymes of the phenylalanine/tyrosine/catecholamine/dopamine pathway that serve as DNA markers for risk modification.

Current research approaches to complex diseases include genome-wide searches for single nucleotide polymorphisms (SNPs occurring every 2-300 bp in human DNA) that associate with the phenotype. Given the connection of Parkinson disease with low dopamine, looking at SNPs near loci encoding enzymes of the phenylalanine/tyrosine/catecholamine/ dopamine pathway would be a reasonable start. If a G for C nucleotide substitution was present in a certain allele, and a majority of those with Parkinson disease were G/G homozygotes or G/C heterozygotes, than the G SNP becomes a DNA marker for Parkinsonism susceptibility—more than 10 such loci have been found (MIM*168601). Another approach is to examine rare familial forms of Parkinsonism (eg, MIM*168601) for insights into disease causation, just as study of familial hypercholesterolemia (MIM*144010) highlighted elevated cholesterol as a risk factor for coronary artery disease.

436. The answer is c. *(Lewis, pp 132-151. Scriver, pp 1667-1724. Murray, pp 264-269.)* Dopamine is produced from L-DOPA (3,4-dihydroxy-L-phenylalanine), which in turn is made from tyrosine. Therapy with the L-DOPA precursor increases dopamine concentrations and improves the rigidity and immobility that occur in Parkinson disease. Stimulation of monoamine oxidase (incorrect answer a) or inhibition of dopamine oxidation (incorrect answer a) would not increase dopamine; incorrect answers b and c involve pathways unrelated to dopamine metabolism. Dopamine is degraded in the synaptic cleft by monoamine oxidases A and B (MAO-A and MAO-B), producing 3,4-dihydroxyphenylacetaldehyde (DOPAC). DOPAC is in turn broken down to homovanillic acid, which can be measured in spinal fluid to assess dopamine metabolism. Inhibitors of MAO-A and MAO-B have some use in treating Parkinson disease. The metabolism of histidine or alanine is not related to that of dopamine, but phenylalanine is a precursor of tyrosine and L-DOPA (small molecules like L-DOPA can cross the blood-brain barrier).

437. The answer is d. *(Lewis, pp 431-438. Scriver, pp 225-258. Murray, pp 396-414.)* A family history is an important precedent for anesthesia, and awareness of individual differences is important when administering any drug. Genetic differences in drug metabolism should be recognized rather than giving false reassurance about undo anxiety, improved anesthetic safety, or assumptions all drug reactions are environmental (incorrect answers a-c, e). Pharmacogenetics is the area of study that examines genetic influences on drug metabolism. The extensive human genetic variation revealed by DNA analysis has important implications for pharmacology, since drug effects often vary according to each patient's unique genome.

438. The answer is b. *(Lewis, pp 430-446. Murray, pp 396-414. Scriver, pp 233-238.)* Unusual reactions to drugs targeting enzymes may be mediated by autosomal recessive mutations, regardless of anesthetic management (incorrect answers a-c, e). Succinylcholine is metabolized by a plasma enzyme formerly called pseudocholinesterase (now called butyrylcholinesterase [BChE] to designate its favored substrate). Approximately 1 in 100 individuals are homozygous for a variant of BChE that has 60% activity, whereas 1 in 150,000 individuals are homozygous for a variant with 33% activity. The latter group exhibits prolonged recovery from succinylcholine-induced anesthesia, a phenotype known as succinylcholine apnea (MIM*177400). As with most enzyme defects, succinylcholine apnea exhibits autosomal recessive inheritance. The parents will be heterozygous for a BChE variant but have not undergone anesthesia to display the phenotype.

439. The answer is b. *(Lewis, pp 267-270. Murray, pp 388-405. Scriver, pp 233-238.)* The Hardy-Weinberg law specifies that the distribution of genotypes, given frequencies of normal (p) and abnormal (q) alleles in an ideal population, will be p^2 for homozygous normal, 2pq for heterozygotes, and q^2 for homozygous abnormal. If the heterozygote frequency for butyrylcholinesterase variant alleles is 4 per 100 = 2pq, then pq = 2/200. Since the frequency of abnormal alleles (q) is usually much less than that of normal (p), one can approximate p to 1 and assume q = 2 per 100 with q = $^4/_{10,000}$ or 1 in 2500. As a simplification, one can calculate carrier rates as the square root of disease incidence for autosomal recessive disorders. The proportion of individuals with susceptibility to severe consequences of anesthesia (1 in 2500) is similar to frequencies of common genetic diseases in Caucasians like cystic fibrosis (MIM*219700) and certainly deserves consideration for genetic screening.

440. The answer is e. *(Scriver, pp 5559-5586. Lewis, pp 399-402. Murray, pp 21-30.)* Serum protein electrophoresis separates proteins according to their structure and charge. Two bands for AAT (α_1-antitrypsin deficiency-MIM*107400) in this male imply that two types of AAT protein with different structures or charges are present. The electrophoresis does not reveal whether the abnormal AAT protein has normal or abnormal activity (incorrect answers a-c). The McKusick number indicates that AAT deficiency is an autosomal dominant, single gene disorder, implying paired alleles at a single AAT locus. The male is thus heterozygous, one allele encoding a normal and the other an abnormal protein (incorrect answer d). The AAT locus is located on chromosome 14 within a family of protease inhibitors called serpins. Altered AAT proteins termed M, S, or Z variants have normal inhibitory activity but are defective in their rates of secretion across the liver membrane into the blood. Lower levels of AAT protein apparently expose lung proteins to damage, causing emphysema. Heterozygotes are usually not affected, so the male may have emphysema because of cigarette smoking or other factors. Homozygous ZZ individuals may have liver disease in addition to lung disease because the abnormally secreted AAT accumulates in liver cells.

441. The answer is b. (*Lewis, pp 82-86. Scriver, pp 3827-3876.*) Metabolic diseases usually exhibit autosomal or X-linked recessive inheritance with autosomal disease likely in this female patient. The child's parents are obligate carriers and there is a one-fourth chance (25% recurrence risk) that their next child will be affected (incorrect answers a, c-e). The symptoms suggest Tay-Sachs disease (MIM*272800), an autosomal recessive disorder involving neurodegeneration and early death that has a higher frequency in Ashkenazi Jewish populations.

442. The answer is b. (*Lewis, pp 82-86. Scriver, pp 3827-3876. Murray, pp 205-211.*) The lysosomal enzyme hexosaminidase A is deficient in Tay-Sachs disease. The enzyme cleaves aminohexose groups from gangliosides, complex lipids formed from ceramide (a derivative of sphingosine). Ceramide is synthesized in the endoplasmic reticulum from palmitoyl coenzyme A (16-carbon acyl-CoA) and serine in a reaction catalyzed by pyridoxal phosphate. Uridine diphosphoglucose (UDP-glucose) or UDP-galactose moieties and sialic acid groups are then added in the Golgi apparatus and the gangliosides contribute to myelin in nerve cells. Neurolipidoses like Tay-Sachs disease lack certain lysosomal enzymes necessary to degrade the gangliosides, causing severe effects on nerve cells (neurodegeneration). A parallel group of disorders called mucopolysaccharidoses result from the absence of lysosomal enzymes that degrade complex carbohydrate chains and their associated proteins (called proteoglycans). Proteoglycans are more widely distributed than gangliosides, occurring in the ground substance of many tissues.

Accumulation of the glycosaminoglycans from these proteoglycans thus causes a wide spectrum of symptoms including coarsening of the face and hair, cardiopulmonary problems, and bony deformities such as kyphosis (beaked spine). There is a specific lysosomal receptor that recognizes mannose 6-phosphate on certain lysosomal enzymes and targets them to lysosomes. Mutations in this receptor can cause increased blood levels and lysosomal deficiencies of several enzymes that are normally targeted to lysosomes. One such disease is I (inclusion) cell disease (MIM*252500). The slow accumulation of abnormal gangliosides in lipidoses and of abnormal proteoglycans in mucopolysaccharidoses causes a characteristic clinical course of normal early development that plateaus and then regresses. The age of regression and life span vary widely among the lysosomal storage diseases, with Tay-Sachs being one of the most severe.

443. The answer is e. (*Lewis, pp 82-86, 267-282. Murray, pp 205-211. Scriver, pp 3827-3876.*) The female is a known carrier of Tay-Sachs disease (MIM*272800) and thus has one normal and one Tay-Sachs allele. The male has a 1 in 30 chance to have this same genotype. Each will have a 1 in 2 chance to transmit their abnormal allele to a future child, giving a joint probability of $\frac{1}{2} \times \frac{1}{2} \times \frac{1}{30} = \frac{1}{120}$ (answers a-d incorrect). The joint probability of two or more independent events equals the product of their separate probabilities.

444. The answer is c. (*Lewis, pp 70-82, 399-402. Scriver, pp 3827-3876.*) The probability that any one sibling is homozygous normal is one-third. The human leukocyte antigen (HLA) cluster on chromosome 6 consists of several loci that are each highly polymorphic. Because the loci are clustered together, their polymorphic products form haplotypes (ie, A1-B8-DR2 on one chromosome and A9-B5-DR3 on another chromosome). Since recombination among HLA loci is unlikely, the chances of two siblings being HLA-identical are essentially those of inheriting the same parental chromosomes, that is, $\frac{1}{4}$. The chance for a sibling to be both homozygous normal for Tay-Sachs disease and HLA-compatible is $\frac{1}{3} \times \frac{1}{4} = \frac{1}{12}$. Since there are three siblings, the total chance is $\frac{1}{12} \times 3 = \frac{1}{4}$.

445. The answer is e. (*Lewis, pp 403-410. Scriver, pp 3827-3876.*) The physician is obligated to describe a patient's disease accurately in the medical record and to share such records with legally entitled entities, such as health insurance companies. Although care should be exercised that records containing confidential information are not shared inappropriately, there was no such breach of confidentiality in this case. If the physician had declined further care without appropriate notice, then this would be a breach of ongoing care. However, insurance companies and managed care plans have excluded patients because of prior conditions or excessive expenses (ie, capitation limits). This does constitute discrimination, and the Genetic Information Nondiscrimination Act (GINA) of 2008 was passed to protect such patients and families. These dilemmas will grow dramatically with the increasing ability to test for genetic diseases and predispositions. Although the administration of exogenous normal enzyme (enzyme therapy) or transplantation to provide a cellular source of normal enzyme has been successful in correcting lysosomal deficiencies, the enzymes fail to cross the blood-brain barrier in sufficient amounts to remit neurological symptoms in patients with lipidoses. This form of enzyme therapy has the advantage of targeting the defective organelle via the mannose 6-phosphate residues on the enzyme. It is very expensive but effective in lipidoses that have few neurological symptoms, such as Gaucher disease (MIM*230800).

446. The answer is a. (*Lewis, pp 396-398. Scriver, pp 3827-3876.*) Most enzymes are expressed in chorionic villi or amniocytes and allow prenatal diagnosis of metabolic disorders through cell culture and enzyme assay. Percutaneous umbilical blood sampling (PUBS), or cordocentesis, offers another strategy if the enzyme is normally present in leukocytes. However, transabdominal aspiration of the umbilical cord is difficult and must be performed later in pregnancy (18+ weeks), with higher risks for inducing abortion (~5%) than CVS (8-10 weeks gestation, ~2-3%), or amniocentesis (14-16 weeks gestation), less than 1 in 1000 risk when performed with ultrasound guidance. Fetal tissues produce α-fetoprotein (AFP) and this protein does not cause any metabolic disorders but is used as an index of fetal tissue differentiation and integrity. Amniotic or maternal serum α-fetoprotein (MSAFP) is most often used to detect, respectively, neural tube defects or chromosomal disorders and would not be useful in a case of normal fetal development with hexosaminidase A deficiency. Measure of α-fetoprotein in maternal serum is combined with 2 to 3 other markers (estriol, human chorionic gonadotropin, α-inhibin) that constitute the triple test or quad screen used to indicate higher risks for fetal chromosome disorders.

447. The answer is c. (*Lewis, pp 91-98. Murray, pp 527-544. Scriver, pp 5287-5312.*) Although a mutation at a single locus generally alters a single gene, the result being the abnormal synthesis or lack of production of a single RNA molecule or polypeptide chain, the results of this mutation may be far-reaching. When there are multiple phenotypic effects involving multiple systems, the result is referred to as pleiotropy. Penetrance is the all-or-none expression of an abnormal genotype, whereas expressivity is the degree of expression of that genotype. Incomplete or reduced penetrance implies that some individuals have a mutant allele with absolutely no phenotypic expression of that allele. Variable expressivity implies that all individuals with a mutant allele have some phenotypic effects, although the severity and range of effects differ in different people. Marfan syndrome (MIM*154700) exhibits pleiotropy of its single-gene mutation by causing lens dislocation, loose connective tissue (joint laxity, tall stature, sternal and vertebral deformities), and fragile aortic tissue that can lead to aortic valve insufficiency or aortic dissection. Individuals with the disease exhibit variable combinations and severity of these symptoms due to variable expressivity of this single gene.

448. The answer is c. *(Lewis, pp 399-402. Scriver, pp 5287-5312. Murray, pp 527-544.)* Mutations in structural proteins often exhibit autosomal dominant inheritance, while mutations in enzymes often exhibit autosomal recessive inheritance. Structural proteins such as collagen or fibrillin must interact to form scaffolds in the extracellular matrix of connective tissue. Mutation at one of the homologous autosomal loci can introduce an abnormal polypeptide throughout the scaffold much like a misshapen brick in a wall—the distorted polypeptide from the abnormal locus subverts that from the normal locus and weakens the connective tissue matrix, causing autosomal dominant disease. Sometimes the abnormal polypeptide complexes with normal polypeptides and causes them to be degraded, a mechanism called protein suicide. The suicidal effects of mutations at some loci are referred to generally as "dominant negative" mutations. Fibrillin is a glycoprotein used to form a scaffold in the connective tissue filaments called microfibrils. It is distributed in the suspensory ligament of the lens of the eye, the aorta, and the bones and joints, accounting for the symptoms of Marfan syndrome (MIM*154700). Similar pathogenetic mechanisms occur in the osteogenesis imperfecta (eg, MIM*166200) with multiple fractures and in the Ehlers-Danlos syndromes (eg, MIM*130060) with skin fragility (scarring) and vascular disease due to mutations in various collagens. The mutations disrupt the α-helix secondary structure of collagens, which is dependent on the glycine-X-Y triplet amino acid repeats;

the distorted collagen polypeptides then disrupt the collagen fibrils with symptoms dependent on its tissue distribution (2 types of fibrillin and more than 15 types of collagen are known).

449. The answer is b. *(Lewis, pp 395-413. Scriver, pp 5241-5286. Murray, pp 527-544.)* The spectrum of mutations in collagen (and fibrillin) disorders is very broad, making it more efficient to evaluate electrophoretic mobility of their polypeptide chains as a clue to structural abnormality. Almost every patient with osteogenesis imperfecta (and other collagen disorders) has a different type of mutation. PCR amplification followed by allele-specific oligonucleotide (ASO) hybridation to detect specific alleles is thus impractical—hundreds of PCR/ASO reactions would be required to screen for all of the possible mutant alleles. Similarly, DNA sequencing would be extraordinarily time consuming and give many false positives due to nucleotide polymorphisms or silent mutations that do not cause structural abnormalities in the polypeptide. Northern blotting would detect mutations that affect RNA processing and generate RNAs of altered size, but these are a small fraction of possible collagen mutations. As DNA chip technology becomes practical, screening for thousands of mutations at a locus may be possible. DNA chips contain thousands of different oligonucleotides embedded on a solid matrix. Hybridization of colored or labeled gene fragments with randomized sequences from that gene on a chip gives signals corresponding to the gene sequences that are present. The chip can then be washed and used again. Hybridization of the chip with suitably digested DNAs from patients and controls can thus detect any variant gene fragment (complementary oligonucleotide). Use of numerous control DNAs would separate true mutant alleles (sequence variants associated with disease) from polymorphisms or silent mutations.

450. The answer is b. *(Lewis, pp 355-377. Scriver, pp 521-524. Murray, pp 454-458.)* The two-hit hypothesis was developed by Knudsen to explain why patients with hereditary retinoblastoma (germ-line mutations [MIM*180200]) have multiple, bilateral tumors while those with sporadic tumors (no family history) have single tumors. A germ-line mutation (first hit) alters one Rb allele and confers enhanced susceptibility to retinoblastoma. A somatic mutation (second hit) inactivating the other homologous Rb allele can then occur in any tissue. If it occurs in the retina, a tumor is born. The multiple tumors thus represent the sites at which somatic mutations have occurred in the retina. In sporadic cases, two somatic mutational events must take place. Since these somatic mutations are relatively rare events, it is extremely uncommon for more than one tumor to develop. It is curious that, although retinoblastoma susceptibility is inherited in a dominant fashion, tumor development is a recessive event, requiring the inactivation of both alleles. Genes such as *Rb* are called tumor suppressor genes, in contrast to oncogenes, in which only one of the two homologous alleles must be altered to initiate malignant transformation. Alteration of an enhancer or promoter site on one Rb allele would thus not be sufficient to cause cancer, since the other Rb allele would not be affected. Obvious chromosome changes such as 13q–are rare compared to other mutations that alter Rb function.

451. The answer is a. (*Lewis, pp 248-261, 355-377. Scriver, pp 521-552. Murray, pp 376-387.*) Chromosome translocations may often promote tumors in somatic cells by placing regulatory genes next to promoters that aberrantly increase their expression. Burkitt lymphoma, a B-cell lymphoma that usually occurs in childhood, often involves reciprocal translocation of chromosomes 8 and 14. The result of this is to place the *c-myc* proto-oncogene from 8q24 into the immunoglobulin heavy chain locus at 14q32. Because immunoglobulin genes are actively transcribed, this move alters the normal regulatory control of c-myc. Another example is the Philadelphia chromosome, a shortened chromosome 22 caused by translocation t(9:22)(q34:q11). This translocation is seen in almost all patients with chronic myelogenous leukemia (CML) and in a percentage of patients with acute lymphoblastic leukemia (ALL). The Philadelphia chromosome is seen with increased frequency in individuals with Down syndrome.

452. The answer is b. (*Lewis, pp 355-377. Scriver, pp 521-552. Murray, pp 388-405.*) Genetic predisposition to cancer is best understood by the Knudsen hypothesis, where two independent mutations or "hits" are required to produce neoplasia of a somatic tissue. In many hereditary cancers, the "first hit" is a germ-line mutation that is transmitted in families. Individuals who inherit this mutation are much more likely to develop cancer through a "second hit" in their somatic cells. The second hit can be any mutation that removes the homologous allele (loss of heterozygosity); mechanisms include missense mutation, chromosome deletion, and chromosome nondisjunction. For tumor suppressor genes like those responsible for neurofibromatosis 1 (MIM*162200) or the Li-Fraumeni syndrome (MIM*114480), the first hit removes one suppressor allele and the second hit removes the homologous suppressor allele. The family in the question is an example of a "cancer family" that exhibits the bone, breast, colon, and blood cancers that are typical of Li-Fraumeni syndrome. The mechanism involves mutations in the *src* tumor suppressor gene.

453. The answer is d. *(Lewis, pp 355-377. Scriver, pp 521-552. Murray, pp 388-405.)* Presymptomatic DNA testing of individuals in cancer families is increasingly available. However, testing of minors is controversial because they may not be old or mature enough to understand the personal, medical, and financial implications. They therefore cannot give truly informed consent. Beneficence is the ethical imperative to do good for patients, while nonmaleficence is the imperative to do no harm. Autonomy refers to a patient's right to make decisions regarding his or her health care, and confidentiality to the privilege of doctor-patient communication.

454. The answer is d. *(Lewis, pp 395-413. Scriver, pp 2863-2914. Murray, pp 429-435, 637-639.)* This male has familial hypercholesterolemia (MIM*143890), an autosomal dominant phenotype defined by studying males who experienced heart attacks at young ages. Mutations in the LDL receptor lead to decreased cellular cholesterol uptake and increased serum cholesterol. Since LDL has a high cholesterol content, the LDL fraction is elevated compared to the HDL fraction on lipoprotein electrophoresis. In normal individuals, the LDL is taken up by its specific receptor and imported via caveolae to the cell interior. Cholesterol then produces feedback inhibition on the rate-limiting enzyme of cholesterol synthesis (hydroxymethylglutaryl-CoA reductase) and also leads to a decrease in the number of LDL receptors. In rare cases, two individuals with familial hypercholesterolemia marry and produce a child with homozygous familial hypercholesterolemia. These children develop severe atherosclerosis and xanthomas (fatty tumors) at an early age.

455. The answer is c. *(Lewis, pp 19-29. Scriver, pp 2863-2914. Murray, pp 446-454.)* Nitroglycerin causes release of nitric oxide (NO), which activates guanyl cyclase, produces cyclic GMP, and causes vasodilation. NO is formed from one of the guanidino nitrogens of the arginine side chain by the enzyme nitric oxide synthase. NO has a short half-life, reacting with oxygen to form nitrite and then nitrates that are excreted in urine. Coronary vasodilation caused by nitroglycerin is thus short-lived, making other measures necessary for long-term relief of coronary occlusion. The neurotransmitter formed by condensation of acetyl-CoA and choline is acetylcholine, which does not play a role in dilation of coronary arteries.

456. The answer is c. *(Lewis, pp 395-413. Scriver, pp 2961-3062. Murray, pp 467-481, 593-608.)* The symptoms are typical of iron-deficiency anemia, in this case caused by increased blood loss through menstruation. Transferrin is a glycoprotein that transports iron among tissues. Its amounts in serum can be measured as the total iron-binding capacity. Under conditions of iron deficiency, the percentage of transferrin saturated with iron (normally about 33%) is decreased. A specific transferrin receptor brings the iron-ferritin complex into cells, and it is regulated in response to iron stores. When iron is deficient, the number of transferrin receptors is increased. Ferritin is a protein that stores iron in tissues and is minimally present in serum unless there is iron excess. About 10% of the hemoglobin released by normal red cell destruction is bound by haptoglobin. The remainder is salvaged from damaged red cells that are degraded in the reticuloendothelial system. Haptoglobins are decreased in hemolytic anemias in which there is increased release of hemoglobin.

457. The answer is d. *(Lewis, pp 333-354. Scriver, pp 3127-3162. Murray, pp 593-608.)* The male has symptoms of hemochromatosis (MIM*235200), an autosomal recessive disorder with increased iron absorption from the small intestine. There is increased serum iron, higher saturation of transferrin, and increased amounts of ferritin-iron complex so that it appears in serum. The red cell lifetime is normal in hemochromatosis, resulting in normal release of hemoglobin and normal serum haptoglobin. Hemochromatosis is caused by mutations at a locus in the histocompatibility region of chromosome 6; the protein product is localized to the small intestine and influences iron absorption by an unknown mechanism.

458. The answer is d. *(Lewis, pp 182-201. Murray, pp 376-387. Scriver, pp 3127-3162.)* The regulation of mammalian gene expression is selective: specific genes are up- or downregulated by controls at the gene dosage, mRNA transcription, mRNA splicing, mRNA stability, or protein function levels. Under conditions of iron deficiency, transferrin receptor mRNA is stabilized so that more protein is synthesized. Regulation thus occurs at the protein translation level, without changes in transferrin mRNA transcription through transcription factors or transferrin receptor activity through interaction with small molecules (allostery) or through phosphorylation by protein kinases. Overall increases in rates of RNA transcription or protein elongation are not employed for gene regulation by mammalian cells.

459. The answer is b. *(Lewis, pp 379-394. Murray, pp 487-505. Scriver, pp 3105-3126.)* This child's kinky hair is a symptom of Menke disease, an alteration in a copper-binding ATPase. Dysfunction of the ATPase imprisons copper in cells and prevents its normal absorption from the intestine. Enzymes that use copper as cofactor have diverse roles in metabolism, including some that modify and degrade amino acids in collagen. This accounts for the connective tissue symptoms (lax joints, thin skin) in Menke disease. Wilson disease (MIM*277900) is also caused by mutations in a copper-binding ATPase that lead to copper storage in the eye (Kayser-Fleischer ring of corneal depositions that give a greenish-brown ring around the iris), liver (causing hepatitis and cirrhosis), and the brain (sometimes causing psychosis). Ceruloplasmin, the major copper transporter in serum, is decreased in both diseases.

460. The answer is e. *(Lewis, pp 248-261. Scriver, pp 3-45.)* Contiguous gene syndromes, also known as microdeletion syndromes, occur when deletions result in the loss of several different closely linked loci. Depending on the size of the deletion, different phenotypes may result. Mutations in the individual genes may result in isolated features that may be inherited in a Mendelian fashion.

461. The answer is c. *(Lewis, pp 70-82. Scriver, pp 5467-5492.)* Polycystic kidney disease (MIM*173900) occurs in two distinctive genetic forms—adult-onset and infantile. Two different genetic loci are involved (locus heterogeneity), causing infantile disease to exhibit autosomal recessive inheritance and adult-onset disease to exhibit autosomal dominant inheritance. Allelic heterogeneity (incorrect answer b) refer to different alleles at the same locus, pleiotropy (incorrect answer a) to multiple effects of a single mutation, multifactorial determination (incorrect answer d) to causation by multiple genes and the environment, and variable expressivity (incorrect answer e) to variable phenotypes for individuals with the same gene mutation. Confusion between these types can occur due to variable expressivity in the adult, dominant form. Occasional onset in young children may occur in adult-type disease. Consistency of early onset, the presence of consanguinity, and the lack of vertical transmission distinguish the infantile, recessive form. Polycystic kidney disease is an example of genetic heterogeneity, in which different mutations may cause similar phenotypes. This may be further divided into allelic and nonallelic (locus) heterogeneity. Allelic heterogeneity implies that there are different mutations at the same locus that both result in similar disease (ie, the many fibrillin mutations in Marfan syndrome [MIM*154700]). In locus heterogeneity, mutations occur at different loci, yet the phenotype is similar. Locus heterogeneity also explains why certain disorders, such as polycystic kidney disease, Charcot-Marie-Tooth disease, sensorineural hearing loss, and retinitis pigmentosa may be inherited in several different fashions. A general rule predicts that the autosomal recessive forms of these diseases will be more severe, the autosomal dominant forms less so. It is especially important to recognize the possibility of genetic heterogeneity when counseling patients in regard to recurrence risks.

462. The answer is a. (*Lewis, pp 70-82. Scriver, pp 2537-2570. Murray, pp 292-301.*) The child has Lesch-Nyhan syndrome (MIM*308000), an X-linked recessive disorder that is caused by HGPRT enzyme deficiency. HGPRT is responsible for the salvage of purines from nucleotide degradation, and its deficiency elevates levels of PRPP, purine synthesis, and uric acid. PRPP is also elevated in glycogen storage diseases due to increased amounts of carbohydrate precursors.

463. The answer is e. (*Lewis, pp 101-106. Murray, pp 292-301. Scriver, pp 2537-2570.*) Polymorphic DNA regions with variable numbers of tandem repeats (VNTRs) yield an assortment of DNA fragment sizes after restriction endonuclease digestion. The visualization of variable fragments (alleles) from a particular VNTR region can be performed by hybridization with a DNA probe after electrophoresis and transfer (Southern blotting). If the VNTR region is near (linked to) a disease locus, the VNTR alleles can be used to determine which accompanying allele at the disease locus is present. Transmission of VNTR allele B to the affected individual III-3 in the figure below Question 463 establishes phase and indicates that the abnormal Lesch-Nyhan (L-N) allele is cosegregating with VNTR allele B in this family. Individual I-1 is an obligate carrier because both II-4 and III-3 received abnormal L-N alleles (the rare chance of two L-N mutations in one family is discounted). Individuals II-2 and II-3 are thus carriers by virtue of inheriting the B allele from their mother. Individual III-2 is not a carrier because she did not inherit the B allele, and her fetus is not at risk for L-N. These conclusions do not reflect the possibility of recombination between the VNTR allele and the abnormal L-N allele. If one of the affected individuals had a common mutant allele that could be detected by direct analysis of the *HGPRT* gene, then fetal DNA analysis could be performed without concern about recombination.

464. The answer is b. (*Lewis, pp 53-62, 248-261. Scriver, pp 3-45.*) The child described in the question has multiple independent anomalies that are characteristic of a syndrome. Although they are likely to be causally related, they do not appear to reflect sequential consequences of a primary embryonic error (incorrect answer a). These problems do not appear to be caused by the breakdown of an originally normal developmental process as in a disruption (incorrect answer c), nor do they appear to be related to a nondisruptive mechanical force as in a deformation (incorrect answer d).

465. The answer is c. (*Lewis, pp 248-261. Scriver, pp 3-45.*) Fluorescent in situ hybridization (FISH) analysis is a technique in which molecular probes that are specific for individual chromosomes or chromosomal regions are used to identify these regions. FISH probes frequently identify chromosomal regions that are submicroscopic and therefore may be useful when standard karyotypic analysis is normal. In this case, the fact that only one signal is present, despite the fact that there are two number 22 chromosomes, indicates that a submicroscopic deletion has occurred. The parental chromosome of origin cannot be determined using this technique unless that parent also carries a similar deletion and his or her chromosomes are evaluated. Submicroscopic deletion at band 22q11 causes a spectrum of disorders ranging from DiGeorge anomaly to Shprintzen syndrome (MIM*192430).

466. The answer is b. (*Lewis, pp 101-106, 333-354. Scriver, pp 193-202. Murray, pp 566-582.*) Individuals affected with autoimmune disorders such as juvenile diabetes mellitus, ankylosing spondylitis, or rheumatoid arthritis often have increased frequencies of particular HLA alleles, termed allele associations. Genetic linkage differs from allele association in that the linking of allele and phenotype depends on the family context; one family may exhibit segregation of the nail-patella phenotype with allele A of the ABO blood group, whereas another family exhibits segregation with allele O. Allele association or linkage disequilibrium implies that the same allele is always seen at higher frequency in affected individuals from different families (eg, HLA-B27 in ankylosing spondylitis). Allele association implies neither a genotype-phenotype relation between allele and disease nor a common chromosomal location for allele and disease. It may indicate a role for the allele in facilitating disease pathogenesis. In contrast, genetic linkage places a disease gene on the chromosome map, facilitating its isolation by positional cloning. Gene mutations in various individuals can then be characterized, allowing genotype-phenotype correlations. HLA testing for autoimmune disorders, like cholesterol testing for heart disease, exemplifies the use of risk factors to modify risks for multifactorial diseases.

467. The answer is c. *(Lewis, pp 267-270. Scriver, pp 4571-4636.)* Under certain conditions, the Hardy-Weinberg law allows one to interconvert genotype and allele frequencies in a population by using the formula $(p + q)^2 = p^2 + 2pq + q^2$. For a locus with two alleles, p represents the frequency of the more common allele, q of the less common allele, and $p + q = 1$. The Minnesota population therefore has $p^2 = {}^7/_8 \times {}^7/_8 = {}^{49}/_{64}$ (4900 individuals) with the AA genotype, $2pq = 2 \times {}^7/_8 \times {}^1/_8 = {}^{14}/_{64}$ (1400 individuals) with sickle trait (AS genotype), and $q^2 = {}^1/_8 \times {}^1/_8 = {}^1/_{64}$ (100 individuals) with sickle cell disease (SS genotype). The African population has a higher frequency of AS and SS genotypes caused by heterozygote advantage for the AS genotype that confers resistance to malaria.

468. The answer is e. *(Lewis, pp 284-299. Scriver, pp 4571-4636.)* Even if all SS individuals were successfully counseled to avoid reproduction, breeding between much more common AS individuals would replenish SS individuals in the population. Note also that an SS individual would only produce SS offspring if they mated with an AS carrier. This stability of populations in accord with the Hardy-Weinberg law is often referred to as the Hardy-Weinberg equilibrium. During the decades of 1900 to 1920 in America, the eugenics movement succeeded in passing laws obligating sterilization of those with mental disabilities. These laws were based on two false premises—the idea that mental retardation is always due to Mendelian transmission (ignoring chromosomal and multifactorial disease) and the idea that elimination of affected people will always change gene frequencies.

469. The answer is c. (*Lewis, pp 395-413. Scriver, pp 1553-1588. Murray, pp 113-120.*) This infant may have galactosemia (MIM*230400), a deficiency of galactose-1-phosphate uridyl transferase (GALT). Galactose from lactose in breast milk or infant formula is phosphorylated by galactokinase, activated to uridine diphosphogalactose (UDP-galactose) by GALT, and converted to UDP-glucose by UDP-galactose epimerase. The elevation of galactose metabolites is thought to cause liver toxicity, and their urinary excretion produces reducing substances. Infants with the signs and symptoms listed are placed on lactose-free formulas until enzyme testing is complete. Deficiencies of epimerase or kinase can cause mild forms of galactosemia.

470. The answer is b. (*Lewis, pp 267-270. Scriver, pp 1553-1588. Murray, pp 113-120.*) The Hardy-Weinberg expansion, $p^2 + 2pq + q^2$, describes the frequency of genotypes for allele frequencies p and q. In the case of rare disorders, ($q^2 < \frac{1}{10,000}$), p approaches 1. The heterozygote frequency 2pq is thus approximately 2q. In this case, $q^2 < \frac{1}{40,000}$, $q < \frac{1}{200}$, and $2q = \frac{1}{100}$. Since carriers are still quite rare compared with normal individuals, the matching of rare recessive alleles is greatly enhanced when there is common descent through consanguinity.

471. The answer is d. (*Lewis, pp 110-126. Scriver, pp 4367-4392. Murray, pp 583-592.*) The mother of the pregnant female (consultand) is an obligate carrier since she has two affected sons with hemophilia. The consultand thus has a one-half chance of receiving the X that carries the abnormal allele and being a carrier. The risk for the consultand's fetus to have hemophilia A is one-half for the consultand to be a carrier × one-fourth (one-half for the fetus to receive the X with the abnormal allele × one-half chance the fetus will be male) or $\frac{1}{2} \times \frac{1}{4} = \frac{1}{8}$. One could use Bayesian analysis in this case since the female's two normal sons favor the chance she received the normal allele from her mother. The conditional probabilities if she were a carrier for having two normal boys is one-fourth, if she were not a carrier 1; multiplying the prior probabilities of one-half by these conditional probabilities yields joint probabilities of $\frac{1}{2} \times \frac{1}{4} = \frac{1}{8}$ that she is a carrier and $\frac{1}{2} \times 1 = \frac{4}{8}$ that she is not a carrier or a Bayesian probability of one-fifth that she is a carrier after incorporating the condition that she had two normal boys.

472. The answer is e. (*Lewis, pp 110-131. Scriver, pp 4367-4392. Murray, pp 583-592.*) Hemophilia A is caused by deficiency of factor VIII and hemophilia B by deficiency of factor IX. Both factors are involved in the intrinsic blood coagulation pathway that results in activation of factor X. Alternatively, factor X can be activated by tissue factors through the extrinsic blood coagulation pathway. Activated factors X and V produce thrombin from prothrombin, which in turn cleaves fibrinogen to produce fibrin monomers. The fibrin monomers are polymerized and cross-linked to produce a fibrin polymer, which interacts with platelets and other factors to produce a blood clot. The genes for factor VIII and factor IX are on the X chromosome, making hemophilia A and B X-linked recessive diseases.

473. The answer is b. (*Lewis, pp 110-126. Scriver, pp 4367-4392. Murray, pp 583-592.*) Chorionic villus sampling (CVS) is performed at 10 to 12 weeks' gestation, before a female is obviously pregnant. This technique preserves the confidentiality of prenatal decisions because diagnostic results are available by 12 to 14 weeks' gestation rather than the 18 to 20 weeks for standard amniocentesis. DNA analysis must be employed because factor VIII is not expressed in chorion or amniotic cells. Percutaneous umbilical blood sampling (PUBS) must be performed later in gestation (>18 weeks). Because some factor VIII gene mutations may give normal amounts of structurally abnormal factor VIII, activity rather than amounts of factor VIII protein must be measured for diagnosis.

474. The answer is c. (*Lewis, pp 110-126. Scriver, pp 5739-5788.*) The predominance of affected males with transmission through females makes this pedigree (figure below Question 474) diagnostic of X-linked recessive inheritance. Individual I-1 is an obligate carrier, as demonstrated by her affected son and grandson. Individual II-2 cannot transmit an X-linked disorder, although his daughters are obligate carriers. Individual II-3 must be a carrier because of her affected son, which results in a one-fourth probability of recurrence of CMT in her offspring. Individual II-5 has a one-half probability of being a carrier with a one-eighth probability for affected offspring. Individual III-4 also has a one-eighth probability of being a carrier; her risk for affected offspring is also one-eighth despite the consanguineous marriage. Individual III-8 has a one-fourth chance of being a carrier and a one-sixteenth chance of having affected offspring. CMT is one of the disorders exhibiting genetic heterogeneity, with autosomal dominant (MIM*118200), autosomal recessive (MIM*214380), and X-linked recessive (MIM*302800) forms.

475. The answer is b. *(Lewis, pp 82-86. Scriver, pp 5759-5788.)* The large fragment could derive from a mutation ablating one flanking restriction site or from extra DNA inserted between the restriction sites. The fact that there are two DNA fragment sizes in the affected individual but one in controls suggests alteration of only one of the two homologous CMT regions on chromosome 17. The production of disease by alteration of one homologous locus (one abnormal allele) causes autosomal dominant inheritance. This form of CMT is caused by a duplication of the *PMP22* gene, a gene encoding a peripheral myelin protein. The extra copy of *PMP22* increases protein abundance and interferes with nerve conduction. DNA duplication is one form of atypical inheritance discovered through DNA analysis.

476. The answer is e. *(Lewis, pp 82-86. Scriver, pp 3-45.)* The Prader-Willi deletion is quite small and is not usually detected by standard metaphase karyotyping. Fluorescent in situ hybridization (FISH) is the most cost-effective and accurate method for detecting the deletion in Prader-Willi syndrome (incorrect answers a-d). Fluorescent DNA probes from the deletion region (chromosome band 15q11) will give two signals on the two chromosomes 15 in normal subjects but only one signal in Prader-Willi patients with one normal and one deleted Chromosome 15. Detection of RNA or DNA fragments from this region would require quantitation to reveal one-half normal amounts, since genes on the homologous 15 chromosome would be normal (incorrect answer b). Standard karyotypes typically display about 300 bands over the 23 chromosomes or about 10 bands on chromosome 10. This is adequate for detecting aneuploidy but inadequate for small (submicroscopic) deletions seen in conditions like Prader-Willi syndrome. Bone marrow samples could provide rapid karyotype results because marrow contains actively dividing cells, avoiding the delays for standard karyotyping because peripheral blood T leukocytes must be stimulated to divide using lectins like phytohemagglutinin. Now a combination of DNA probes for the chromosomes involved in common trisomies (13, 18, 21, X, and Y) is used to evaluate chromosomes in white blood cell nuclei, giving results without the requirement of cell division (rapid FISH). Although the nuclear chromosomes are not clumped as they would be in metaphase of cell division, counting of the fluorescent signals for each chromosome provides a preliminary diagnosis (eg, three signals for chromosome 21 in a child with trisomy 21 or Down syndrome).

477. The answer is d. (*Lewis, pp 248-261. Scriver, pp 3-45.*) This child has several minor anomalies, a major anomaly that affects the genitalia, and developmental delay. These multiple affected and embryologically unrelated body regions suggest a syndrome rather than a sequence. Because of the multiple anomalies and developmental delay, the first diagnostic test to be considered is a karyotype rather than a test for specific organ function, such as serum testosterone.

478. The answer is c. (*Lewis, pp 127-128, 248-261. Scriver, pp 3-45. Murray, pp 388-405.*) Because both parents are heterozygous for the D15S8 locus (mother with alleles 1 and 2, father with alleles 3 and 4) as distinguished by different migration (different sizes) during gel electrophoresis, the child (C) has only the maternal alleles 1 and 2 and must have received both of mother's chromosomes 15 (answers a, b, e incorrect; nonpaternity possible as in answer d but less probable in this context). Angelman syndrome with seizures, severe mental disability, and a normal appetite is quite different from Prader-Willi syndrome with mild disability and insatiable appetite (never feel full). Patients with Angelman syndrome lack maternal imprinting of the chromosome 15q11 region while those with Prader-Willi lack the paternal imprint. This deficiency can arise by deletion (60% in Prader-Willi, ~5% of Angelman), origin of both chromosomes 15 from one parent (uniparental disomy), or failure of imprinting (the latter causes occur in ~30% of Prader-Willi but in the majority of Angelman patients). DNA methylation testing (maternal vs. paternal imprinting is reflected by the pattern of 5-methyl-cytosines on DNA) is the most sensitive test for these disorders, revealing a maternal 15 imprinting pattern (deletion or absence of paternal chromosome 15 as in Prader-Willi), paternal 15 imprinting pattern (deletion or absence of maternal chromosome 15 as in Angelman), or both maternal and paternal 15 imprinting patterns (normal result).

479. The answer is d. (*Lewis, pp 379-394. Scriver, pp 3-45 Murray, pp 388-405.*) DNA fingerprinting is used in both paternity and forensic analyses and relies on highly variable DNA polymorphisms called variable numbers of tandem repeats (VNTRs). The multicopy repeats include $(CA)_n$ and minisatellite sequences that are present throughout the genome. The usual VNTR probe is directed against single-copy DNA that flanks these repeats and yields multiple restriction fragment sizes that reflect the number of intervening repeats. The hypothetical probes D7Z5 and D20Z1 shown in the question (figure below Question 479) recognize VNTR loci on chromosomes 7 and 20 that yield at least three alleles. Because the child's two alleles for D7Z5 (and D20Z1) match those of the mother and father, correct maternity and paternity are established with a degree of error equal to the chance that these allele combinations would occur in an unrelated individual. In practice, at least five VNTR probes are employed so that the odds for paternity (or nonpaternity) are very high indeed.

480. The answer is c. (*Lewis, pp 379-394. Scriver, pp 3-45. Murray, pp 388-405.*) Informed consent requires that the patient be informed of all adverse effects that might result from a procedure. Evidence for nonpaternity may result from various types of DNA analysis and should be discussed with the concerned parties at the time of blood collection. Some physicians speak to the mother and father separately about this issue to maximize the opportunity for independent decision making.

481. The answer is b. (*Lewis, pp 127-128. Scriver, pp 3-45. Murray, pp 388-405.*) In rare cases, two chromosomes from one parent rather than one from each is present in the conceptus, leading to disease if this chromosome is subject to genomic imprinting. The mechanism for uniparental disomy appears to involve generation of a trisomic conceptus (eg, two chromosomes 15 from mother, one from father) followed by correction to a disomic cell early in embryogenesis. The correction may involve loss of the paternal chromosome 15, and the more viable disomic cell with two maternal chromosome 15s forms most of the fetus and resulting child. Since chromosomes 7, 11, 14, 15, and 16 are imprinted in humans (DNA methylation patterns different according to maternal versus paternal origin), maternal uniparental disomy 15 results in lack of the paternal chromosome 15 imprint and Prader-Willi syndrome. Deletion of the Prader-Willi region on the chromosome 15 from father is another mechanism that causes Prader-Willi syndrome (incorrect answer c), and rare translocations can inactivate the same region (incorrect answer d). Two cell lines with different DNA or chromosome structure in the germline can account for successive children with dominant diseases (eg, Marfan syndrome) born to normal parents (incorrect answer a). Anticipation refers to increasing severity of disease with vertical transmission (in subsequent generations—incorrect answer e).

In humans and other mammals, the source of genetic material may be as important as its content. Mice manipulated to receive two male pronuclei develop as abortive placentas, whereas those receiving two female pronuclei develop as abortive fetuses. The different impact of the same genetic material according to whether it is transmitted from mother or father is due to genomic imprinting. The term imprinting is borrowed from animal behavior and refers to parental marking during gametogenesis—the physical basis may be DNA methylation or chromatin phasing. Both maternally derived and paternally derived haploid chromosome sets are thus necessary for normal fetal development. This is why parthenogenesis does not occur in mammals. The imprint is erased in the fetal gonads and reestablished based on fetal sex.

482. The answer is a. *(Lewis, pp 248-261. Scriver, pp 3-45. Murray, pp 388-405.)* A missing band suggests an interstitial (internal) deletion rather than removal of the distal short or long arm (known as a terminal deletion). The shorthand notation 15q⁻ implies a terminal deletion of the long arm of chromosome 15. Pericentric (surrounding the centromere) or paracentric (not including the centromere) inversions result from crossover of a chromosome with itself and then breakage and reunion to produce an internal inverted segment. Interstitial deletion 15q11q13 is seen in approximately 60% of patients with Prader-Willi and 5% of patients with Angelman syndromes. Other patients with these syndromes inherit both chromosomes 15 from their mother (Prader-Willi) or both from their father (Angelman's), a situation known as uniparental disomy. Genomic imprinting of the 15q11q13 region is different on the chromosome inherited from the mother than on the chromosome inherited from the father. The normal balance of maternal and paternal imprints is thus disrupted by deletion or uniparental disomy, leading to reciprocal differences in gene expression that present as Angelman or Prader-Willi syndromes.

483. The answer is c. *(Lewis, pp 91-98. Scriver, pp 3-45.)* Anticipation refers to the worsening of the symptoms of disease in succeeding generations. The famous geneticist L. S. Penrose dismissed anticipation as an artifact, but the phenomenon has been validated by the discovery of expanding trinucleotide repeats. Steinert myotonic dystrophy is caused by unstable trinucleotide repeats near a muscle protein kinase gene on chromosome 19; the repeats are particularly unstable during female meiosis and may cause a severe syndrome of fetal muscle weakness and joint contractures. Variable expressivity could also be used to describe the family in the question, but the concept implies random variation in severity rather than progression with succeeding generations. Diseases that involve triplet repeat instability exhibit a bias for exaggerated repeat amplification during meiosis (eg, females with the fragile X syndrome or myotonic dystrophy and males with Huntington chorea). The explanation for this bias is unknown.

484. The answer is a. *(Lewis, pp 132-151. Scriver, pp 3-45.)* Spina bifida is a defect of neural tube development that can be partially prevented by encouraging preconceptional folic acid supplementation in females desiring to become pregnant. Examination for subtle evidence of dysmorphology in children with major birth defects is necessary to rule out a syndrome. Syndromes often exhibit Mendelian or chromosomal inheritance.

485. The answer is c. *(Lewis, pp 132-151. Scriver, pp 193-202.)* When present as an isolated anomaly, spina bifida (meningomyelocele) exhibits multifactorial inheritance. Chromosomal inheritance with imbalance of chromosome segments usually produces a pattern of multiple birth defects (a syndrome) with concurrent mental disability (incorrect answer b). Maternal inheritance refers to transmission from the mother as with mitochondrial DNA mutations (incorrect answer d). Atypical inheritance (incorrect answer e—genomic imprinting, trinucleotide repeat instability, mitochondrial inheritance) has not been implicated in neural tube defects.

486. The answer is c. *(Lewis, pp 132-151. Scriver, pp 193-202.)* The parent's next child will be related to the child with spina bifida as a first-degree relative (parent-child, siblings), having 50% of their genes in common. Sharing of these genes that are now shown to confer polygenic susceptibility to spina bifida (by birth of an affected child) means that the second child will have a much higher (3%) chance for spina bifida than the general 1 in 1000 risk in the Caucasian population. However, the polygenic component of multifactorial determination can be moderated by changing the environmental component; reducing the risk for spina bifida in the second child to 1% through preconception counsel and ensuring mother takes folic acid supplementation (incorrect answers a, b, d, e). Second-degree relatives have 25% of their genes in common (parent-grandchild, aunt/uncle-niece/nephew). Risk for multifactorial disorders (diabetes, schizophrenia, most common diseases including isolated birth defects) drop off sharply with degrees of relationship as shown in the example of spina bifida. Had the child had a rare pattern of birth defects that includes spina bifida, then a Mendelian disorder could be possible and with recurrence risks as high as 25% from autosomal recessive inheritance.

487. The answer is c. *(Lewis, pp 395-413. Scriver, pp 193-202.)* Any defect of the fetal skin may elevate the amniotic α-fetoprotein (AFP) level, causing a parallel rise of this substance in the maternal blood. Neural tube defects such as anencephaly or spina bifida elevate the AFP in amniotic fluid or maternal serum; other causes of increased AFP include fetal kidney disease with leakage of fetal proteins into amniotic fluid. Mild forms of spina bifida or meningomyelocele may be covered by the skin, so that the AFP is not elevated, and maternal serum AFP is less sensitive than amniotic fluid AFP for such cases. Ultrasound is required to detect covered neural tube defects that do not leak fetal AFP into the amniotic fluid and maternal blood. Acetylcholinesterase is an enzyme produced at high levels in neural tissue that is somewhat more specific than AFP for neural tube defects; it is used for confirmation rather than as a primary prenatal test. Chorionic villus biopsy is performed at about 10 weeks after the last menstrual period (LMP) and amniocentesis at 14 to 16 postmenstrual weeks. Because conception often occurs 2 weeks prior to the LMP, distinction between postconceptional and postmenstrual timing is important for early stages of pregnancy. Neural tube defects are usually localized, multifactorial anomalies rather than part of a malformation syndrome that can result from chromosomal aberrations. For this reason, documentation of the fetal karyotype by chorionic villus biopsy or amniocentesis does not influence the risk for neural tube defects.

488. The answer is e. *(Lewis, pp 396-398. Scriver, pp 3-45.)* Genetic counseling is an essential component of every prenatal diagnostic test. Couples must understand their risks and options before selecting a prenatal diagnostic procedure. There must also be adequate provisions for explaining the results. Because additional obstetric procedures, such as pregnancy termination, may follow prenatal diagnosis, obstetricians need to be comprehensive and thorough with the genetic counseling process.

489. The answer is d. *(Lewis, pp 82-86. Scriver, pp 2297-2326. Murray, pp 193-199.)* Metabolic disorders almost always involve enzyme deficiencies and are thus autosomal or X-linked recessive inheritance. Assuming that nonpaternity or an unusual method of inheritance is not operative, the parents of a child with an autosomal recessive condition are obligate heterozygotes. Therefore, their risk of having a child with medium chain acyl-coenzyme A (CoA) dehydrogenase deficiency (MCAD) is one-fourth or 25% for each future pregnancy.

490. The answer is a. *(Lewis, pp 82-86. Scriver, pp 2297-2326. Murray, pp 193-199.)* Catastrophic metabolic disease often begins after the first few feedings, when the baby is exposed to nutrients that cannot be metabolized and are toxic. Often there are misguided attempts to encourage feeding, which further poison the child. Inborn errors of carbohydrate, amino acid, or organic/fatty acid metabolism can present in the newborn period. They are characterized by a similar pattern of symptoms that include spitting up, vomiting, exaggeration of the usual physiologic jaundice, lethargy progressing to coma, hypoglycemia, acidosis, hyperammonemia, and, in the case of maple syrup urine disease or isovaleric acidemia, unusual odors. Disorders of fatty acid oxidation worsen during fasting to cause carnitine depletion, failure of fatty acid oxidation, and excretion of dicarboxylic acid intermediates. Deficiencies in medium chain fatty acid oxidation are milder, and may present after a period of illness with calorie deprivation in children aged 2 to 6 years. Urea cycle disorders worsen during fasting (catabolic breakdown) or protein feeding, producing excess ammonia, rapid breathing, and respiratory alkalosis. Galactosemia worsens on exposure to lactose-containing formula, producing hypoglycemia, liver failure, and excretion of urinary sugars (reducing substances). Tyrosinemia and maple syrup urine disease are amino acid disorders that worsen after protein feeding and produce elevated levels of tyrosine or branch-chain amino acids (leucine, isoleucine, valine). Tyrosinemia is associated with severe liver failure and maple syrup urine disease with severe acidosis due to conversion of excess amino acids to ketoacids.

491. The answer is d. *(Lewis, pp 82-86. Scriver, pp 2297-2326. Murray, pp 193-199.)* Propionic acidemia (MIM*232000) results from a block in propionyl-CoA carboxylase (PCC), which converts propionic to methylmalonic acid. Excess propionic acid in the blood produces metabolic acidosis with a decreased bicarbonate and increased anion gap (the serum cations sodium plus potassium minus the serum anions chloride plus bicarbonate). The usual values of sodium (~140 mEq/L) plus potassium (~4 mEq/L) minus those for chloride (~105 mEq/L) plus bicarbonate (~20 mEq/L) thus yield a normal anion gap of approximately 20 mEq/L. Low bicarbonate of 6 to 8 mEq/L yields an elevated gap of 32 to 34 mEq/L, a "gap" of negative charge that is supplied by the hidden anion (propionate in propionic acidemia). Biotin is a cofactor for PCC and its deficiency causes some types of propionic acidemia. Vitamin B_{12} deficiency can cause methylmalonic aciduria because vitamin B_{12} is a cofactor for methylmalonyl coenzyme A mutase. Glycine is secondarily elevated in propionic acidemia, but no defect of glycine catabolism is present.

492. The answer is b. (*Lewis, pp 82-86. Scriver, pp 2297-2326. Murray, pp 193-199.*) In treating inborn errors of metabolism that present acutely in the newborn period, aggressive fluid and electrolyte therapy and caloric supplementation are important to correct the imbalances caused by the disorder. Calories spare tissue breakdown that can increase toxic metabolites. Because many of the metabolites that build up in inborn errors of metabolism are toxic to the central nervous system, hemodialysis is recommended for any patient in stage II coma (poor muscle tone, few spontaneous movements, responsive to painful stimuli) or worse. Dietary therapy should minimize substances that cannot be metabolized—in this case fatty acids, because the oxidation of branched-chain fatty acids results in propionate. Antibiotics are frequently useful because metabolically compromised children are more susceptible to infection.

493. The answer is c. (*Lewis, pp 82-86. Scriver, pp 2297-2326.*) The proband in this case has inherited the A allele from one parent and the B allele from the other (figure below Question 493). However, it is impossible to determine which allele came from which parent. The fetus has the same genotype as his affected brother. However, it cannot be determined if he inherited these alleles from the same parents as the affected boy and is thus affected, or from the opposite parents and is thus an unaffected non carrier. It can be said that he is definitely not an unaffected carrier. Assuming no recombination has occurred, the risk for the fetus to be affected is one-half, or 50%.

494. The answer is c. (*Lewis, pp 395-413. Scriver, pp 175-192.*) Genetic screening requires not only a highly accurate diagnostic test but also one that can be adapted to testing of large numbers of individuals. Key for neonatal screening is that the disease can be ameliorated because of early diagnosis—some countries have tried screening for Duchenne muscular dystrophy (MIM*310200) but most do not because there is no treatment advantage from early diagnosis. Neonatal screening is set up so there will be more false positives than false negatives; this requires some work for pediatricians in obtaining and interpreting repeat screens, but is considered far preferable to missing a child with preventable disease consequences. The Guthrie test was the first to allow screening of large populations, as exemplified by the test for phenylketonuria (PKU-MIM*261600): infant blood from a heel or finger stick is placed on filter paper discs and mailed to the central screening laboratory. Discs are arrayed on agar plates containing a competitive inhibitor of bacterial growth (thienylalanine), which must be overcome by sufficient amounts of phenylalanine for bacterial colonies to be visible. Rapid scanning of agar plates with hundreds of filter discs is thus possible by eye, and discs surrounded by bacterial growth constitute a positive result. A recent problem for newborn screening is the trend toward early infant discharge (24 hours or less). If the infant blood sample is obtained too early before adequate dietary intake, blood levels of phenylalanine or other metabolites may not be elevated and a false negative result will be obtained. Many hospitals request that parents return with their infant for proper screening. The supplemental newborn screen by tandem mass spectrometry can be justified because the aggregate incidence of its 30 detected disorders is 1 in 5 to 6000, well above that for currently screened metabolic disorders such as PKU (1 in 10-12,000) and galactosemia (1 in 40,000).

495. The answer is b. (*Lewis, pp 393-412. Scriver, pp 5121-5188. Murray, pp 402-421.*) Multiple polymerase chain reaction (PCR) primers targeting regions of the cystic fibrosis gene known to contain mutations (multiplex PCR) are used for cystic fibrosis screening of adults and newborns. Comparative genomic hybridization (CGH), also known as microarray analysis, uses DNA arrays or chips containing 40-100,000 DNA segments affixed to microbeads or glass slides, hybridized in duplicate to control and patient DNAs, and passed through machines for reading of excess hybridization (duplicated DNA segments) or deficiencies (deleted DNA segments— incorrect answer e). Microarray analysis essentially provides a high resolution karyotype and is defining subtle chromosome aberrations in patients with disorders like autism or learning disabilities. Fluorescent in situ hybridization may employ control and test labeled DNA probe to highlight their specific locus on a chromosome, showing two signals for individuals with paired autosomes. An absence of test signal on one chromosome when the control signal is present shows there is a submicroscopic deletion as in the DiGeorge or Williams syndromes (incorrect answer a). Subtelomere FISH analysis extends this to many DNA probes, highlighting all 44 autosome and the two X chromosome ends—subtle rearrangements will shift the position of the FISH signal, and deletions or duplications involving a target region will yield a missing or extra signal (incorrect answer b). Southern analysis is labor intensive and has limited use in this era of automated allele detection and DNA sequencing (incorrect answer d).

Advances in rapid DNA sequencing may soon allow screening for multiple genetic diseases in patients, detecting DNA markers of risk or mutations that cause disease—an example is the threefold coverage of DNA pioneer James Watson's DNA in several weeks for a million dollars (50 years from discovering DNA structure to a genome sequence for the discoverer!). Complicating the clinical applications of total genomic sequencing (personalized medicine, prenatal or newborn screening) is the enormous amount of variation; distinguishing diseases from traits and false from true positives will be enormously difficult. Another problem is exemplified by current expanded newborn screening where as many as 60 inborn errors of metabolism can be detected, many of which cannot be treated effectively. Such detection violates the prime justification for screening: early or presymptomatic diagnosis should benefit the patient through treatment or planning.

496. The answer is c. (*Lewis, pp 287-299, 395-413. Scriver, pp 1667-1724. Murray, pp 248-261.*) Decreased melanin can occur in PKU because melanin is produced from phenylalanine and tyrosine. The defect in most children with PKU is deficiency of phenylalanine hydroxylase. Rare children have deficiency of biopterin cofactor due to a defect in its synthetic enzyme that is also autosomal recessive. Phenylalanine is converted to tyrosine by phenylalanine hydroxylase, so deficient tyrosine can occur in children on restrictive diets.

497. The answer is c. (*Lewis, pp 248-261. Scriver, pp 4077-5016.*) A peripheral blood karyotype provides the most reliable examination of the sex chromosomes. A bone marrow karyotype is more rapid (it uses rapidly dividing bone marrow cells) but usually has less resolution for defining subtle X and Y chromosome rearrangements. A buccal smear would theoretically show one Barr body in females (representing inactivation of one X chromosome) and none in males. In practice, this test is not very reliable and is rarely used. Detection of material of the Y long arm by polymerase chain reaction (PCR) would be useful but does not examine the Y short arm that contains the sex-determining region.

498. The answer is a. (*Lewis, pp 248-261. Scriver, pp 4077-5016. Murray pp 429-435.*) The dot-blot demonstrates hybridization of the proband's DNA with the DXS14 and SRY DNA probes and suggests the diagnosis of a genetic male. The presence of a Y rules out the possibility of the proband being a genetic female but not the rare occurrence of 46,XX/46,XY mosaicism. Gender assignment is not based solely on genetic testing but must include surgical and reproductive prognoses for male versus female adult function. For these reasons, the patient with ambiguous genitalia is a medical emergency that requires delicate management until gender assignment is agreed on. In the past, individuals judged not to have adequate phallic tissue for reconstruction of normal male genitalia underwent appropriate surgery for female gender assignment. However, recent follow-up studies suggest that at least some XY individuals who had feminizing surgery including orchiectomy have developed a male sexual identity. These findings make management more complex in that sexual identity may be at least partly determined during fetal life.

499. The answer is b. (*Lewis, pp 248-261, 379-394. Scriver, pp 4077-5016. Murray pp 429-435.*) True hermaphroditism implies the presence of both male and female genitalia in the same patient and is extremely rare. Male pseudohermaphroditism implies a genetic male with incomplete development of his genitalia, as in the proband. Causes can range from abnormalities of the pituitary-adrenal-gonadal hormone axis to local defects in tissue responsiveness to testosterone. The XY female and XX male refer to phenotypically normal individuals whose genetic sex does not match their phenotypic sex. Examples include testicular feminization and pure gonadal dysgenesis (XY females) and offspring of fathers with Y translocations that inherit a cryptic SRY region without a visible Y chromosome (XX males).

500. The answer is a. (*Lewis, pp 248-261, 379-394. Scriver, pp 4077-5016. Murray pp 379-394.*) Sex steroids are synthesized from cholesterol by side-chain cleavage (employing a P450 enzyme) to produce pregnenolone. Pregnenolone is then converted to testosterone in the testis, to estrogen in the ovary, and to corticosterone and aldosterone in the adrenal gland. The enzymes 3β-hydroxysteroid dehydrogenase, 21-hydroxylase, 11β-hydroxylase, and 18-hydroxylase modify pregnenolone to produce other sex and adrenal steroids. Deficiencies in adrenal 21-hydroxylase can thus lead to inadequate testosterone production in males and produce ambiguous external genitalia. Such children can also exhibit low sodium and high potassium due to deficiency of the more distal steroids corticol and aldosterone. 5β-Reductase converts testosterone to dihydrotestosterone, and its deficiency produces milder degrees of hypogenitalism without salt wasting. Deficiency of the androgen receptor is called testicular feminization, producing normal looking females who may not seek medical attention until they present with infertility.

Appendix

METABOLIC-GENETIC DISORDERS INCLUDED AS EXAMPLES IN QUESTIONS

Disorder	Abnormality/ Deficiency	Clinical Information	Question Numbers
DNA repair disorders			
Xeroderma pigmentosum	DNA repair defect with UV light sensitivity (MIM*278700)	Skin ulcers healing with brown pigment, photosensitivity retinal disease	2, 18, 29
HNPCC (MIM*120435)	DNA mismatch repair defect (HNPCC-MIM*120435)	No colonic polyps, high incidence colon cancer	13, 20
Cockayne syndrome (MIM*216400)	DNA repair/transcription factor defect	Growth failure, rapid aging, sunken eyes, sparse hair, old-age diseases as child	12
Cancers and cancer syndromes			
Acute lymphocytic leukemia (MIM*187040)	Multifactorial with specific T- or B-cell markers	Anemia, fatigue, bone pain—first effective chemotherapy now curing > two-thirds of patients	31
Breast-ovarian cancer (MIM*113705)	BRCA1 and BRCA2 genes	AD breast-ovarian cancer with early onset compared to multifactorial breast cancer	24
Burkitt lymphoma (MIM*113970)	Translocations involving MYC oncogene	Lymphoid proliferation (lymphoma) with secondary bone and immune disease	94, 451
Chronic myelogenous leukemia (MIM*608232)	Philadelphia chromosome (translocation 9/22)	Increased white blood cell count, bone marrow failure, chronic infections	5, 79

Gardner syndrome (MIM*175100)	Adenomatous polyposis coli (APC) gene	Unusual teeth, retinal lesions, multiple colon polyps, early-onset colon cancer	7, 20, 402
Li-Fraumeni syndrome (MIM*114480)	p53 oncogene	Predisposition to breast and colon cancers	452-453
Prostate cancer (MIM*176807)	Multifactorial	Most common cancer in males	
Retinoblastoma (MIM*180200)	Rb tumor suppressor gene; origin of two-hit hypothesis	Retinal tumors	17, 450
Wilms tumor (MIM*194070)	WT-1 tumor suppressor gene	Renal tumors, sometimes with aniridia, genital anomalies, retardation (WAGR)	84, 86, 460
Triplet repeat amplification			
Fragile X syndrome (MIM*309550)	Fragile X mental retardation (FMR-1) gene	MR, long face, prominent ears and jaw, loose connective tissue, large testes	1, 11
Huntington chorea (MIM*143100)	Huntington gene	Tremors, staccato and slurred speech, degeneration	1, 386
Chromosomal and imprinting disorders			
Angelman syndrome (MIM*105830)	Deletion or abnormal parental origin at 15q11	Severe MR, seizures, jerking movements	482
Cri-du-chat syndrome	46,XX,5p- or 46,XY,5p-	MR, growth failure, microcephaly, cat-like cry, multiple congenital anomalies	400

(Continued)

METABOLIC-GENETIC DISORDERS INCLUDED AS EXAMPLES IN QUESTIONS (Continued)

Disorder	Abnormality/Deficiency	Clinical Information	Question Numbers
Down syndrome	Trisomy 21 or translocation (2%-3% eg, 46,XX,(t14;21)	MR, short stature, eye, heart, thyroid, GI defects, atlantoaxial instability	394-395, 398-399
Klinefelter syndrome	47,XXY karyotype	Tall stature, gynecomastia, small testes, infertility; behavior differences	389
Prader-Willi syndrome (MIM*176270)	Deletion or abnormal parental origin at 15q11	MR, early hypotonia, later hyperphagia, and obesity	6, 477-4799
Rett syndrome (MIM*312750)	MECP protein	MR, gradual neurodegeneration, unusual hand wringing movements	26
Shprintzen-DiGeorge spectrum	Submicroscopic deletion at band 22q11 (eg, MIM*192465)	MR, heart, palate, parathyroid, immune defects; schizophrenia in adults	464-465
Triple X syndrome	47,XXX karyotype	MR, variable short stature, occasional somatic defects	390
Turner syndrome	45,X, 46,XX/45,X mosaicism, ring X, etc	Short stature, web neck, broad chest, ovarian dysgenesis, infertility	393, 395, 397-398
XYY syndrome	47,XYY karyotype	Tall stature, variable cognitive disability, and behavior differences	391
Disorders of membrane proteins			
Cystic fibrosis (MIM*219700)	CFTR	Lung disease and pancreatic insufficiency due to viscous mucous	3, 37, 333, 385, 409, 432, 495
Diabetes insipidus (MIM*125800)	Aquaporin	Water loss, hyperosmolar serum with hypernatremia, extreme thirst, polyuria	98

Disorders of carbohydrate metabolism

Disorder	Defect	Clinical/biochemical features	Pages
Diabetes mellitus (MIM*222100)	Multifactorial—insulin deficiency	Hyperglycemia, glucosuria, increased fat oxidation, ketoacidosis	4, 69, 97, 108, 177, 191, 280, 284, 345-346, 377, 382, 466
Essential pentosuria (MIM*260800)	Xylulose reductase	Pentose in urine without pathology	181
Galactosemia (MIM*230400)	Galactose-1-phosphate uridyl transferase	Neonatal illness with cataracts, jaundice, liver disease, reducing substances in urine	176, 469-470
Glucose-6-phosphate dehydrogenase deficiency (MIM*305900)	Enzyme of pentose phosphate shunt	Hemolytic anemia, particularly with exposure to antimalarial drugs or fava beans	77, 175, 188, 211
Hereditary fructose intolerance (MIM*229600)	Liver aldolase B	Hypoglycemia, acidosis, liver disease	166, 178, 196
Hypoglycemia	Multifactorial	Jittery babies; anxiety, tremors, fainting spells in adults	187
Liver GSD (see Table 6)	Defective glycogen breakdown or synthesis	Hypoglycemia, enlarged liver, elevated uric acid, cholesterol	123, 173, 179, 180, 200, 203-204, 339, 379, 401

(Continued)

METABOLIC-GENETIC DISORDERS INCLUDED AS EXAMPLES IN QUESTIONS (Continued)

Disorder	Abnormality/ Deficiency	Clinical Information	Question Numbers
Muscle GSD (see Table 6)	Defective glycogen breakdown or synthesis	Muscle cramps, fatigue with exercise	168, 179, 200, 206
Type II GSD (see Table 6)	Lysosomal α-glucosidase (Pompe-MIM*232300)	Short PR interval on ECG, lethal cardiomyopathy with heart failure	183
Complex carbohydrate (mucopolysaccharide, glycosaminoglycan) storage diseases			
Hunter syndrome (MIM*309900)	Iduronate sulfatase; type II mucopolysaccharidosis	Same as Hurler, males only, clear corneas	81, 130, 272, 404
Hurler and Scheie syndromes (MIM*252800)	Iduronidase; type I mucopolysaccharidosis	Neurodegeneration, cloudy corneas, coarse facies, hepatosplenomegaly	78, 130, 272
I-cell disease (MIM*252500)	Lysosomal transporter	Similar to Hurler, inclusion cells in fibroblasts	121
Fatty acid oxidation disorders and organic acidemias			
Carnitine deficiencies (eg, MIM*212140)	Carnitine transporters	Muscle weakness, heart and liver failure due to defective fatty acid oxidation	228, 239
MCAD deficiency (MIM*201450)	Medium chain CoA dehydrogenase	Lethargy, nonketotic hypoglycemia, heart and liver failure with fasting	228, 246, 249, 263, 339, 356, 489-490
Propionic acidemia (MIM*232000)	Propionyl-CoA carboxylase	Acidosis with anion gap, hypoglycemia, moderate hyperammonemia, lethargy	491-492

Disease	Defect	Clinical features	References
Lipid storage diseases			
Gaucher disease (MIM*231000)	Glucosylceramide β-glucosidase	Organomegaly; fractures	78, 80
Tay-Sachs disease (MIM*272800)	Hexosaminidase A	Cherry red spot of the retina, exaggerated infantile startle reflex, neurodegeneration	272, 423, 441-445
Niemann-Pick disease (MIM*257220)	Sphingomyelinase	Organomegaly, neurodegeneration	268
Lipid transport diseases			
Abetalipoproteinemia (MIM*200100)	ApoB protein	Retinal changes, anemia with acanthocytes, low serum β-lipoprotein	54-55, 82-83
Familial hypercholesterolemia	LDL receptors	Xanthomas, hypercholesterolemia, early onset of atherosclerosis	266, 269-270, 282, 454-455
Familial hypertriglyceridemia	Abnormal VLDL metabolism	Hypertriglyceridemia, atherosclerosis	262
Hemoglobinopathies and anemias			
α-Thalassemia-MR syndrome	Altered transcription factor for the α-globin locus	Mental retardation, coarse facies, hypotonia, anemia	93
Hemoglobin lepore (MIM*141900)	Rearrangement of β-globin cluster	Anemia	34
Hexokinase deficiency (MIM*235700)	Hexokinase	Anemia	174, 241

(Continued)

METABOLIC-GENETIC DISORDERS INCLUDED AS EXAMPLES IN QUESTIONS (Continued)

Disorder	Abnormality/ Deficiency	Clinical Information	Question Numbers
Sickle cell anemia (MIM*603903)	β-Globin point mutation	Anemia, vessel occlusion with pain and sequestration crises	15, 36, 41, 92, 112, 433, 467-468
Spherocytosis (MIM*182900)	Ankyrin erythrocyte protein	Anemia with small spherical red blood cells (spherocytes)	99
Thalassemias (eg, MIM*141900)	Imbalance of α- or β-globin chains	Severe anemia, growth failure, transfusion iron toxicity; bone changes	39, 43-46, 48, 51, 53, 58, 91, 113

Disorders of porphyrin, nucleic acid, or bile acid metabolism

Bile acid synthesis disorders	Heme and bile degradative enzymes (eg, MIM*214950)	Liver disease, cholestatic jaundice with elevated bile acids	353
Gout (hyperuricemia)	Multifactorial disease	Hyperuricemia with joint nodules (tophi), kidney crystals, and joint pain	184, 296
Lesch-Nyhan syndrome (MIM*300322)	HGPRT	MR, self-mutilation to the degree of chewing off lips and fingers	291-292, 462-463
Neonatal jaundice	Multifactorial disease (unconjugated bilirubin)	Excess bilirubin produces yellow skin and yellow whites of eyes (sclerae)	257
Orotic aciduria (MIM*258900)	Uridine monophosphate synthase	Megablastic anemia unresponsive to vitamin B_{12}	290
Porphyrias (one form AD-MIM*176100)	Heme biosynthesis enzyme defects	Episodic abdominal pain, psychosis, skin rash	258, 295

Disorders of amino acid metabolism

Albinism (MIM*203100)	Melanin synthesis	Pale skin and hair, nystagmus due to altered crossover of optic nerves	16, 418
Alkaptonuria (MIM*203500)	Homogentisic acid oxidase	Blackened urine on standing, black cartilage with arthritis (ochronosis)	116
Cystinosis (MIM*219800)	Lysosomal transporter	Childhood growth failure with eye and renal disease	105, 276
Gyrate atrophy (MIM*258870)	Ornithine aminotransferase	Retinal degeneration with vision and neurologic problems	76
Hartnup disease (MIM*234500)	Renal neutral amino acid transporter	Tryptophan and niacin deficiency with pellagra (rash, neurologic symptoms)	253, 318
Histidinemia (MIM*235800)	Histidine degrading enzyme	No symptoms or speech delay	128
Homocystinuria (MIM*236300)	Cystathionine synthase, others	Marfanoid habitus with tall stature, joint laxity, hernias, scoliosis, flat feet	251, 319, 405
Hyperprolinemia (MIM*239500)	Proline degrading enzyme	No symptoms or speech delay	128
Maple syrup urine disease (MIM*248600)	Branched-chain amino acid dehydrogenase	Seizures, acidosis, neurologic damage, death without low protein diet	126
Phenylketonuria (MIM*261600)	Phenylalanine hydroxylase	Mousy odor, pale skin, blond hair	106, 267, 421, 496
Urea cycle disorders	Citrullinemia (215700)	Neonatal lethargy, seizures, coma due to hyperammonemia	95, 120, 244-247, 294

(Continued)

METABOLIC-GENETIC DISORDERS INCLUDED AS EXAMPLES IN QUESTIONS (Continued)

Disorder	Abnormality/ Deficiency	Clinical Information	Question Numbers
Mitochondrial disorders			
Kearns-Sayre syndrome (MIM*530000)	Mitochondrial DNA point mutation	Ptosis, ataxia, muscle weakness	23
Respiratory chain disorders (eg, Leigh syndrome, MIM*256000)	Several encoded by mitochondrial or nuclear DNA	Low muscle tone, mental retardation, optic symptoms, lactic acidosis, ragged red fibers in muscle	197, 208-209, 231, 329
Disorders primarily affecting the nervous system			
Charcot-Marie-Tooth disease (eg, MIM*118200)	Peripheral myelin protein 22 in some forms	Peripheral neuropathy with characteristic "stepping" gait due to foot drop	411, 474-475
Deafness (eg, MIM*220290)	Many single gene forms, most commonly recessive	Sensorineural deafness	8, 132
Hallervorden-Spatz disease (MIM*234200)	Pantothenic acid kinase	Insidious loss of cognitive and neural function, neurodegeneration	310
Menkes disease (MIM*309400)	Copper-transporting ATPase	Kinky hair, neurologic devastation, seizures, hypotonia, skeletal changes	81, 459
Retinitis pigmentosa (eg, MIM*180100)	Many genes, all Mendelian mechanisms	Variable onset of vision loss, beginning with night blindness	412-413
Succinyl choline apnea (MIM*177400)	Butyrylcholinesterase	Inability to recover from succinylcholine paralysis during anesthesia	438-439

Developmental disabilities, birth defects, and birth defect syndromes

Achondroplasia (MIM*100800)	Fibroblast growth factor receptor-3	Dwarfism, short proximal limbs (rhizomelia), hydrocephalus, scoliosis	408, 422
Autism spectrum disorders	Many gene mutations and chromosome changes	Behavior complex with poor communication, social interaction, and repetitive behaviors, often accompanying mental disability	1, 32
Cardiomyopathy (MIM*160760)	Cardiac myosin	Dilated heart with weakening cardiac muscles, sudden death from arrhythmia	124
Cleft lip/cleft palate	Multifactorial disease	Cleft of lip and/or palate, ear infections	424
Crouzon syndrome (MIM*123500)	Fibroblast growth factor-1	Premature fusion of the cranial sutures (craniosynostosis), no limb anomalies	406
Ectrodactyly (MIM*183500)	Several genes including sonic hedgehog	Split hand-split foot or lobster claw anomaly	403
Epidermolysis bullosa	Adhesive proteins of skin	Multiple blisters, similar to burns	115
Fetal warfarin syndrome	Multifactorial, defects in vitamin K synthesis	Short "fleur-de-lys" nose and skeletal changes	311
Hemophilia A (MIM*306700)	Factor VIII	Coagulopathy often presenting after circumcision, joint damage	471–473
Holoprosencephaly (eg, MIM*157170)	Many single gene and chromosome aberrations	Failure of forebrain development with facial cyclopia to midline cleft lip/palate	90, 341
Hydrocephalus	Multifactorial	Enlarged cerebral ventricles with macrocephaly	431

(Continued)

METABOLIC-GENETIC DISORDERS INCLUDED AS EXAMPLES IN QUESTIONS (Continued)

Disorder	Abnormality/ Deficiency	Clinical Information	Question Numbers
Incontinentia pigmenti (MIM*308300)	Unknown	Skin lesions—vesicles, scaling, pigment patches—sparse hair, absent teeth	416
Marfan syndrome (MIM*154700)	Fibrillin	Tall stature, myopia, dislocated lens, high palate, heart defects, scoliosis, flat feet	114, 117, 447-478
Osteogenesis imperfecta (MIM*155210)	Type I collagen	Multiple fractures, deafness, blue-gray sclerae, large skull with wormian bones	103, 118, 132, 242, 414, 449
Osteopetrosis (MIM*259730)	Carbonic anhydrase	Hardened, sclerotic bones and renal transport defect with acidosis	101
Pyloric stenosis (MIM*179010)	Multifactorial	Narrowing of pylorus with vomiting and hyperchloremic alkalosis	104, 417
Retinoic acid embryopathy	Prenatal exposure to retinoids (eg, Accutane)	Brain, eye, limb, and craniofacial defects, usually with severe MR	89
Roberts syndrome (MIM*268300)	Unknown	Cleft palate and congenital limb amputations	10, 19
Spina bifida	Multifactorial	Failure of caudal neural tube closure with lower limb paralysis and incontinence	484-487
Stickler syndrome (MIM*108300)	Type II collagen	Retinal detachment, lax joints, arthritis, short stature	75, 119

Disorder	Mechanism	Features	Pages
Waardenburg syndrome (MIM*193500)	PAX genes	Deafness, hypertelorism, central white patches of hair (poliosis) and skin	419
Zellweger syndrome (MIM*214100)	Paroxysmal protein defects	Severe hypotonia, large fontanelle, liver disease, MR, short life span	283
Endocrine disorders			
Addison disease (eg, MIM*103230)	Multifactorial due to adrenal insufficiency	Hypokalemia, hypoglycemia, muscle weakness, hypotension, fainting spells	342, 349
Ambiguous genitalia	Multifactorial, many single gene disorders	Incomplete development or sex reversal of external genitalia	497-500
Testicular feminization	Testosterone receptor (MIM*300068)	Female phenotype without uterus and ovarian tubes, infertile, XY karyotype	338
Cushing syndrome	Multifactorial due to ACTH or cortisol excess	Truncal obesity, "buffalo hump," striae of skin, hypertension, potassium loss	340
Diabetes insipidus	Multifactorial due to vasopressin (ADH) defect	Excessive thirst, dehydration, hypernatremia	98, 341, 428
Immune disorders			
AIDS (MIM*609423)	Viral infection with genetic susceptibility	Immune deficiency	25
Adenosine deaminase deficiency (MIM*102700)	Adenosine deaminase with stem cell immune defects	Viral, fungal, and bacterial infections due to B- and T-cell deficiencies	27, 73

(Continued)

METABOLIC-GENETIC DISORDERS INCLUDED AS EXAMPLES IN QUESTIONS (Continued)

Disorder	Abnormality/ Deficiency	Clinical Information	Question Numbers
Bruton agammaglobulinemia (MIM*300300)	Tyrosine kinase gene; deficiency of B-cells that fight bacterial infections	Severe and recurrent bacterial infections when maternal antibodies are cleared from system (age 3-6 months).	40, 111
Toll-like receptor deficiency (MIM*603030)	Defective toll-like receptors on white blood cells	Susceptibility to bacterial infections	21
Organ system disorders			
Alcoholism	Multifactorial disease	Liver disease, cirrhosis, deficiencies of vitamins B_1 and B_{12}, psychosis	169, 172, 264, 316, 330
α_1-Antitrypsin deficiency (MIM*107400)	Proteinase inhibitor PI, mutant S and Z alleles	Childhood liver and adult pulmonary disease	35, 57, 72, 170, 440
Cholera	Bacterial infection with *Vibrio cholerae*	Diarrhea, dehydration, shock	237
Crohn disease	Multifactorial	Inflammatory bowel disease with bloody diarrhea, cramping, malabsorption	304
Ethylene glycol intoxication	Environmental poisoning	Acidosis, liver failure	259
Polycystic kidney disease (eg, MIM*173900)	Polycystin—dominant and recessive forms	Cysts in kidneys and liver with propensity to strokes	461

Multiple sclerosis	Multifactorial with abnormal CNS lipids	Waxing and waning neurologic symptoms with incoordination, ataxia, depression	261
Prematurity	Multifactorial	Lung and liver immaturity, deficient fatty acid and iron stores	260
Disorders of vitamin and mineral metabolism			
Multiple carboxylase deficiency (MIM*253260)	Biotinidase	Intermittent acidosis, hair loss, skin rashes, neutropenia	312
Hemochromatosis (eg, MIM*235200)	Proteins encoded by *HFE*, *HFE2A*, *HFE 2B* genes	Abnormal iron transport and storage with accumulation in heart and liver	303, 457-458
Mineral deficiencies (see Table 10)			324
Vitamin deficiencies (see Table 9)			230, 286, 301, 305-308, 314, 316, 318, 320-322, 325-328, 332-337

*Online Mendelian Inheritance in Man (MIM) number provided for single gene disorders—some multifactorial or chromosomal diseases will have an MIM number to list genes implicated in pathogenesis/susceptibility; HNPCC, hereditary nonpolyposis colorectal cancer; AD, autosomal dominant; AR, autosomal recessive; MR, mental retardation; GI, gastrointestinal; CFTR, cystic fibrosis transmembrane conductance regulator; GSD, glycogen storage diseases; ACTH, adrenocortical hormone; ADH, antidiuretic hormone; HGPRT, hypoxanthine-guanine phosphoribosyltransferase; AIDS, acquired immunodeficiency syndrome.

Bibliography

Lewis R. *Human Genetics: Concepts and Applications*. 9th ed. New York, NY: McGraw-Hill: 2010.

*McKusick VA. *Mendelian Inheritance in Man*. 13th ed. Baltimore: Johns Hopkins University Press; 1996.

Murray RK, Bender DA, Botham KM, Kennelly PJ, Rodwell VW, Weil PA. *Harper's Illustrated Biochemistry*. 28th ed. New York, NY: McGraw-Hill; 2009.

Scriver CR, Beaudet AL, Sly WS, Valle D. *The Metabolic and Molecular Bases of Inherited Disease*. 8th ed. New York, NY: McGraw-Hill; 2001.

The primary references cited in the key concepts and answers include the Murray and Scriver textbooks, which are more directed toward biochemistry, and the Lewis textbook that is more directed toward medical genetics. The Murray text has added a relevant section on biochemical case histories and the Lewis text has superb historical and patient perspectives on genetic disease.

Many genetic diseases cited in this book include a six-digit McKusick number preceded by MIM to indicate Online Mendelian Inheritance in Man (OMIM at www.ncbi.nlm.nih.gov/omim/) that references more than 5000 genetic diseases. For all but the most recently entered disorders, the digit at the beginning of the McKusick number provides the inheritance mechanism as follows: MIM*154700 designates autosomal dominant Bender inheritance (Marfan syndrome), MIM*219700 autosomal recessive diseases (cystic fibrosis), MIM*310200 X-linked recessive diseases (Duchenne muscular dystrophy), MIM*480000 Y-linked diseases (so far only gene loci, in this case sex-determining region on the Y = SRY), and MIM*530000 mitochondrial DNA–encoded diseases (Kearns-Sayre syndrome). The reader may enter "OMIM" in their search engine, go to Online Mendelian Inheritance in Man, designate the disease name or symptom of interest, and access the relevant entries. For the more common disorders, there is a link to www.genetests.org in the upper right corner of the entry that will indicate any laboratories doing DNA testing for that disease.

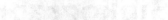

Index

Note: Page numbers followed by "t" indicate table and page numbers followed by "f" indicate figure.